Understanding Medical Cannabis

This accessible text provides trainee human service providers and those currently working in the field with a comprehensive, cutting-edge overview of topics related to the medical and therapeutic use of cannabis.

Employing an interdisciplinary, biopsychosocial framework, the book explores the different biological, cultural, and policy contexts of medical cannabis from a wide range of perspectives including practitioners, academics, and medical cannabis advocates. This book bridges the gap between theory and practice and underscores the urgent need for expanded and rigorous scientific research as medical cannabis is increasingly legalized, that may result in new cannabis-based medicines and help in identifying what health risks cannabis use may present.

Chapters are both evidence-based and practical, weaving in learning objectives, review questions, and varied case examples, all of which will prepare students and professionals for the reality of working with medical cannabis consumers.

Joanne Levine, DSW, MSW, MPH, is an associate professor and associate department chair, School of Health and Human Services, SUNY Empire State College. She developed and co-teaches the first multidisciplinary course in SUNY on medical cannabis.

Understanding Medical Cannabis

Critical Issues and Perspectives for Human Service Professionals

Edited by Joanne Levine

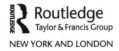
Routledge
Taylor & Francis Group

NEW YORK AND LONDON

First published 2021
by Routledge
52 Vanderbilt Avenue, New York, NY 10017

and by Routledge
2 Park Square, Milton Park, Abingdon, Oxon, OX14 4RN

Routledge is an imprint of the Taylor & Francis Group, an informa business

Library of Congress Cataloging-in-Publication Data
Names: Levine, Joanne, editor.
Title: Understanding medical cannabis : critical issues and perspectives
for human service professionals/edited by Joanne Levine.
Description: New York, NY: Routledge, 2021. |
Includes bibliographical references and index. |
Summary: "This accessible text provides trainee human service providers
and those currently working in the field with a comprehensive, cutting-edge
overview of topics related to the medical and therapeutic use of cannabis.
Chapters are both evidence-based and practical, weaving in learning objectives,
review questions, and varied case examples, all of which will prepare students
and professionals for the reality of working with medical cannabis consumers"–
Provided by publisher.
Identifiers: LCCN 2020039039 (print) | LCCN 2020039040 (ebook) |
ISBN 9780367360993 (hardback) | ISBN 9780367361013 (paperback) |
ISBN 9780429343803 (ebook)
Subjects: LCSH: Cannabis–Therapeutic use. | Marijuana–Therapeutic use.
Classification: LCC RM666.C266 U53 2021 (print) | LCC RM666.C266 (ebook)
| DDC 615.7/827–dc23
LC record available at https://lccn.loc.gov/2020039039
LC ebook record available at https://lccn.loc.gov/2020039040

ISBN: 978-0-367-36099-3 (hbk)
ISBN: 978-0-367-36101-3 (pbk)
ISBN: 978-0-429-34380-3 (ebk)

Typeset in Sabon
by Deanta Global Publishing Services, Chennai, India

Contents

Contributors

Michael J. Balick, PhD, is Vice President for Botanical Sciences, Director of the Institute of Economic Botany and Senior Philecology Curator at The New York Botanical Garden in Bronx, New York. His research and teaching have focused on ethnobotany, the relationship between plants, people and culture, in particular the indigenous and contemporary uses of plants as medicines, poisons, and foods.

Kimberly Balko, PhD, RN, is an Associate Professor in the School of Nursing and Allied Health at SUNY Empire State College. Her nursing career encompasses over 40 years in various areas of nursing with expertise including long term health care, End-of-Life Nursing Education Consortium (ELNEC) Train the Trainer Program and co-development of an Interdisciplinary Palliative Care course.

Courtney V. Collins is a doctoral student at the Morgridge College of Education at the University of Denver and Education Director at the Realm of Caring; an independent high impact non-profit in Colorado Springs, Colorado that is redefining the way we talk about cannabis, collaborate on research, provide education, and empower people to lead better lives.

Stephen M. Dahmer, MD, is a board-certified family physician whose passion for health and healing has taken him around the globe. A fellow of the Arizona Center for Integrative Medicine, for over two decades he has studied the relationships between plants and people, working closely with diverse cultures and documenting their uses of plants and other integrative therapies. He practices Family Medicine in New York and serves as Chief Medical Officer of Vireo Health, a physician-founded, patient-focused medical cannabis company. Dr. Dahmer is also an Assistant Clinical Professor of Family Medicine and Community Health at the Icahn School of Medicine at Mount Sinai Medical Center, New York, New York.

Bonni S. Goldstein, MD, is the owner and Medical Director of Canna-Centers Wellness & Education in Los Angeles, California. A trained pediatrician who practiced Pediatric Emergency Medicine for many years, Dr. Goldstein began seeing chronically ill patients for use of medical cannabis in 2008 after witnessing its beneficial effects in a loved one. She has a special interest in treating children with epilepsy, autism, and cancer.

Kim Hewitt, PhD, is a Full Professor of American History and American Studies at SUNY Empire State College. She is a cultural studies scholar whose research pursuits include psychedelic studies, body studies, mental health, and spirituality.

Heather Jackson is the Co-Founder/Board President of the Realm of Caring Foundation, Inc., Colorado Springs, Colorado and has been leading a movement to change the way we think about cannabis and the people who use it through furthering research and creating a global community. Jackson is nationally and internationally recognized as an author, researcher, and speaker but, most importantly, as mother to a boy who transitioned from hospice to health using medical cannabis.

Joanne Levine, DSW, MSW, MPH, is an Associate Professor, School of Health and Human Services, SUNY Empire State College. Her research and teaching interests include the psychosocial issues experienced by medical marijuana consumers including medical refugees. She is the author of textbooks on human service practice and the Internet and publishes and presents widely on topics including distance education, gerontology, and mental health.

Cathleen Lewandowski, PhD, MSW, is Director and Professor, Cleveland State University School of Social Work and Director of the Center for Behavioral Health Sciences which conducts interdisciplinary research to improve substance abuse and mental health treatment. Her academic and research interests include children and family services, substance abuse treatment, veterans' issues, and program implementation and development. She is a former Lieutenant Colonel in the Army Reserves, serving as a Social Work Officer, was deployed in 2004 with a combat stress unit to Iraq, and led a combat stress team. She is actively engaged in training and educating students, social workers, and other behavioral health professionals on best practices to support veterans' readjustment. Dr. Lewandowski has widely published in substance abuse, veterans' issues, and child welfare including (2018) *Child Welfare: An Integrative Approach, Oxford Press.*

Lynn McNall, MS, RN, CNE, is an Associate Professor in the School of Nursing and Allied Health at SUNY Empire State College. Her nursing career encompasses over 30 years working as a certified oncology nurse caring for patients in areas of medical and radiation oncology, research coordinator, and staff development education with an oncology focus.

Paul Seaborn, MBA, PhD, is an Assistant Professor in the Management Area at the McIntire School of Commerce, University of Virginia. His research and teaching interests encompass strategic management, public policy, consulting, and the business of cannabis. He created the first-ever Business of Marijuana course at the University of Denver in 2017.

Gary Starr, MD, is a board-certified emergency medicine physician who practices in Minnesota. He has served for over 5 years as Chief Medical Officer and Chief Quality Officer for multiple companies engaged in standards development for and the manufacture and clinical utilization of cannabinoid-based therapies. Dr. Starr has lectured extensively on cannabinoid-related medical topics and has led dozens of pharmacists in treating tens of thousands of patients with cannabinoid therapies. He graduated from the University of Cincinnati College of Medicine, and completed his residency in emergency medicine at the University of Chicago, and his residency in family medicine at Saint Louis University.

Heather Trela is the Director of Operations and a Fellow at the Rockefeller Institute of Government, the public policy research arm of the State University of New York. Her research focuses on federalism issues with an emphasis on marijuana policy.

Sherry Yafai, MD, is boarded in Emergency Medicine since 2009 after completing her training at University of California at San Diego. Dr. Yafai pivoted away from Emergency Medicine in 2017 and began working in Cannabis Medicine opening The Releaf Institute in Santa Monica, California. Since that time, she has helped over 1,000 patients using cannabis products, including dozens of narcotic reductions with non-smokable cannabis. Dr. Yafai is the author of the monthly column in Emergency Medicine News, *The Case for Cannabis.*

Introduction

Medical Cannabis: Critical Issues and Perspectives for Human Service Professionals

Joanne Levine

> *Leaving behind jobs, family, and friends, the parents of a child strug-*
> *gling with intractable epilepsy relocate to a state where medical can-*
> *nabis is legal.*
>
> *An elderly cancer patient undergoing chemotherapy seeks relief from*
> *nausea and vomiting; despite feeling embarrassed and ashamed, she asks*
> *her health care provider for a medical cannabis recommendation.*
>
> *A combat veteran experiencing flashbacks and nightmares from Post-*
> *Traumatic Stress Disorder (PTSD) seeks an alternative treatment to*
> *antidepressants; some members of his veterans' support group describe*
> *how medical cannabis helps relieve their debilitating symptoms.*

Over the course of many centuries, diverse cultures have used cannabis and cannabis extracts as medicine. Yet, the current sociopolitical landscape in the United States reflects tensions arising from legal gray areas, federal prohibitions, and stigmas associated with cannabis use. Portrayals of cannabis users depicted in stoner films such as Cheech and Chong's *Up in Smoke* and *Dazed and Confused* contrast sharply with the real lives of those legally eligible to obtain cannabis for medical use. To qualify, patients must have a diagnosed ailment that is on their state's list of qualifying conditions including catastrophic diseases such as AIDS, cancer, Parkinson's disease, chronic pain, amyotrophic lateral sclerosis, post-traumatic stress condition, multiple sclerosis, and epilepsy.[1]

Despite prohibitions and controversies, human service professionals are encountering growing numbers of clients actively using, or seeking to use, cannabis as medicine. Many countries now allow the use of medical cannabis, including the United States, where currently 34 states, the District of Columbia, and four territories have legalized cannabis for either medical or

---

1 Current cannabis laws and regulations in the United States by state are available at: https://
  public.findlaw.com/cannabis-law/cannabis-laws-and-regulations/medical-marijuana-laws-by
  -state.html

recreational use, or both.[2] Nonetheless, cannabis remains federally illegal in the United States, with a Schedule 1 drug status of the Controlled Substances Act.[3] Paralleling this widespread legalization of medical cannabis, is the urgent need to increase awareness for expanded and rigorous scientific research which may result in new cannabis-based medicines and identify what health risks cannabis use may present. Of note, multiple efforts in the United States to reschedule cannabis under the Controlled Substances Act have been unsuccessful and it remains classified as having high potential for abuse and no accepted medical value. This keeps in place significant restrictions on biomedical research. When armed with proper knowledge, human service professionals are uniquely poised to advocate for changes that will expeditiously move research efforts forward.

Education on both the pros and cons of medical cannabis use is also essential for human service professionals so they may provide appropriate services and care. Human service professionals must ask themselves how they can be best prepared and best informed to competently support and advise clients when it comes to cannabinoid therapy use. To this end, using a biopsychosocial framework, this book explores critical issues by bringing together multiple and distinct perspectives and expertise of practitioners, academics, and medical cannabis advocates. Since events are progressing so rapidly, it is difficult to keep up with all the advances. Hopefully, by the time this book comes out, there will be new and helpful developments in policy, research, and practice. Topics covered include:

- the historical and contemporary medicinal uses of cannabis in various cultural contexts and medical systems with a focus on specific delivery forms and diseases;
- the impact of U.S. federal policy on marijuana on financial institutions, taxation, economic development, cannabis businesses, environmental concerns, and social justice;
- a comprehensive overview of the Endocannabinoid System and the discoveries that elucidated its crucial role in health;
- medical cannabis treatment for adult, pediatric, and palliative care patients, including current research, indications for use, risk factors, public health concerns, and future directions;
- case studies from the front lines: medical cannabis refugees, a veteran, and a child welfare worker;
- advocacy by medical cannabis refugees;
- a glossary of key terms and an appendix with resources.

2 An overview of cannabis laws and policies in various international jurisdictions are provided at: https://www.theworldlawgroup.com/writable/documents/news/6.25.2020-Final-Cannabi si-Guide.pdf
3 For the entire Controlled Substances Act see: https://www.dea.gov/controlled-substances-act

Below are overviews of the chapters which are thematically grouped.

Part One: The Context of Cannabis: Culture, Clashes and Commerce (Chapters 1–4) discusses the juxtaposition of *Cannabis sativa* L. (cannabis) with cultural, historical, political, and economic contexts. The landscape of cannabis is explored from ancient times through to the present day. While this book focuses on medical cannabis, it is impossible to disaggregate it from issues also pertaining to recreational usage, including the impact of U.S. federal policy on financial institutions, environmental concerns, and social justice.

Ethnobotanical Origins of Cannabis as a Medicine (Stephen Dahmer, MD, and Michael Balick, PhD) discusses the historical and contemporary medicinal uses of cannabis in various cultural contexts and medical systems with a focus on specific delivery forms and diseases. *Historical and Cultural Context of Marijuana in the United States* (Kim Hewitt, PhD) charts the history of and attitudes towards marijuana use from colonial times to the present. *Clash of Laws: How States are Legalizing Marijuana in the Shadow of a Federal Prohibition* (Heather Trela) describes the evolution of federal marijuana policy and the impact of federal policy in the United States on financial institutions, taxation, economic development, environmental concerns, and social justice. *The Business of Cannabis* (Paul Seaborn, PhD) examines the unique business environment for cannabis. Discussion includes the creation of a wide variety of cannabis businesses in the United States and countries, including Uruguay and Canada, and thoughts on the future outlook of the cannabis industry.

Part Two: Cannabis as Medicine: Research, Practice and Future Directions (Chapters 5–9) opens with an overview of the endocannabinoid system and the clinical endocannabinoid deficiency that could potentially be the underlying commonality of numerous disease states. Medical cannabis treatments for adult, pediatric, and palliative care patients are discussed including case reports from cannabis specialty medical practitioners. These include the emerging uses of cannabis-based medications as alternatives for pain management and as a method for opiate reduction. Risk and protective factors to help understand the progression from cannabis use to cannabis use disorder are also covered. These chapters underscore the urgent need for expanded biomedical research.

The Endocannabinoid System (Gary Starr, MD and Stephen Dahmer, MD) explores the evidence supporting the endocannabinoid system's rightful place within the Western medical paradigm and promoting strong interest to identify its future therapeutic potentials. *Medical Cannabis for Children and Adolescents* (Bonnie S. Goldstein, MD) reviews the latest understanding of the pediatric endocannabinoid system in both healthy and diseased states and includes a care report from the author's cannabis specialty medical practice. Although still considered controversial, the use of phytocannabinoid medicines for pediatric medical conditions is now considered an option in many states in the United States and in European countries. *Medical Cannabis for Adults: Current Uses and Future Directions* (Sherri Yafai, MD) provides a general overview on indications for the medical use of cannabis for adults, including the use of both FDA- and DEA-approved medications and cannabis formulations available in local dispensaries throughout the United States. This chapter also looks at a potential future for cannabis as a treatment strategy for the current opiate crisis, and includes case reports from the author's medical practice. *Medical Cannabis and Palliative Care* (Lynn McNall, MS, RN, CNE and Kimberly Balko, PhD, RN) explores the use of medical cannabis in the palliative care setting and uses a case study approach to understand how barriers such as stigma may impact a plan of care.

Benefits and disadvantages related to the physical and psychosocial aspects of chronic illness and end-of-life care are also examined. Finally, *Risk and Protective Factors for Cannabis Abuse* (Cathleen Lewandowski, PhD) discusses the diagnostic criteria used to diagnose cannabis use disorder using the DSM V and the ICD 10 and 11. The biological, psychological, social, and environmental factors associated with cannabis use disorder are explored.

Part Three: In Their Own Voice (Chapter 10) presents *Lessons from the Realm of Caring Foundation: Case Studies, Research, and Practical Knowledge* (Heather Jackson and Courtney Collins). This chapter includes case studies based on the real-life experiences of diverse medical cannabis consumers and their caregivers, including those of the chapter's co-author Heather Jackson, mother of a son who uses medical cannabis to control his life-threatening seizures. She is also the co-founder and former Chief Executive Officer of the non-profit Realm of Caring Foundation (Colorado Springs, Colorado) which provides practical information, financial aid for medical cannabis, and research-based education on hemp, CBD, medical marijuana, and THC.[4] The complex professional challenges that can arise due to existing codes of ethics and legalities are also explored from the perspective of a Colorado-based human service worker.

Finally, as readers explore these critical issues and perspectives, they are encouraged to remain aware of underlying themes regarding social justice. Some of the many questions to consider include: How can legalization address racial and economic justice concerns? How will changes in drug policies and legislation affect the communities traditionally most affected by cannabis prohibition? How can legal and regulatory policies thwarting research be changed so that there can be discovery of the best and most effective uses for marijuana as medicine? How can equity be ensured in the

---

4 See Chapter 10 and the Appendix of this book for additional information about the Realm of Caring Foundation.

growing marijuana industry? How do we ensure the health and well-being of our communities?

The core values of human service professions are based on service, social justice, and the dignity and worth of the individual and human relationships[5]. In their historic role as advocate, human service professionals are strongly encouraged to enter this important and timely debate to ensure that their core professional values are heard. They are further challenged to publicly ask questions such as those above and press for responses from governmental and private entities involved in making policy and enacting legislation.

---

5 For the current (2017) National Association of Social Workers Code of Ethics see: https://www.socialworkers.org/about/ethics/code-of-ethics

The Context of Cannabis: Culture, Clashes and Commerce

Chapter 1

Cannabis Ethnomedicine

Stephen Dahmer and Michael Balick

Introduction

Ethnobotany, the largest subdiscipline of ethnobiology, is generally defined as the "science of people's interaction with plants" (Dunlap & Turner, 1995). Ethnomedicine refers to the study of traditional medical practices and is concerned with the cultural interpretation of health, diseases, and illness, as well as the healthcare-seeking process and traditional healing practices (Krippner, 2003). *Cannabis sativa* L. (cannabis) (Figure 1.1) has a long history of traditional use as a medicine by many cultures around the world, dating back 6,000 years (Small, 2015). In addition to medicinal use, this versatile plant was recognized long ago as a source of food and fiber. This long-shared history with humans has been rife with debate claiming the plant and its flowers both pariah and panacea, both scourge and benefactor, both hoax and soothing medicine (Hudson & Puvanenthirarajah, 2018; Abel, 1980; www.nationalacademies.org, 2017).

Cannabis is an herbaceous annual plant with ancient origins mainly in Western or Central Asia (Russo et al., 2008, Small, 2015) and is arguably one of the most multipurpose ethnobotanical resources as fiber (stalks), food (seeds), medicine (flowers), and recreational/religious purposes (Piluzza et al., 2013). Its versatility ranges from the manufacturing of fish nets, ropes, textiles, paper, bricks, parachutes, and American flags (Onaivi, 2002) to being touted as useful for 25,000 products "ranging from dynamite to Cellophane" (Small & Marcus, 2002). It has been referred to as the oldest known cultivated fiber plant (Schultes et al., 2001), with some suggesting that its use goes back 8,500 years ago in China (Cherney & Small 2016).

The discovery of where cannabis affects the human biological system—the endocannabinoid system (ECS)—combined with a recent surge in acceptance and legitimacy of this plant, has led to an explosion of research regarding potential medical applications of cannabis and the cannabinoid components that it produces (Treister-Goltzman et al., 2019). However, despite this recent popularity, the plant has been a part of healing traditions

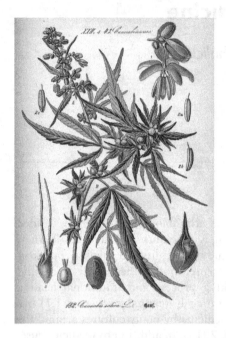

Figure 1.1   Thomé, O.W., *Flora von Deutschland Österreich und der Schweiz, Tafeln*, vol. **2**: t. 182 (1885) Source: plantillustrations.org

in many cultures throughout time and across the globe, ever-present in periods of favor and absolute disdain.

Although cannabis has often been framed as a "scapegoat" for drug abuse and xenophobia (Steen, 2010), it provides a contemporary mirror for modern medicine, rooted in an extensive history that reflects on the definition of the term "medicine." Cannabis may also offer a renewed possible argument and path for the use of whole plant botanicals in the western medicine paradigm. Understanding the history of human use of cannabis as medicine may not only help prioritize research on potential therapeutic applications, challenging the single molecule pharmaceutical approach, but also potentially help avoid pitfalls in our relationship with a psychoactive plant that has potential for abuse.

This chapter will take the reader through the topsy-turvy history of the cannabis plant as medicine, including both historical and contemporary medicinal uses of cannabis in various cultural contexts and medical systems. Clarke and Merlin (2016), Mechoulam (1986), and Russo (2007) offer additional, comprehensive resources that consider cannabis's evolution and widespread, diverse use by humans, and readers can find information on cannabis and its use in treating specific conditions in Chapters 3 and 4.

Plants as Medicine

Plants play an essential role in contemporary medicine, both at the primary care level and for specialized therapies. Today about 80% of the world's population rely heavily on plants and plant extracts for healthcare (Setzer et al., 2006). In addition, of the top 150 proprietary drugs used in the United States, 57% contain at least one major active compound currently or once derived from plants (Grifo & Rosenthal, 1997). The global market for herbal medicine has been valued at more than $60 billion U.S. dollars in annual sales (WHO, 2003). In the past, the traditional medicinal uses of plants have been a successful criterion used by the pharmaceutical industry in finding new therapeutic agents for the various fields of biomedicine (Cox, 1994), although this is less so today, where approaches depend more heavily on technology.

Cannabis was among the first plants cultivated by early people who adopted a more sedentary lifestyle, perhaps as much as 10,000 years ago (Russo et al., 2008). This led to selections of plants grown to obtain nutritious starch-containing food, tough water-resistant fibers, and euphoric and medicinal substances (Fort, 2012; Sauer, 1952). Cannabis continued to accompany the progress of the first human societies in the changes that occurred after the glacial Pleistocene epoch; sophisticated plaited basketry based on cannabis found at Czech Paleolithic sites is perhaps the world oldest archaeological evidence of cannabis use (Adovasio et al., 1996). Its use as an intoxicant likely solidified its use as a medicine and fostered its spread rapidly from Asia to the entire world.

Medicinal plants, despite serving as the foundation of traditional healing therapies for centuries, have not maintained a prominent visible status in the contemporary western medical paradigm. This institutionalized marginalization has also contributed to confusion and strong contradictory opinions about the value of plants, in particular cannabis and its use as a medicine. On one hand, it is argued that if cannabis were unknown, and bioprospectors were suddenly to find it in some remote mountain crevice, its discovery would no doubt be hailed as a medical breakthrough. Scientists would praise its potential for treating everything from pain to cancer and marvel at its rich pharmacopoeia because many of its chemicals mimic essential molecules in the human body (Craker, 2006). On the other hand, a gullible Googler could easily believe that we are on the brink of a miracle cure (Sides, 2015).

Cannabis: The Name

Marijuana, hashish, dope, bud, ganja, reefer, and whacky tabacky are among the many names given to cannabis throughout history. Few substances exhibit the wide variation of names afforded *Cannabis sativa*, reflecting our intimate and longstanding history with this plant and including more than

1,200 slang terms, with more than 2,300 names for individual chemovars or "strains." "Cannabis" comes from the Latin word "cannabis" and the earlier Greek word κάνναβις (OED 2018) and is the scientific name given to the plant *Cannabis sativa* and its variants from which the drug is produced. It is argued that lawmakers adopted the foreign-sounding word "marijuana" precisely because they wanted to underscore that it was a Latino, particularly Mexican "vice" and thereby boost support among xenophobes for laws prohibiting the drug (National Hispanic Caucus, 2017).

The taxonomy of cannabis remains in debate by some taxonomists. Three arguments persist: supporting the idea that the genus *Cannabis* is made up of one (monotypic) highly variable species (*Cannabis sativa* L.); supporting the concept of two species; and supporting the concept of three species (polytypic) (Schultes et al., 1974; Small & Cronquist, 1976; Small, 2015) based upon morphological, geographical, ecotypic or chemotypic differences. The three hypothetical species include: *Cannabis sativa* Linnaeus, *Cannabis indica* Lamarck, and *Cannabis ruderalis* Janisch, each circumscribing several biotypes or subspecies (Clarke & Merlin, 2006; Small, 2015).

Most recently, *Cannabis* specialist Small (2015) suggested that there be considered a single but variable species, *Cannabis sativa*, divided into six groups based on their chemical composition, fiber and oil content, and evidence of hybridization. Schultes, et al. (1974) and Anderson (1980) suggested that there are three species differing fundamentally in terms of height and content of psychoactive molecules. This chapter refers only to cannabis to simplify the discussion, but it is imperative to note that naming for such a complex plant is especially important in deciphering medicinal value. A valuable delineation for medical purposes includes Δ-9-tetrahydrocannabinol (THC)-predominant (Type I cannabis), mixed THC: cannabidiol (CBD) (Type II), and CBD-predominant (Type III cannabis) (Lewis et al., 2018).

Cannabis: The Plant

Cannabis is a dioecious, rarely monoecious, autumn-flowering, short-day photoperiod, anemophilous (wind-pollinated) annual plant of the family Cannabinaceae, that can reach up to five meters in height (Clarke & Merlin, 2016; Farag & Kayser, 2017). It has been described as a sun-loving plant that thrives in open, nitrogen-rich environments, including rubbish piles created by humans (Small, 2015) and as a rapidly growing, highly adaptable, herbaceous species that spread widely around the world (Abel, 1980). Cannabis speciation occurred during the early Pleistocene epoch, and domestication occurred more than a few million years later in the same region (Clarke & Merlin, 2016). As a result of protracted coevolution and its relationship with humans, it has been postulated that cannabis has become a stronger, more adaptable, diversified, and widely-cultivated plant (McPartland & Guy, 2004).

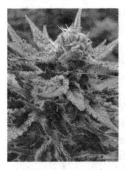

Figure 1.2 Cannabis Glandular Trichomes—from the Greek τρίχωμα (trichōma) meaning "hair" Source: Photograph © Stephen Dahmer, MD

Phytocannabinoids are predominantly, if not entirely, synthesized and sequestered in microscopic structures called trichomes (Mahlberg et al., 1984) (Figure 1.2). Most of the essential oils (monoterpenes and sesquiterpenes) found in cannabis are also located in these glandular structures (Malingré et al., 1975). When considering medical applications, it is important to recognize the importance of the female species, as physiologically active compounds are mostly present in the resin secreted from the trichomes of female plants.

Cannabis grows vertically and produces new leaves mostly in pre-flowering phase, along with the production of new branches and nodes. During its growth, the plant requires a moderate level of environmental and soil humidity and a good light intensity. The form of the plant varies according to the climate and variety. In the wild, it most commonly grows as a persistent weed at the edge of the cultivated fields on soil with high nitrogen content (Brown, 1998).

Food as Medicine

When reviewing plants as medicine it is easy to focus on a purely pharmaceutical approach, e.g., as a drug treating a symptom or condition, and overlook the important role of plants as food and medicine. Since the beginning of human civilization, people have used plants as food and medicine, and the value of the two uses are sometimes combined into the concept of food-medicines (Vandebroek and Balick 2012). Both food and medicinal plants have interventional uses, especially in indigenous and local traditions. Food can be used as medicine and vice versa. This key ancient tradition in various areas of the world is especially pertinent today (Etkin & Ross 1982). Throughout history, many things were purely medicines, but medicines often became food if people learned to like them; many foods became merely medicines when people stopped relishing them; and all foods were considered to have medicinal value, positive or negative, with important effects on health (Anderson, 1988).

This concept of food as medicine applies to the traditional use of cannabis in other parts of the world as well. Historical claims of cannabis's medicinal efficacy relate to absorption of phytocannabinoids (the physiologically active compounds found only in *Cannabis sativa*) into the bloodstream via swallowing as well as via inhalation. Chinese medical traditions, for example, hold that diet is the most important determinant of one's health, and there are often no distinct boundaries between foods and medicine. Chinese physicians used the seeds of cannabis mainly for their vegetable oils and proteins. The seeds are rich in γ-linoleic acid (Anwar et al., 2006), and physicians recommended this topically for eczema and psoriasis, and orally for inflammatory diseases (Jeong et al., 2014). Nutritionally, the seeds of cannabis are a vegetarian source of omega-3 fatty acids and other valuable essential fatty acids necessary for human health and found in the plant in ratios that support health. The seeds are a complete source of protein (which contain all the essential amino acids) and a potent source of multiple essential minerals, including magnesium, phosphorus, iron, and zinc (Deferne & Pate 1996; Samir et al., 1998; Corleone, 2014). In addition to an appreciable amount of protein (19%), the seeds contain an impressive array of enzymes, including lipase, maltase, amylase, urease, and tryptase which may be the main reasons for their medicinal activity (Keys, 1997).

The Thousand and One Molecules

Cannabis has been called the plant of the thousand and one molecules due to its tremendous chemical complexity, containing a plethora of chemically active compounds, including cannabinoids, terpenoids, flavonoids, alkaloids, carotenoids, sterols, vitamins, and fatty acids (Andre et al., 2016). Currently, 538 natural compounds have been identified from cannabis, and more than 100 of these are identified as compounds unique to the plant—all known as phytocannabinoids—because of the shared chemical structure (Hanuš et al., 2016).

The most physiologically active compounds are the cannabinoids, terpenophenolic compounds that form mainly in the trichome cavity of the female flowers (Taura et al., 2007; Brenneisen, 2007) (Figure 1.3), and epidermal glandular protuberances covering the leaves, bracts, and stems of the plant (Happyana et al., 2013; Huchelmann et al., 2017).

We are only beginning to understand the chemical make-up of the cannabis plant. New non-cannabinoid and cannabinoid constituents in the plant are being discovered with great frequency. From 2005 to 2015, the number of cannabinoids identified in the whole plant increased from 70 to 104, and other known compounds in the plant increased from ~400 to ~650 (Radwan

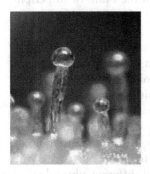

Figure 1.3 Close up of *Cannabis* resin glands that secrete an aromatic essential oil containing the active compounds in this plant including terpenoids and cannabinoids Source: Photograph © Marcus Richardson, from Clarke, R.C. and Merlin M.D. 2016. Cannabis: Evolution and Ethnobotany. University of California Press, Berkeley, CA

et al., 2015). THC levels are also shifting, with breeding of different strains yielding plants and resins with dramatic increases in THC content over the past decade, from ~ 3% to 12–16% or higher (weight for weight or percent THC weight/per dry weight of cannabis) and differing in different countries (Radwan et al., 2008).

Cannabinoids: Endo, Phyto and Synthetic

The cannabinoids are examples of secondary metabolites, which are defined as organic compounds not directly involved in the normal structural growth, development, or reproduction of an organism (Potter, 2014). It is important to note that cannabinoids are divided into three main categories (Figure 1.4): (a)

Varieties of Cannabinoids

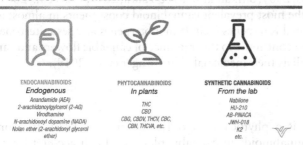

ENDOCANNABINOIDS
Endogenous
Anandamide (AEA)
2-arachidonoylgylcerol (2-AG)
Virodhamine
N-arachidonoyl dopamine (NADA)
Nolan ether (2-arachidonyl glycerol ether)

PHYTOCANNABINOIDS
In plants
THC
CBD
CBG, CBDV, THCV, CBC,
CBN, THCVA, etc.

SYNTHETIC CANNABINOIDS
From the lab
Nabilone
HU-210
AB-PINACA
JWH-018
K2
etc.

Figure 1.4 Cannabinoids: endocannabinoid, phytocananbinoids, and synthetic cannabinoids Source: Structured diagram © Stephen Dahmer, MD

endocannabinoids are neurotransmitters produced in the brain or in peripheral tissues and act on cannabinoid receptors ; (b) phytocannabinoids are cannabinoid compounds produced by the cannabis plant; and (c) synthetic cannabinoids, synthesized in the laboratory, are structurally analogous to phytocannabinoids or endocannabinoids and act by similar biological mechanisms.

Animals produce compounds with properties similar to those of the cannabinoids that occur in plants (the phytocannabinoids) called endocannabinoids. These appear to operate on almost every part of an animal's body and brain, producing effects similar to other phytocannabinoids. In addition to the naturally occurring cannabinoids, many synthetic cannabinoids have been produced by researchers. These compounds do not necessarily exist naturally in plants, but have both similar and different physiological and pharmacological properties to naturally occurring cannabinoids. From a chemical point of view, phytocannabinoids have a lipid structure featuring alkylresorcinol and monoterpene moieties in their molecules (Hanus, 2009; Hill et al., 2012) and are classified as neutral cannabinoids (without carboxyl group) and cannabinoid acids (with carboxyl group).

Examples of synthetic cannabinoids include the FDA-approved medications. Cesamet (nabilone; Meda Pharmaceuticals Inc, Somerset, NJ) and Marinol (dronabinol; Δ9-tetrahydrocannabinol; AbbVie Inc, North Chicago, IL), as well as the illicit market products K2 and Spice. Illicit synthetic cannabinoids have been described as dangerous chemicals with unpredictable composition and human toxicity (Kemp et al., 2016).

Proponents of plant medicine call attention to differing binding at receptor sites between naturally occurring and synthetic cannabinoids. Synthetic cannabinoids as chemicals bind more strongly to the cannabinoid receptor in the brain, but also may interact with other receptors in the brain that cannabis does not. Cannabinoid synthase enzymes are responsible for the generation of cannabinoid acids: CBGA generates cannabidiolic acid (CBDA), cannabichromenic acid (CBCA), and Δ-9-tetrahydrocannabinolic acid (D9-THCA) (Sirikantaramas & Taura, 2017).

The phytocannabinoids can be divided into 10 subclasses, as reported by many authors (Hanus, 2009; Sirikantaramas & Taura, 2017; Izzo et al., 2009). THC and CBD are the most prevalent cannabinoid constituents in almost all cannabis plants. Cannabis terpenes include monoterpenes and sesquiterpenes, which are volatile and contribute to the fragrance of cannabis flowers and cannabis products as well as their medicinal value (Zager et al., 2019).

CBD

Cannabidiol (CBD) is a phytocannabinoid discovered in 1940. It is one of 113 identified cannabinoids in cannabis plants and can account for up to 40% of the plant's extract (Samir et al., 1998). Unlike THC, CBD has negligible affinity for the CB1 and CB2 receptors, and recent studies have suggested that it is an allosteric modulator and an indirect antagonist of cannabinoid receptors, with the ability to potentiate the effect of THC (Laprairie et al., 2015). As of 2019, clinical research on cannabidiol included studies of anxiety, cognition, movement disorders, and pain, but there is insufficient, high-quality evidence that it is effective for these conditions. EPIDIOLEX (Epidiolex, GW Pharmaceuticals, Cambridge, UK), is the first prescription pharmaceutical formulation of highly purified, plant-derived cannabidiol (CBD) and was approved by the U.S. Food and Drug Administration (FDA) on June 25, 2018.

THC

THC is the predominant psychoactive cannabinoid in the plant, responsible for its euphoriant properties, as well as most established medical benefits and the plant's troubled history. It has partial agonist activity at CB1 and CB2 and induces a variety of sensory and psychological effects, including: mild reverie and euphoria; heightened sensory awareness, creativity, and empathy; impaired short-term memory; altered sense of time and space; enhanced appetite and sexual desire; occasional drowsiness; and a tendency to enhance introspection—although these effects vary among individuals depending on their age, dosage, strain consumed, and frequency of use (Zablocki et al., 1991). Traditionally, THC content in the plant used both as a medicine and recreationally has been much higher than the other cannabinoids (Hanus, 2009).

Entourage

Historically, in plant-derived or herbal medications, chemists have identified the molecule responsible for the pharmacological activity. Often then administered in higher dosages, these molecules form the basis of the modern pharmaceutical industry. A widely held and user-reported belief is that the benefit of smoking the whole plant product provides more relief than isolated cannabinoids, a belief referred to as the "entourage effect" (Russo, 2011), whereby the whole is greater than the sum of the parts. This issue lies at the crux of botanical medicine because it is a motivating force for whole cannabis plant to be used for medical purposes in lieu of isolated compounds.

Various explanations support the greater medicinal efficacy resulting from the delivery of whole plant combinations. One is simply the additive inherent medicinal value of minor cannabinoids and terpenoids. Another is the facilitation of the passage of cannabinoids through the blood-brain barrier and/or enhancing their permeability at the cellular level. Finally, there is the observation that CBD, or other chemical constituents, may also ease THC-induced side effects and the combination results in a more satisfying net effect (Russo & Guy, 2006). Full spectrum standardized extract allows multiple cannabinoids to simultaneously affect certain health conditions in a complementary way, and the use of an isolated cannabinoid may not provide the full benefit available from the plant (Pertwee, 2008).

Supportive of this effect are the arguments that CBD also potentiates the pharmacologic effects of THC—enhancing the level of CB1 receptor expression in the brain, decreasing anxiety component of THC effects, and patients reporting overall more pleasurable effects. Without the synergistic effect of CBD, THC arguably could have lower efficacy and a greater degree of negative side effects (Atakan, 2012).

Further research is needed to prove or disprove the validity and potential mechanism/s of action of the widely held belief and self-reporting that whole plant cannabis is superior to isolated compounds because of synergism between various components.

Similar examples exist elsewhere in botanical medicine. Valerian (*Valeriana officinalis* L.) has been used to treat insomnia in Europe and Asia for centuries and, despite identification of many molecules in the plant, we have been unable to pin down one or even a small number of molecules that are responsible for all of the reported pharmacological activity (McClatchey et al., 2009). Valerian, along with cannabis, is suspected to be an example where a high number of active molecules are acting in concert. This complexity triggers a primary problem in medical research: The plant material used by so many of the studies that have been conducted differ so dramatically from the traditionally developed products that many of the more recent and best controlled research studies were fundamentally flawed (Taibi et al., 2007).

From Plants to Humans

When moving beyond plant utility as fiber or specifically as a source of nutrition, it is interesting to ask why a plant would produce compounds that have physiological activity in the human body. Why might plant molecules interact with and modulate key regulators of mammalian physiology in ways that are beneficial to health? The affinity of psychoactive phytochemicals within the hominid nervous system may also indicate some kind of mutualistic coevolution, with ancient humans seeking and perhaps cultivating plant psychotropics to facilitate survival, by alleviating starvation, fatigue, and pain (Sullivan & Hagen 2002).

One interesting theory is that animals may have retained the ability to sense stress-induced molecules produced by plants in the context of certain environmental stresses (xenohormesis). Heterotrophs (animals and fungi) sense chemical cues synthesized by plants in response to stress, providing advance warning about deteriorating environmental conditions and allowing heterotrophs prepare for adversity while conditions are still favorable. These compounds modulate key pathways in humans that control inflammation, the energy status of cells, and cellular stress responses in a way that is predicted to increase health and survival of the organism (Howitz & Sinclair 2008).

As noted earlier, the glandular trichomes enclose secondary metabolites as phytocannabinoids, responsible for the defense and interaction with herbivores and pests and terpenoids, which generate the typical smell of the cannabis (Andre et al., 2016). The overlap of stress for both plants and humans, and the plant production of specific compounds in relation to stress is an interesting hypothesis. THC, the main component of the trichomes resin, plays a protective function due to its viscous and hydrophobic nature and low volatility (Pate, 1994).

Stressful conditions that often increase plant secondary compounds include sparse rainfall, low humidity, and sunny climate—often generating a plant rich in psychoactive components. In addition, cannabis pollen growing under conditions of decreased humidity has an increased phytocannabinoid content. Scientists have also found that phytocannabinoid contents of cannabis are influenced by certain extreme environmental conditions of humidity, temperature, radiation, soil nutrients, and parasites (Russo, 2011). Phytocannabinoids and several terpenes, present in cannabis leaves and flowers, serve as a barrier to water loss, as observed in analogy to the waxy coatings of the cacti and other succulent plants (Pate, 1994).

Terpenes and phytocannabinoids can block other sources of environmental stress such as attacks by bacteria, fungi, and insect, or competition with surrounding vegetation. In particular, female cannabis plants, often noted for their aromatic quality and many of the terpenes produced (pinene, limonene, terpineol, and borneol), are known to possess insect-repellent properties and may help to suppress growth of surrounding vegetation (McPartland, 1997). In addition, temperature has a role in determining the cannabinoid amount, but only through its association with environmental humidity.

Selection and breeding of cannabis further reinforce the means by which humans exert the most control over its evolution as a domesticated crop plant, and lie at the heart of the human-cannabis relationship (Small, 2015), as well as heavily influencing the chemical composition of the plants and how that might impact health. THC and aromatic psychoactive secretions are evolutionarily significant because these attracted early human attention, and at least in modern times, remain the primary impetus for the continued breeding and worldwide dispersal of cannabis cultivars (Pollan, 2002). If inherent value has any relation to risk-taking on the part of the caretakers, despite any plant containing >0.3% THC being almost universally illegal, humans across the globe continue to risk consequences of propagating the plant. In a study from 2006, cannabis production was estimated to have a value of $35.8 billion, exceeding the value of corn ($23.3 billion) and wheat ($7.5 billion) combined (Small & Marcus, 2002).

Early Cannabis Use as Medicine

For as long as there has been the phenomenon known as civilization, people have used mind-altering substances, and this almost certainly began in prehistory and spread with migrations. It can be argued that in ancient cultures, there may have been no distinction between medicine and mind-altering drugs. As documented with other psychoactive plants, shamans from Iquitos in Peru used a drink (ayahuasca) based on two plants, *Banisteriopsis caapi* and *Psychotria viridis*, during shamanic rites, capable of generating psychedelic effects (Luna, 1984). These two plants were considered "teachers" because the shamans (Don Emilio Andrade Gomez, Don Alejandro Vasquez Zarate, Don Celso Rojas and Don Jose Coral More) using these, among others, could heal the diseases of people who employed these in their village, often accompanied by fasting and certain melodies. This "plant-teacher" approach has also been argued by other authors (VanPool, 2009; Mafimisebi & Oguntade, 2010; Jauregui et al., 2011; Armijos et al., 2014) and could explain the use of cannabis in the religious rituals of early human societies. Clarke and Merlin (2016) argued that the discovery of cannabis psychoactivity may be considered as an unintentional event. The western-centered viewpoint of American researchers maintains that perhaps the accidental burning of cannabis plants, triggered by natural events, revealed its psychotropic nature.

Recent advances in identifying traces of organic fats, waxes, and resins invisible to the eye have allowed scientists to pinpoint the presence of various substances with a degree of accuracy previously unthinkable. For example, the Yamnaya people, who swept out of Central Asia about 5,000 years ago, appear to have carried cannabis to Europe and the Middle East. In 2016, a team from the German Archaeological Institute and the Free University (both in Berlin) found residues and botanical remains of the plant at Yamnaya sites across Eurasia. The challenge is determining whether the Yamnaya, and other earlier cultures, used cannabis simply to make hemp for rope or also smoked and/or ingested it (Ren et al., 2019).

Southeast Asia

Several Neolithic pieces of evidence found in Taiwan suggest that cannabis was used 12,000 years ago for several different purposes (Li, 1973) and played a significant role in early cordage and textile manufacturing. Historically, Central Asia and South-East Asia have been proposed as potential regions for the natural origin and/or primary domestication of cannabis and may have played a vital role in its evolution (Stevens et al., 2016; Jiang et al., 2006). Recent evidence from analysis of excellent preservation of whole plant cannabis, including seeds from the 2,700 year old Yanghai Tombs near Turpan, Xinjiang-Uighur Autonomous Region, China, allowed an unprecedented level of modern botanical investigation through biochemistry

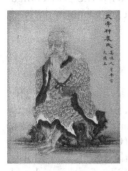

Figure 1.5 Emperor Shen Nung Source: Xu Jetian / Public domain

and genetics to conclude that the cannabis plant was cultivated for psychoactive purposes and offers the most compelling physical evidence to date for the use of cannabis for its medicinal or mystical attributes (Russo et al., 2008).

The medical use of cannabis dates back about 5,000 years ago, when the emperor Shen Nung (Figure 1.5), defined king and "father" of Chinese agriculture, drew up the first Chinese pharmacopoeia. According to ancient text, cannabis was prescribed for fatigue, rheumatism, and malaria (Abel, 1980). It was also utilized as an anesthetic during surgery, including for the emperor Shen Nung in 2737 BC (Merlin, 1972). Cannabis elixirs were incorporated into certain Taoist religious ceremonies, often associated with the Hemp Maid, or Ma Gu, as described in the religious text *The Secret of the Golden Flower* (Abel, 1980).

India

Cannabis was carried into the South Asian subcontinent between 2000 and 1000 BC, most likely as part of the series of Aryan invasions (Zuardi, 2006). In India, herbal medicine dates back several thousand years to the "Rig-Veda." This led to a system of healthcare known as Ayurvedic medicine. *Cannabis sativa* was depicted extensively in the ancient Sanskrit Vedic poems, particularly the Atharvaveda, or "Science of Charms" (Bennett et al., 1995), in which it is celebrated as one of "five kingdoms of herbs ... which release us from anxiety."

Ayurvedic medicinal traditions used the drug extensively, typically mixed with other herbs (Warf, 2014). In India, cannabis came into its own both as a narcotic and a medicine, largely because its association with religion gave it all the virtues conferred by holiness (Touw, 1981). It is mentioned in the Bhagavad-Gita as sharpening the memory and alleviating fatigue and continues to have spiritual connotations with the god Ganga (cognate with Ganges), from which the widespread term ganja is derived (Bennett et al., 1995).

Greeks and Romans

Cannabis was also well known among the ancient Greeks and Romans. The historian Herodotus (ca. 400 BC) mentioned its use among the Indians, and Diodorus Siculus (ca. 60 BC) reported that the ancient Egyptian women used cannabis to reduce pain and improve their mood (Carod-Artal, 2013). In the 5th century BC, in the first western mention of the plant, Herodotus famously noted in *The Histories* that in Macedonia "The Scythians howl with joy for the vapour bath" (Benet, 1975), referring to the practice of shamanic chanting following the heating of cannabis seeds on stones and inhaling the fumes under small tents as part of purification ceremonies (Warf, 2014).

In addition, the Roman historian Pliny the Elder recounted the use of cannabis roots for easing pain (Ryz et al., 2017). In the same period, Pedacius Dioscorides, a Greek physician, classified different plants, including cannabis, and described their useful benefits (Riddle, 2011). He reportedly prescribed it for toothaches and earaches, remedies that persisted through the medieval era (Warf, 2014).

The Roman physician, Claudius Galen (131–201 AD), considered highly influential in the Ancient and Middle Ages, also wrote some notes about cannabis. In particular, he described a practice, diffused among Roman aristocrats, to conclude their lunch with a cannabis-based dessert (Butrica, 2002). He noted that cannabis was widely consumed throughout the empire and astutely argued that overuse caused sterility (Clarke & Merlin 2016; Payne et al., 2019).

Egypt

Semitic peoples in the Middle East who acquired cannabis from Aryan cultures include the Assyrians, Egyptians, and Hebrews, who burned it as incense as early as 1000 BC. While exact origins of cannabis use are unclear in Egypt, cannabis pollen was recovered from the tomb of Ramses II, who governed 67 years during the 19th dynasty, and several mummies contain trace cannabinoids (Warf, 2014). Around 60 BC, Assyrian clay tablets and Egyptian Ebers Papyrus document ancient Egyptian women using cannabis for pain management and to improve their mood (Scurlock & Andersen, 2005; Epstein, 2010). According to evidence in ancient texts and glyphs, *Cannabis sativa* was used to treat fatigue, rheumatism, and malaria, as well as numerous other common maladies. The tomb of an Egyptian Pharaoh, Ramses II, was discovered with a mummy containing particles of kief, tiny crystals that cover the cannabis plant. According to the medieval Muslim botanist Ibn al-Baytar, a second wave of cannabis introduction into Egypt occurred in the mid-12th century as the result of the emigration of mystic devotees from Syria (Khalifa, 1975).

Middle East

The cultivation and use of cannabis in the classical Arab world has been the topic of some speculation. Cannabis arrived in the Middle East between 2000 and 1400 BC (Aldrich, 1997), perhaps as part of the broader Aryan infiltration of the region. Medieval Arab doctors considered it a sacred medicine (Rosenthal, 1971). The discovery of hashish was allegedly attributable to Haydar, founder of a Sufi order in the mid-12th century, who used it to enhance ecstatic religious states (Abel, 1980). Sufi mystics are known to have used hashish regularly, and played a key role in spreading it throughout the Middle East (Warf, 2014). In the medieval Arabic culture, the use of cannabis was associated with disadvantaged social conditions. The term hashish became famously associated with the ashishin, or the Assassins. An example is a myth of "Old Man of the Mountains" and the followers of Hasan, the "ashishin," as written in the chronicles by Marco Polo (Fleischhauer, 1956).

Europe

The various forms of cannabis were known to medieval Europe. In particular, Italians began the first large-scale cultivation and commercialization of the plant in the Mediterranean area. Assertive efforts by the British and Portuguese colonial governments from the 16th to the 19th centuries to promote cannabis use were linked to the worldwide commodification of labor power and the production of a quiescent labor force (Angrosino, 2003). Cannabis played an important, if largely unacknowledged, role in the British Empire (Mills, 2005). The British learned about smoking cannabis from their Indian subjects, notably from Irish physician William Brooke O'Shaughnessy (O'Shaughnessy, 1840), employed in India as Professor of Chemistry and Materia Medica in Calcutta, who conducted a series of experiments with cannabis in the 1830s and concluded it had no negative medicinal effects.

He observed the use of cannabis in Indian traditional medicine for the treatment of spastic and convulsive disorders such as ëhydrophobiaí (rabies), tetanus, cholera, and delirium tremens, and consequently sent supplies of the material to a pharmaceutical firm in London for analysis and clinical trials (Kalant, 2001). The extracts of cannabis were adopted into the British Pharmacopoeia and later into the American Pharmacopeia and were widely used in the English-speaking world as sedative, hypnotic, and anticonvulsant agents in the late 19th and early 20th centuries (Walton, 1938; Mikuriya,

1969). In addition, in the English medicine of the 19th century, cannabis was introduced as an analgesic, anti-inflammatory, anti-emetic, and anti-convulsant (Aldrich, 1997).

While in England the use of cannabis focused on medical purposes, in France, the psychoactive effects of cannabis were pursued (Kalant, 1972). The popularity of hashish in Europe arose in the aftermath of the Napoleonic invasion of Egypt in 1798, when returning soldiers brought hashish with them to France (Warf, 2014). The myth of the Orient that pervaded the 19th century also brought with it the development of private hashish consumer clubs. Many Romantic artists and writers frequented these clubs such as Théophile Gautier, Charles Baudelaire, Honoré de Balzac, Alexandre Dumas, and Gustave Flaubert (Levinthal, 1999).

In 1830, the French physician Jacques Joseph Moreau studied the effects of cannabis in mental illness. He thought that the voluptuary use of cannabis could generate sensations common to the hallucinations and delusions in psychotic individuals (Moreau, 1973). Conversely, cannabis was not known in the Americas until the arrival and settlement of the first European colonists. During this period cannabis was used primarily for the strength and the resistance of its fibers.

New World

More recently, 19th-century English doctors prescribed cannabis to reduce pain, inflammation, nausea, and seizures, and to soothe difficulties of menstruation. In the early 20th century, American cannabis use was concentrated among Mexican Americans in the southwestern part of the country (Bonnie & Whitebread, 1970).

Despite the benefits described above, it was strongly prohibited in the twentieth century due to its remarkable psychoactive effects. It was removed from the British Pharmacopoeia in 1932 and included as a banned substance for therapeutic use in the Act of the Parliament of the United Kingdom, Misuse of Drugs Regulation Act in 1971 (Hall, 2008). The Mexican Revolution of 1910–1911 introduced a new chapter in the historical geography of American cannabis. Waves of immigrants fleeing the violence washed across the southwestern United States, bringing the herb with them. Many early prejudices against cannabis were thinly veiled racist fears of its smokers, often promulgated by reactionary newspapers such as those owned by the Hearst chain. Mexicans were frequently blamed for smoking "marijuana," property crimes, seducing children, and engaging in murderous sprees (Warf 2014).

It is well documented how the initial panic over cannabis in the 1930s was socially constructed by the media and government influence on public opinion (see Chapter 6). In a shock to the human historical trend, both England and the United States moved to prohibit its use in the 1930s, creating steep barriers for its therapeutic use and an enduring smokescreen for the memory of its historical continuity. In 1937, production, possession or transfer of cannabis was forbidden in the United States due to "The Marihuana Tax Act" federal law (Bonnie & Whitebread, 1970).

From a pharmacological point of view, the western medicine approach to cannabis shifted significantly with the biochemical identification of the molecules and endogenous systems responsible for its potential human physiologic effects. In 1964, Gaoni and Mechoulam opened the way for studying cannabinoids by isolating and synthesizing the main phytocannabinoid, THC (Mechoulam & Gaoni, 1965).

In the 1980s, Pfizer worked on the development of synthetic ligands of cannabinoid receptors. Subsequently, the cannabinoid type-1 (CB1) receptor was first discovered in 1990, and then the cannabinoid type-2 (CB2) receptor in 1993. Moreover, in the 1990s the two endogenous CB receptor ligands, arachidonoylethanolamine and 2-arachidonylglycerol, were also discovered (Pertwee, 2009). Finally, around the same time, Di Marzo and colleagues coined the term "endocannabinoid system," which comprises endogenous ligands, receptors, and synthesis and degradation enzymes (Di Marzo et al., 1994). Chapter 2 provides an in-depth look at the endocannabinoid system.

All these discoveries related to cannabis have contributed to the identification of new synthetic molecules that are able to modulate the endocannabinoid system in inflammation, pain, and metabolic processes (Lazzari et al., 2017; Mastinu et al., 2018; Tambaro et al., 2014; Bonini et al., 2016). This has led to both FDA-approved medicines as earlier discussed, as well as an extensive and dangerous illicit market. It is important to note that neither medicine nor science drives present day cannabis opinion and attitudes; rather, the media plays a large role in shaping cannabis laws and the general public's attitudes toward cannabis (Stringer & Maggard, 2016).

Cannabis and Health

The use of different preparations of cannabis can be found in folk medicine traditions and old herbals of the Middle East, East and South Asia, Europe, Africa, and the New World. Its historical use is associated with therapeutic strategies for many diseases and symptoms. Mechoulam provided a list of 20 medicinal applications of *Cannabis* by traditional societies (Mechoulam, 1986) and it is reportedly his interest in these historical uses that triggered his extensive research in cannabinoid chemistry and physiology.

A discussion of cannabis and health cannot be complete without the mention of "set and setting." The relationship between mind-altering and medicinal use in ritual contexts is also often assumed by the person consuming cannabis or celebrating its symbolic therapeutic potency. The set and setting hypothesis basically holds that the effects of psychedelic drugs are dependent first and foremost upon set (personality, preparation, expectation, and intention of the person having the experience) and setting (the physical, social, and cultural environment in which the experience takes place) Hartogsohn, 2017). These "nondrug parameters of psychopharmacology," as it was sometimes called in the 1960s (Felman, 1963) has been debated extensively over the past century, yet it has still not been answered in full.

ECS is involved in various disorders, including metabolic and neuroinflammatory pathologies. Especially in the brain, cannabinoids modulate hunger/satiety and neuroinflammation, and in the periphery, are involved in the peripheral metabolic reactions of liver, fat, muscles, and anti-inflammatory response in the blood cells. Due to the diffuse presence of the ECS in the brain and periphery and multifold activity in human physiology, its activation or inhibition regulates several pathophysiological phenomena and has grounds to serve as potentially one of the greatest breakthroughs in human health in the 21st century (Mastinu et al., 2018).

Apart from the potential treatment of symptoms and mitigation of disease, the mechanism of cannabis exists as a potential "tonic" when used in the correct dose for everyday life. An adaptogen is a plant or other substance that increases endurance, longevity, resistance, health, or generally protects the body from stressful situations (Darbinyan et al., 2007). This category, as with many others of traditional medicines, is inconsistent with the dominant paradigm of biomedicine, and is thus difficult to test as a pharmacological hypothesis. Cannabis, with many similar attributes, may serve a role in the health-supporting or "wellness" sphere of medicine akin to the earlier discussion of xenohormesis.

Cannabis and Harm

As we review the rich history of the use of cannabis and medicine, it is also important to be aware of the concerns related to the more widespread use of the plant. Cannabinoids are associated with an increased risk of short-term adverse events such as asthenia, balance problems, confusion, dizziness, disorientation, diarrhoea, euphoria, drowsiness, dry mouth, fatigue, hallucination, nausea, somnolence, vomiting, and anxiety (Whiting et al., 2015; Lim et al., 2017).

The addictive potential of cannabis is low, compared to nicotine, alcohol, and other drugs of abuse. The risk of dependence increases with duration and frequency of use, consumption of high potency THC products, and co-use of other substances (Jager, 2012). Cannabis Use Disorder is a DSM-V diagnostic category, but controversy still exists regarding the existence of a clinically significant cannabis withdrawal syndrome. Withdrawal symptoms have been described as: restlessness, loss of appetite, and irritability and insomnia. Symptoms can last for up to 10 days (Budney et al., 1999). Despite the controversy surrounding the plant, millions of dollars have gone to studying its potential for harm (NIDA, 2016). Similar to questions related to medicinal benefit, many questions remain open with numerous contradictory negative effects. Health professionals should be aware of adverse health effects of cannabis use and which populations are at most risk (Volkow et al., 2014).

Cannabis and Spirituality

For centuries, the spiritual aspects of health and sickness have been an integral component of the ethnomedicinal inquiry, which is an aspect of healing often ignored by western medicine. Like the plant itself, many difficulties exist in validating the impact of spirituality on health using existing scientific principles and experiments. Nonetheless, cannabis has also been recognized as a sacred plant by several religions over the centuries (Touw, 1981).

Indeed, the holy texts of Asiatic cultures referred to it as a plant with sacred virtues and considered it a part of religious rituals. In India and Tibet, Hinduism and tantric Buddhism traditions used flowers and resins of cannabis to facilitate the meditation and communication with the spirits (Schultes & Hoffman, 1992). There is a Buddhist legend about the ability of the bhang, a particular cannabis preparation, to have been the only source of nourishment for Siddhartha Gautama during his six years of asceticism (Touw, 1981). According to some authors, the word cannabis was present in Semitic languages such as Hebrew, and it appears several times throughout the Old Testament. In fact, in some passages of Exodus, Isaiah, Jeremiah, and Ezekiel, the use of cannabis as incense and sacred oil is cited (Bennett, 2011; Bonini et al., 2018).

Research and Future Ethnomedicinal Inquiry

Many questions remain open with numerous contradictory therapeutic effects reported. The disconnect between the willingness of some states to regulate, sell, and tax cannabis and the federal reluctance to allow research to progress leaves more and more people without the knowledge to make informed, science-based choices. Future research will help to fill in the tremendous gaps in our knowledge related to cannabis and potentially help direct those hoping to use it responsibly in the mitigation of disease and fostering wellness.

A criticism of ethnomedicine is that chemical composition, dosages, and toxicity of the plants used in ethnomedicine are not clearly defined (Lowe 2000). As we have seen for both cannabis and valerian, among others, this poses a major hurdle for acceptance in the current medical paradigm. For this and many other reasons, plant medicine has long been ignored by many biomedical practitioners. Considered "dirty" compounds that interact with numerous endogenous proteins, there is additional concern for negative "off-target" effects of plant medicines when compared to a molecule that specifically targets one protein (Howitz & Sinclair, 2008).

What we do not know about the cannabinoids and their interaction with the ECS far eclipses what we do know. Is there legitimacy to the theory of entourage? Is there a real correlation on the voluptuary use of cannabis and psychiatric diseases such as schizophrenia? Why is the action of individual phytocannabinoids not always comparable with the consumption of cannabis? At what level does the activation of CB1 receptors improve/worsen cognitive functions? How might this affect driving? Furthermore, how can some CB1 agonist compounds act on memory consolidation mechanisms? Can CB1 antagonists as be used regulators of energy metabolism?

We also know that cannabis is a complex mixture of hundreds of chemicals affecting human physiologic processes such as energy metabolism, pain, and inflammation in many formulations of unknown concentrations, pharmacological effects, and side effects. Arguments exist and continue to gather improved research substantiation that favors the administration of whole plant medicines over single molecules. These real challenges force us to look at reductionist models in evaluation of this plant versus new modalities that could help inform the use of a complex whole plant medicine.

Multiple barriers prohibit a better understanding of this complex plant and its role in human health. The challenges for researchers studying this plant have long been overly burdensome from both a political and scientific perspective. It is often difficult for researchers to gain access to the quantity, quality, and type of cannabis product necessary to address specific research questions on the health effects of cannabis use (NASEM, 2017). Reinforcing the active debate on the positive/negative effects of cannabis products will further condition the government to lower barriers to high-quality research.

Imagine developing a randomized control trial that included over 800 different medicines. This seeming impossibility is only the tip of the iceberg for cannabis research. As a psychoactive substance, any research with a THC-containing product is difficult to categorize as placebo. Astutely renamed the "meaning response" (Moerman & Jonas, 2002), placebo contributes to the overall therapeutic effects of virtually all medicines, in addition to the pharmacotherapeutic actions of medicines. When considering psychoactive cannabis and cannabinoids, there may be a molecular aspect via CB1/ CB2 receptor activation/modulation to the meaning response. Therefore, rather than being either a placebo or a drug, cannabis might be a drug both conveying and inducing a meaning response (Gertsch, 2018).

Even more challenging is the wide range of products, doses, and routes of administration. Accumulating evidence is not focused on a single product but is spread out across many products, often without a common denominator to reinforce the power of the disparate research. The majority of research that is funded is related to harm, primarily focused on bud/flower (with high THC, minimal if any CBD), and not focused on medical use. Hope exists in the marked change we have seen in a brief period of time, in large part triggered by the resurgence of cannabis popularity. In 2018, for the first time in the USA at the federal level, a derivative of cannabis was approved by the Food and Drug Administration for the treatment of two epilepsy disorders (U.S. FDA, 2018). The U.S. Food and Drug Administration recently reinforced its support of cannabis drug development via regulatory pathways (Voelker, 2020).

Extensive pharmacological studies are still needed to better understand the clinical relevance and applications of non-psychoactive cannabinoids in the prevention and treatment of life-threatening diseases. Cannabinoid medicine chemically standardized and administered clinically under medical supervision is a markedly different set and setting than illicit or even recreational use. It is likely that future research will reveal new classes of receptors, new binding sites, and potential new mechanisms for treating a wide range of illnesses that traditional medicines have been treating for centuries.

Finally, cannabis is alerting us to the idea that illness, in contrast to disease, is patient defined and is often culturally bound. Modern medicine is slowly beginning to see the value of the illness-based approach in treating patients (Eisenberg, 1977; Green et al., 2002). Evaluating "efficacy" may therefore be more complex and require a keen understanding of culture (Murdock, 1980), as well as more sophisticated research tactics to effectively study complex medicines that go beyond a "bucket of pills" (McClatchey et al., 2009).

Conclusion

Cannabis is a fascinating, versatile plant whose mystery far overshadows known facts related to its medicinal impact on humans despite a near 6,000 year history as a medicine. Cannabis use has been alternately promoted and demonized, forming shifting, contingent, and contested islands of morality situated between competing discourses of legitimacy and illegitimacy (Thompson et al., 2007). Looking at historical, botanical, chemical, and ethnopharmacological knowledge from the first human communities to current medical applications reinforces the utility and versatility of cannabis, placing it in various forms and environments on every continent. These reflections may also help us decipher next steps in the best utilization of this plant and its 1,001 molecules.

The current resurgence of cannabis serves to reinforce the role of plants in the modern western medical paradigm and encourage new ways to approach both illness and health. According to data released by the World Health Organization (WHO), ethnomedicine has maintained its popularity in all regions of the developing world and its use is rapidly expanding in the industrialized countries. For cannabis to earn its place in modern medicine, and to find the answers to the many questions this plant has raised for the human species related to both health and harm, current research limitations will need to be lifted. Potentially, new mechanisms of scientific evaluation will need to continue to evolve to better understand complex relationships with complex medicines. Promising examples of this evolution includes crowd-sourcing human data, FDA paths of real-world evidence, large-scale high-quality observational studies, and silicon quantum computers (Tucker & Shen, 2005; Jarow et al., 2017). Contingent on future changes related to research on cannabis, this plant may foster a future chapter of ethnomedicine where the stigmatized weed moves from fringe to well-studied and accepted medicine, potentially providing safer relief for patients based on solid science. Solid science may also definitively show that harm outweighs benefits, solidifying the stigma as legitimate. Cannabis has played a crucial role in human history and cultural evolution, and further research and clinical experience will guide us in making appropriate decisions for its future, purely based on sound medical science rather than emotion or politics.

References

Abel, E. L. (1980). *Marihuana*. Springer US. https://doi.org/10.1007/978-1-4899-2189-5

Adovasio, J. M., Soffer, O., & Klíma, B. (1996). Upper palaeolithic fibre technology: Interlaced woven finds from Pavlov I, Czech Republic, c. 26,000 years ago. *Antiquity, 70*(269), 526–534. https://doi.org/10.1017/S0003598X0008368X

Aldrich, M. (1997). *History of therapeutic cannabis: Cannabis in medical practice: A legal, historical and pharmacological overview of the therapeutic use of marijuana* (pp. 35–55) (M. L. Mathre, Ed.). Jefferson, NC: McFarland & Company.

Anderson, E. N. (1988). *The food of China*. New Haven, CT: Yale University Press.

Anderson, L. C. (1980). Leaf variation among cannabis species from a controlled garden. *Botanical Museum Leaflets, Harvard University, 28*, 61–69.

Andre, C. M., Hausman, J.-F., & Guerriero, G. (2016). Cannabis sativa: The plant of the thousand and one molecules. *Frontiers in Plant Science, 7*. https://doi.org/10.3389/fpls.2016.00019

Angrosino, M. (2003). Rum and Ganja: Indenture, drug foods, labor motivation, and the evolution of the modern sugar industry in Trinidad. In W. Jankowiak & D. Bradburd (Eds.), *Drugs, labor, and colonial expansion* (pp. 101–116). Tucson, AZ: University of Arizona Press.

Anwar, F., Latif, S., & Ashraf, M. (2006). Analytical characterization of hemp (Cannabis sativa) seed oil from different agro-ecological zones of Pakistan. *Journal of the American Oil Chemists' Society, 83*(4), 323–329. https://doi.org/10.1007/s11746-006-1207-x

Armijos, C., Cota, I., & González, S. (2014). Traditional medicine applied by the Saraguro yachakkuna: A preliminary approach to the use of sacred and psychoactive plant species in the southern region of Ecuador. *Journal of Ethnobiology and Ethnomedicine, 10*(1), 26. https://doi.org/10.1186/1746-4269-10-26

Atakan, Z. (2012). Cannabis, a complex plant: Different compounds and different effects on individuals. *Therapeutic Advances in Psychopharmacology, 2*(6), 241–254. https://doi.org/10.1177/2045125312457586

Benet, S. (1975). Early diffusion and folk uses of hemp. In Rubin (Ed.), *Cannabis and culture* (pp. 39–49). The Hague and Paris: Mouton Publishers.

Bennett, C. (2011). Early/ancient history. In J. Holland (Ed.), *The Pot Book: A complete guide to cannabis, its role in medicine, politics, science, and culture* (pp. 17–26). Rochester: Park Street Press.

Bennett, C., Osburn, L., & Osburn, J. (1995). *Green gold the tree of life: Marijuana in magic & religion*. Access Unlimited.

Bonini, S. A., Mastinu, A., Maccarinelli, G., Mitola, S., Premoli, M., La Rosa, L. R., ... Memo, M. (2016). Cortical structure alterations and social behavior impairment in p50-deficient mice. *Cerebral Cortex*, 26(6), 2832–2849. https://doi.org/10.1093/cercor/bhw037

Bonini, S. A., Premoli, M., Tambaro, S., Kumar, A., Maccarinelli, G., Memo, M., & Mastinu, A. (2018). Cannabis sativa: A comprehensive ethnopharmacological review of a medicinal plant with a long history. *Journal of Ethnopharmacology*, 227, 300–315. https://doi.org/10.1016/j.jep.2018.09.004

Bonnie, R., & Whitebread, C. (1970). The forbidden fruit and the tree of knowledge: An inquiry into the legal history of American marijuana prohibition. *Virginia Law Review*, 56(6), 971–1203.

Brenneisen, R. (2007). Chemistry and analysis of phytocannabinoids and other cannabis constituents. In M. A. ElSohly (Ed.), *Marijuana and the cannabinoids* (pp. 17–49). New York: Humana Press. https://doi.org/10.1007/978-1-59259-947-9_2

Brown, D. T. (Ed.) (1998). *Cannabis: The genus cannabis*. Boca Raton: CRC Press. https://doi.org/10.1201/9780203304228

Budney, A. J., Novy, P. L., & Hughes, J. R. (1999). Marijuana withdrawal among adults seeking treatment for marijuana dependence. *Addiction*, 94(9), 1311–1322. https://doi.org/10.1046/j.1360-0443.1999.94913114.x

Butrica, J. L. (2002). The medical use of cannabis among the Greeks and Romans. *Journal of Cannabis Therapeutics*, 2(2), 51–70. https://doi.org/10.1300/J175v02n02_04

Carod-Artal, F. J. (2013). Psychoactive plants in ancient Greece. *Neurosciences and History*, 1, 28–38.

Carroll, R. (2004). Under the influence: Harry Anslinger's role in shaping America's drug policy. In J. Erlen & J. Spillane (Eds.), *Federal drug control: The evolution of policy and practice* (pp. 61–99). Bingham, NY: Haworth Press.

Cherney, J., & Small, E. (2016). Industrial hemp in North America: Production, politics and potential. *Agronomy*, 6(4), 58. https://doi.org/10.3390/agronomy6040058

Clarke, R. C., & Merlin, M. D. (2016). *Cannabis: Evolution and ethnobotany*. Berkeley, CA: University of California Press.

Committee on the Health Effects of Marijuana. An Evidence Review and Research Agenda, Board on Population Health and Public Health Practice, Health and Medicine Division, & National Academies of Sciences, Engineering, and Medicine (2017). *The health effects of cannabis and cannabinoids: The current state of evidence and recommendations for research* (p. 24625). Washington, DC: National Academies Press. https://doi.org/10.17226/24625

Corleone, J. (2014, January 11). *What are the benefits of hemp seeds?* Retrieved from Livestrong.com, after March 2, 2020.

Cox, P. A. (1994). The ethnobotanical approach to drug discovery: Strengths and limitations. *Ciba Foundation Symposium*, 185, 25–36; discussion 36–41.

Craker, P. L. (2006, April 27). Reefer madness: Marijuana is medically useful, whether politicians like it or not. *The Economist*. Retrieved from https://www.economist.com/, after March 2, 2020.

Darbinyan, V., Aslanyan, G., Amroyan, E., Gabrielyan, E., Malmström, C., & Panossian, A. (2007). Clinical trial of *Rhodiola rosea* L. extract SHR-5 in the treatment of mild to moderate depression. *Nordic Journal of Psychiatry*, *61*(5), 343–348. https://doi.org/10.1080/08039480701643290

Deferne, J. L., & Pate, D. W. (1996). Hemp seed oil: A source of valuable essential fatty acids. *Journal of the International Hemp Association*, *3*(1), 4–7.

Di Marzo, V., Fontana, A., Cadas, H., Schinelli, S., Cimino, G., Schwartz, J.-C., & Piomelli, D. (1994). Formation and inactivation of endogenous cannabinoid anandamide in central neurons. *Nature*, *372*(6507), 686–691. https://doi.org/10.1038/372686a0

Eisenberg, L. (1977). Disease and illness distinctions between professional and popular ideas of sickness. *Culture, Medicine and Psychiatry*, *1*(1), 9–23. https://doi.org/10.1007/BF00114808

Epstein, H. A. (2010). A natural approach to soothing atopic skin. *Skinmed*, *8*(2), 95–97.

Etkin, N. L., & Ross, P. J. (1982). Food as medicine and medicine as food. *Social Science and Medicine*, *16*(17), 1559–1573. https://doi.org/10.1016/0277-9536(82)90167-8

Farag, S., & Kayser, O. (2017). The cannabis plant: Botanical aspects. In *Handbook of cannabis and related pathologies* (pp. 3–12). Elsevier. https://doi.org/10.1016/B978-0-12-800756-3.00001-6

Felman, P. E. (1963). Non-drug parameters of psychopharmacology: The role of the physician. M. Rinkel (Ed.), *Specific and non-specific factors in psychopharmacology* (pp. 149–158). New York: Philosophical Library.

Fleischhauer, W. (1956). The old man of the mountain: The growth of a legend. *Symposium: A Quarterly Journal in Modern Literatures*, *9*(1), 79–90. https://doi.org/10.1080/00397709.1956.10113536

Fort, J. (2012). Synthesis between demic and cultural diffusion in the neolithic transition in Europe. *Proceedings of the National Academy of Sciences*, *109*(46), 18669–18673. https://doi.org/10.1073/pnas.1200662109

Gertsch, J. (2018). The intricate influence of the placebo effect on medical cannabis and cannabinoids. *Medical Cannabis and Cannabinoids*, *1*(1), 60–64. https://doi.org/10.1159/000489291

Green, A. R., Carrillo, J. E., & Betancourt, J. R. (2002). Why the disease-based model of medicine fails our patients. *The Western Journal of Medicine*, *176*(2), 141–143.

Grifo, F., & Rosenthal, J. (Eds.) (1997). *Biodiversity and human health*. Washington, DC: Island Press.

Hall, W. D. (2008). The contribution of research to the development of a national cannabis policy in Australia. *Addiction*, *103*(5), 712–720. https://doi.org/10.1111/j.1360-0443.2008.02169.x

Hanuš, L. O. (2009). Pharmacological and therapeutic secrets of plant and brain (endo)cannabinoids. *Medicinal Research Reviews*, *29*(2), 213–271. https://doi.org/10.1002/med.20135

Hanuš, L. O., Meyer, S. M., Muñoz, E., Taglialatela-Scafati, O., & Appendino, G. (2016). Phytocannabinoids: A unified critical inventory. *Natural Product Reports*, *33*(12), 1357–1392. https://doi.org/10.1039/C6NP00074F

Happyana, N., Agnolet, S., Muntendam, R., Van Dam, A., Schneider, B., & Kayser, O. (2013). Analysis of cannabinoids in laser-microdissected trichomes of medicinal Cannabis sativa using LCMS and cryogenic NMR. *Phytochemistry*, *87*, 51–59. https://doi.org/10.1016/j.phytochem.2012.11.001

Hartogsohn, I. (2017). Constructing drug effects: A history of set and setting. *Drug Science, Policy and Law*, *3*, 205032451668332, https://doi.org/10.1177/2050324516683325

Hill, A. J., Williams, C. M., Whalley, B. J., & Stephens, G. J. (2012). Phytocannabinoids as novel therapeutic agents in CNS disorders. *Pharmacology and Therapeutics*, *133*(1), 79–97. https://doi.org/10.1016/j.pharmthera.2011.09.002

Howitz, K. T., & Sinclair, D. A. (2008). Xenohormesis: Sensing the chemical cues of other species. *Cell*, *133*(3), 387–391. https://doi.org/10.1016/j.cell.2008.04.019

Huchelmann, A., Boutry, M., & Hachez, C. (2017). Plant glandular trichomes: Natural cell factories of high biotechnological interest. *Plant Physiology*, *175*(1), 6–22. https://doi.org/10.1104/pp.17.00727

Hudson, R., & Puvanenthirarajah, N. (2018). Cannabis for pain management: Pariah or panacea? University of Western Ontario Medical Journal, 87(1), 58–61. https://doi.org/10.5206/uwomj.v87i1.1922

Izzo, A. A., Borrelli, F., Capasso, R., Di Marzo, V., & Mechoulam, R. (2009). Non-psychotropic plant cannabinoids: New therapeutic opportunities from an ancient herb. *Trends in Pharmacological Sciences*, *30*(10), 515–527. https://doi.org/10.1016/j.tips.2009.07.006

Jarow, J. P., LaVange, L., & Woodcock, J. (2017). Multidimensional evidence generation and FDA regulatory decision making: Defining and using "real-world" data. *JAMA*, *318*(8), 703. https://doi.org/10.1001/jama.2017.9991

Jauregui, X., Clavo, Z. M., Jovel, E. M., & Pardo-de-Santayana, M. (2011). "Plantas con madre": Plants that teach and guide in the shamanic initiation process in the East-Central Peruvian Amazon. *Journal of Ethnopharmacology, 134*(3), 739–752. https://doi.org/10.1016/j.jep.2011.01.042

Jeong, M., Cho, J., Shin, J.-I., Jeon, Y.-J., Kim, J.-H., Lee, S.-J., … Lee, K. (2014). Hempseed oil induces reactive oxygen species- and C/EBP homologous protein-mediated apoptosis in MH7A human rheumatoid arthritis fibroblast-like synovial cells. *Journal of Ethnopharmacology, 154*(3), 745–752. https://doi.org/10.1016/j.jep.2014.04.052

Jiang, H.-E., Li, X., Zhao, Y.-X., Ferguson, D. K., Hueber, F., Bera, S., … Li, C.-S. (2006). A new insight into Cannabis sativa (Cannabaceae) utilization from 2500-year-old Yanghai Tombs, Xinjiang, China. *Journal of Ethnopharmacology, 108*(3), 414–422. https://doi.org/10.1016/j.jep.2006.05.034

Kalant, H. (2001). Medicinal use of cannabis: History and current status. *Pain Research and Management*, *6*(2), 80–91. https://doi.org/10.1155/2001/469629

Kalant, O. J. (1972). Report of the Indian Hemp Drugs Commission, 1893–94: A critical review. *International Journal of the Addictions*, *7*(1), 77–96. https://doi.org/10.3109/10826087209026763

Kemp, A. M., Clark, M. S., Dobbs, T., Galli, R., Sherman, J., & Cox, R. (2016). Top 10 facts you need to know about synthetic cannabinoids: Not so nice spice. *The American Journal of Medicine*, *129*(3), 240–244.e1. https://doi.org/10.1016/j.amjmed.2015.10.008

Keys, J. D. (1997). *Chinese herbs: Their botany, chemistry and pharmacodynamics : With special sections on mineral drugs, drugs of animal origin, 300 Chinese prescriptions, toxic herbs*. Charles E. Tuttle Publishing. North Clarendon, VT: Charles E. Tuttle Publishing.

Khalifa, A. (1975). Traditional patterns of hashish use in Egypt. In V. Rubin (Ed.), *Cannabis and culture* (pp. 195–205). The Hague: Mouton Publishers.

Krippner, S. (2003). *Models of ethnomedicinal healing*. Paper presented at the ethnomedicine conferences, April 26–27 and October 11–12, Munich, Germany.

Laprairie, R. B., Bagher, A. M., Kelly, M. E. M., & Denovan-Wright, E. M. (2015). Cannabidiol is a negative allosteric modulator of the cannabinoid CB $_1$ receptor: Negative allosteric modulation of CB $_1$ by cannabidiol. *British Journal of Pharmacology*, 172(20), 4790–4805. https://doi.org/10.1111/bph.13250

Lazzari, P., Serra, V., Marcello, S., Pira, M., & Mastinu, A. (2017). Metabolic side effects induced by olanzapine treatment are neutralized by CB1 receptor antagonist compounds co-administration in female rats. *European Neuropsychopharmacology*, 27(7), 667–678. https://doi.org/10.1016/j.euroneuro.2017.03.010

Levinthal, C. F. (1999). *Drugs, behavior, and modern society*. Boston, MA: Allyn and Bacon. Boston, MA: Allyn and Bacon.

Lewis, M., Russo, E., & Smith, K. (2018). Pharmacological foundations of cannabis chemovars. *Planta Medica*, 84(04), 225–233. https://doi.org/10.1055/s-0043-122240

Li, H.-L. (1973). An archaeological and historical account of cannabis in China. *Economic Botany*, 28(4), 437–448. https://doi.org/10.1007/BF02862859

Lim, K., See, Y. M., & Lee, J. (2017). A systematic review of the effectiveness of medical cannabis for psychiatric, movement and neurodegenerative disorders. *Clinical Psychopharmacology and Neuroscience*, 15(4), 301–312. https://doi.org/10.9758/cpn.2017.15.4.301

Lowe, H. I. C. (2000). *Jamaica's ethnomedicine: Its potential in the healthcare system*. Kingston, Jamaica: Canoe Press, University of the West Indies. Kingston, Jamaica.

Luna, L. E. (1984). The concept of plants as teachers among four mestizo shamans of Iquitos, Northeastern Peru. *Journal of Ethnopharmacology*, 11(2), 135–156. https://doi.org/10.1016/0378-8741(84)90036-9

Mafimisebi, T. E., & Oguntade, A. E. (2010). Preparation and use of plant medicines for farmers' health in Southwest Nigeria: Socio-cultural, magico-religious and economic aspects. *Journal of Ethnobiology and Ethnomedicine*, 6(1), 1. https://doi.org/10.1186/1746-4269-6-1

Mahlberg, P. G., Hammond, C. T., Turner, J. C., & Hemphill, J. K. (1984). Structure, development and composition of glandular trichomes of Cannabis Sativa L. In E. Rodriguez, P. L. Healey, & I. Mehta (Eds.), *Biology and chemistry of plant trichomes* (pp. 23–51). Springer US. https://doi.org/10.1007/978-1-4899-5355-1_2

Malingré, Th., Hendriks, H., Batterman, S., Bos, R., & Visser, J. (1975). The essential oil of *Cannabis sativa*. *Planta Medica*, 28(5), 56–61. https://doi.org/10.1055/s-0028-1097829

Mastinu, A., Premoli, M., Ferrari-Toninelli, G., Tambaro, S., Maccarinelli, G., Memo, M., & Bonini, S. A. (2018). Cannabinoids in health and disease: Pharmacological potential in metabolic syndrome and neuroinflammation. *Hormone Molecular Biology and Clinical Investigation*, 36(2). https://doi.org/10.1515/hmbci-2018-0013

McClatchey, W. C., Mahady, G. B., Bennett, B. C., Shiels, L., & Savo, V. (2009). Ethnobotany as a pharmacological research tool and recent developments in CNS-active natural products from ethnobotanical sources. *Pharmacology and Therapeutics*, *123*(2), 239–254. https://doi.org/10.1016/j. pharmthera.2009.04.002

McKenna, D. J. (1995). Plant hallucinogens: Springboards for psychotherapeutic drug discovery. *Behavioural Brain Research*, *73*(1–2), 109–116. https://doi. org/10.1016/0166-4328(96)00079-4

McKenna, T. (1993). *Food of the gods: The search for the original tree of knowledge : A radical history of plants, drugs and human evolution*. New York: Bantam Press.

McPartland, J. M. (1997). Cannabis as repellent and pesticide. *Journal of the International Hemp Association*, *4*, 87–92.

McPartland, J. M., & Guy, G. W. (2004). The evolution of Cannabis and coevolution with the cannabinoid receptor—A hypothesis. In Guy, G. W., Whittle, B. A., & Robson, P. J. (Eds), *The medicinal use of Cannabis and Cannabinoids* (pp. 71–101). London: Pharmaceutical Press.

Mechoulam, R. (1986). The pharmacohistory of Cannabis sativa. In R. Mechoulam (Ed.), *Cannabinoids as therapeutic agents* (pp. 1–19). Boca Raton, FL: CRC Press.

Mechoulam, R., & Gaoni, Y. (1965). A total synthesis of dl-Δ ^{1}-tetrahydrocannabinol, the active constituent of Hashish[1]. *Journal of the American Chemical Society*, *87*(14), 3273–3275. https://doi.org/10.1021/ja01092a065

Merlin, M. D. (1972). *Man and marijuana: Some aspects of their ancient relationship*. Vancouver, BC: Fairleigh Dickinson University Press.

Mikuriya, T. H. (1969). Marijuana in medicine: Past, present and future. *California Medicine*, *110*(1), 34–40.

Mills, J. (2005). *Cannabis britannica: Empire, trade and prohibition 1800–1928*. Oxford: Oxford University Press.

Moerman, D. E., & Jonas, W. B. (2002). Deconstructing the placebo effect and finding the meaning response. *Annals of Internal Medicine*, *136*(6), 471. https:// doi.org/10.7326/0003-4819-136-6-200203190-00011

Moreau, J. J. (1973). *Hashish and mental illness*. New York, NY: Raven Press.

Murdock, G. P. (1980). *Theories of illness: A world survey*. University of Pittsburgh Press. Retrieved from http://books.google.com/books?id=q1JqAAAAMAAJ

National Hispanic Caucus of State Legislators (2017). *Providing a legal framework when jurisdictions decide to decriminalize, commercialize and tax Cannabis*. Retrieved from https://nhcsl.org/resources/resolutions/2017/2017-12/, after June 25, 2018.

NIDA (2016). *NIH research on marijuana and cannabinoids*. Retrieved from https:// www.drugabuse.gov/drugs-abuse/marijuana/nih-research-marijuana-cannabino ids, after March 2, 2020.

OED Online (2018). *Cannabis*. Retrieved from http://www.oed.com/view/Entry/ 27087?redirectedFrom=cannabis#eid, after March 2, 2020.

Onaivi, E. S. (Ed.) (2002). *The biology of marijuana: From gene to behavior*. Boca Raton: CRC Press. https://doi.org/10.1201/9780203219133

O'Shaughnessy, W. B. (1840). On the preparations of the Indian hemp, or gunjah (Cannabis indica), their effects on the animal system in health, and their utility in the treatment of tetanus and other convulsive diseases. *British and Foreign Medical Review*, *10*(19), 225–228.

Pate, D. W. (1994). Chemical ecology of *cannabis*. *Journal of the International Hemp Association*, 2(29), 32–37.

Payne, K. S., Mazur, D. J., Hotaling, J. M., & Pastuszak, A. W. (2019). Cannabis and male fertility: A systematic review. *Journal of Urology*, 202(4), 674–681. https://doi.org/10.1097/JU.0000000000000248

Pertwee, R. G. (2008). The diverse CB1 and CB2 receptor pharmacology of three plant cannabinoids: Delta9-tetrahydrocannabinol, cannabidiol and delta9-tetrahydrocannabivarin. *British Journal of Pharmacology*, 153(2), 199–215. https://doi.org/10.1038/sj.bjp.0707442

Pertwee, R. G. (2009). Cannabinoid pharmacology: The first 66 years: Cannabinoid pharmacology. *British Journal of Pharmacology*, 147(Suppl.1), S163–S171. https://doi.org/10.1038/sj.bjp.0706406

Piluzza, G., Delogu, G., Cabras, A., Marceddu, S., & Bullitta, S. (2013). Differentiation between fiber and drug types of hemp (Cannabis sativa L.) from a collection of wild and domesticated accessions. *Genetic Resources and Crop Evolution*, 60(8), 2331–2342. https://doi.org/10.1007/s10722-013-0001-5

Pollan, M. (2002). *The botany of desire: A plant's-eye view of the world* (Paperback ed.). Random House.

Potter, D. J. (2014). A review of the cultivation and processing of cannabis (*Cannabis sativa* L.) for production of prescription medicines in the UK: Cultivation and processing of cannabis for production of prescription medicines. *Drug Testing and Analysis*, 6(1–2), 31–38. https://doi.org/10.1002/dta.1531

Radwan, M. M., ElSohly, M. A., El-Alfy, A. T., Ahmed, S. A., Slade, D., Husni, A. S., ... Ross, S. A. (2015). Isolation and pharmacological evaluation of minor cannabinoids from high-potency *Cannabis sativa*. *Journal of Natural Products*, 78(6), 1271–1276. https://doi.org/10.1021/acs.jnatprod.5b00065

Radwan, M. M., ElSohly, M. A., Slade, D., Ahmed, S. A., Wilson, L., El-Alfy, A. T., ... Ross, S. A. (2008). Non-cannabinoid constituents from a high potency Cannabis sativa variety. *Phytochemistry*, 69(14), 2627–2633. https://doi.org/10.1016/j.phytochem.2008.07.010

Ren, M., Tang, Z., Wu, X., Spengler, R., Jiang, H., Yang, Y., & Boivin, N. (2019). The origins of cannabis smoking: Chemical residue evidence from the first millennium BCE in the Pamirs. *Science Advances*, 5(6), eaaw1391. doi: 10.1126/sciadv.aaw1391.

Riddle, J. M. (2011). *Dioscorides on pharmacy and medicine*. Austin, TX: University of Texas Press.

Rosenthal, F. (1971). *The herb: Hashish versus medieval Muslim society*. Leiden, Netherlands: Brill Publishers.

Russo, E. B. (2007). History of cannabis and its preparations in saga, science, and sobriquet. *Chemistry and Biodiversity*, 4(8), 1614–1648. https://doi.org/10.1002/cbdv.200790144

Russo, E. B. (2011). Taming THC: Potential cannabis synergy and phytocannabinoid-terpenoid entourage effects: Phytocannabinoid-terpenoid entourage effects. *British Journal of Pharmacology*, 163(7), 1344–1364. https://doi.org/10.1111/j.1476-5381.2011.01238.x

Russo, E., & Guy, G. W. (2006). A tale of two cannabinoids: The therapeutic rationale for combining tetrahydrocannabinol and cannabidiol. *Medical Hypotheses*, 66(2), 234–246. doi: 10.1016/j.mehy.2005.08.026.

Russo, E. B., Jiang, H.-E., Li, X., Sutton, A., Carboni, A., del Bianco, F., … Li, C.-S. (2008). Phytochemical and genetic analyses of ancient cannabis from Central Asia. *Journal of Experimental Botany, 59*(15), 4171–4182. https://doi. org/10.1093/jxb/ern260

Ryz, N. R., Remillard, D. J., & Russo, E. B. (2017). Cannabis roots: A traditional therapy with future potential for treating inflammation and pain. *Cannabis and Cannabinoid Research, 2*(1), 210–216. https://doi.org/10.1089/can.2017.0028

Samir, A. R., ElSohly, H. N., ElKashoury, E. A., & ElSohly, M. A. (1998). Fatty acids of cannabis seeds. *Phytochemical Analysis, 7*(6), 279–283.

Sauer, C. O. (1952). *Agricultural origins and dispersals.* New York: American Geographical Society.

Schultes, R. E. (1973). Man and marihuana. *Natural History, 82*(7), 58–64.

Schultes, R. E., Hofmann, A., & Rätsch, C. (2001). *Plants of the gods: Their sacred, healing, and hallucinogenic powers* (Rev. and expanded ed.). Rochester, VT: Healing Arts Press.

Schultes, R. E., Klein, W. M., Plowman, T., & Lockwood, T. E. (1974). Cannabis: An example of taxonomic neglect. *Botanical Museum Leaflets, Harvard University, 23*, 337–367.

Schultes, R. E., & Von Reis, S. (2008). *Ethnobotany: Evolution of a discipline.* Portland, OR: Timber Press.

Scurlock, J. A., & Andersen, B. R. (2005). *Diagnoses in Assyrian and Babylonian medicine: Ancient sources, translations, and modern medical analyses.* Champaign, IL: University of Illinois Press.

Sides, H. (June, 2015). High Science. *National Geographic, 227* (6), 30–57..

Setzer, M. C., Werka, J. S., Irvine, A. K., Jackes, B. R., & Setzer, W. N. (2006). Biological activity of rainforest plant extracts from far north Queensland, Australia. In L. Williams (Ed.), *Biologically active natural products for the 21st Century* (pp. 21–46). Trivandrum: Research Signpost.

Sirikantaramas, S., & Taura, F. (2017a). Cannabinoids: Biosynthesis and biotechnological applications. In S. Chandra, H. Lata, & M. A. ElSohly (Eds.), *Cannabis sativa L. - Botany and biotechnology* (pp. 183–206). Springer International Publishing. https://doi.org/10.1007/978-3-319-54564-6_8

Small, E. (2015). Evolution and classification of Cannabis sativa (marijuana, hemp) in relation to human utilization. *The Botanical Review, 81*(3), 189–294. https:// doi.org/10.1007/s12229-015-9157-3

Small, E., & Cronquist, A. (1976). A practical and natural taxonomy for cannabis. *Taxon, 25*(4), 405–435. https://doi.org/10.2307/1220524

Small, E., & Marcus, D. (2002). Hemp: A new crop with new uses for North America. In J. Janick & A. Whipkey (Eds.), *Trends in new crops and new uses* (pp. 284–326). Alexandria, VA: ASHS Press.

Steen, R. J. (2010). *Marijuana as scapegoat, cannabis as medicine: A cognitive-rhetorical analysis of a Canadian drug-policy problem.* https://doi. org/10.14288/1.0069939

Steinberg, M. K., Hobbs, J. J., & Mathewson, K. (Eds.) (2004). *Dangerous harvest: Drug plants and the transformation of indigenous landscapes.* Oxford: Oxford University Press.

Stevens, C. J., Murphy, C., Roberts, R., Lucas, L., Silva, F., & Fuller, D. Q. (2016). Between China and South Asia: A Middle Asian corridor of crop dispersal and agricultural innovation in the Bronze Age. *The Holocene*, 26(10), 1541–1555. https://doi.org/10.1177/0959683616650268

Stringer, R. J., & Maggard, S. R. (2016). Reefer madness to marijuana legalization: Media exposure and American attitudes toward marijuana (1975–2012). *Journal of Drug Issues*, 46(4), 428–445. https://doi.org/10.1177/0022042616659762

Sullivan, R. J., & Hagen, E. H. (2002). Psychotropic substance-seeking: Evolutionary pathology or adaptation? *Addiction*, 97(4), 389–400. https://doi.org/10.1046/j.1360-0443.2002.00024.x

Taibi, D. M., Landis, C. A., Petry, H., & Vitiello, M. V. (2007). A systematic review of valerian as a sleep aid: Safe but not effective. *Sleep Medicine Reviews*, 11(3), 209–230. https://doi.org/10.1016/j.smrv.2007.03.002

Tambaro, S., Casu, M. A., Mastinu, A., & Lazzari, P. (2014). Evaluation of selective cannabinoid CB1 and CB2 receptor agonists in a mouse model of lipopolysaccharide-induced interstitial cystitis. *European Journal of Pharmacology*, 729, 67–74. https://doi.org/10.1016/j.ejphar.2014.02.013

Taura, F., Sirikantaramas, S., Shoyama, Y., Shoyama, Y., & Morimoto, S. (2007). Phytocannabinoids inCannabis sativa: Recent studies on biosynthetic enzymes. *Chemistry and Biodiversity*, 4(8), 1649–1663. https://doi.org/10.1002/cbdv.200790145

Thompson, L., Pearce, J., & Barnett, J. R. (2007). Moralising geographies: Stigma, smoking islands and responsible subjects. *Area*, 39(4), 508–517. https://doi.org/10.1111/j.1475-4762.2007.00768.x

Touw, M. (1981). The religious and medicinal uses of *cannabis* in China, India and Tibet. *Journal of Psychoactive Drugs*, 13(1), 23–34. https://doi.org/10.1080/02791072.1981.10471447

Treister-Goltzman, Y., Freud, T., Press, Y., & Peleg, R. (2019). Trends in publications on medical cannabis from the year 2000. *Population Health Management*, 22(4), 362–368. https://doi.org/10.1089/pop.2018.0113

Tucker, J. R., & Shen, T.-C. (2005). The road to a silicon quantum computer. In H. O. Everitt (Ed.), *Experimental aspects of quantum computing* (pp. 105–113). Springer US. https://doi.org/10.1007/0-387-27732-3_8

United States Food and Drug Administration (2018). *FDA approves first drug comprised of an active ingredient derived from marijuana to treat rare, severe forms of epilepsy.* Retrieved from https://www.fda.gov/news-events/press-announcements/fda-approves-first-drug-comprised-active-ingredient-derived-marijuana-treat-rare-severe-forms, after June 25, 2018.

Vandebroek, I., & Balick, M. J. (2012). Globalization and loss of plant knowledge: Challenging the paradigm. *PLOS ONE*, 7(5), e37643. https://doi.org/10.1371/journal.pone.0037643

VanPool, C. S. (2009). The signs of the sacred: Identifying shamans using archaeological evidence. *Journal of Anthropological Archaeology*, 28(2), 177–190. https://doi.org/10.1016/j.jaa.2009.02.003

Jager, G. (2012). Cannabis. In J. Verster, K. Brady, M. Galanter, & P. Conrod (Eds.), *Drug abuse and addiction in medical illness*. New York: NY: Springer. Publishing Company.

Voelker, R. (2020). FDA says it supports cannabis drug development via regulatory pathways. *JAMA*, 323(7), 600. https://doi.org/10.1001/jama.2020.0833

Volkow, N. D., Baler, R. D., Compton, W. M., & Weiss, S. R. B. (2014). Adverse health effects of marijuana use. *New England Journal of Medicine*, *370*(23), 2219–2227. https://doi.org/10.1056/NEJMra1402309

Walton, R. P. (1938). *Marihuana America's new drug problem*. New York: JB Lippincott Publishers.

Warf, B. (2014). High points: An historical geography of cannabis. *Geographical Review*, *104*(4), 414–438. https://doi.org/10.1111/j.1931-0846.2014.12038.x

Whiting, P. F., Wolff, R. F., Deshpande, S., Di Nisio, M., Duffy, S., Hernandez, A. V., ... Kleijnen, J. (2015). Cannabinoids for medical use: A systematic review and meta-analysis. *JAMA*, *313*(24), 2456. https://doi.org/10.1001/jama.2015.6358

World Health Organization (2003). *Traditional medicine*. Retrieved from http://www.who.int/mediacentre/factsheets/fs134/en/, after March 2, 2020.

Zablocki, B., Aidala, A., Hansell, S., & White, H. R. (1991). Marijuana use, introspectiveness, and mental health. *Journal of Health and Social Behavior*, *32*(1), 65–79.

Zager, J. J., Lange, I., Srividya, N., Smith, A., & Lange, B. M. (2019). Gene networks underlying cannabinoid and terpenoid accumulation in cannabis. *Plant Physiology*, *180*(4), 1877–1897. https://doi.org/10.1104/pp.18.01506

Zuardi, A. W. (2006). History of cannabis as a medicine: A review. *Revista Brasileira de Psiquiatria*, *28*(2), 153–157. https://doi.org/10.1590/S1516-44462006000200015

Chapter 2

History and Cultural Context of Marijuana in the United States

Kim Hewitt

Introduction

Cannabis, or marijuana, has a complex history in the United States. It is the most frequently used illicit substance in the United States; although currently, various forms of legalization have blurred the term "illicit." Understanding the history of cannabis in the United States can help us consider the variety of attitudes toward the use of the plant today and very specifically help us understand resistance to marijuana research and legalization of marijuana. Reform movements pushing to decriminalize marijuana have alternated with more stringent policies, paralleling the rise and fall of political conservatism and liberalism. Even use of the word "marijuana" has come and gone. While popular slang terms by which users refer to the plant (Mary Jane, muggles, ganja, pot, weed, Santa Maria) have changed through time, terms used by those who seek to demonize the plant have also changed. Although cannabis is now the preferred term among medical users and those who seek more lenient laws, this essay will use the term marijuana interchangeably with cannabis.

A Global History View

Cannabis originated in central Asia, and due to its hardy nature and popularity, has spread across the globe. Humans have cultivated and used various forms of cannabis for a very long time. There is evidence that cannabis was used both medicinally and for spiritual purposes in non-Western cultures, including ancient Mesopotamia, China, and even among ancient Hebrews (Bennett, 2010). Because we produce substances in our brains and bloodstreams that mimic cannabinoids and have endocannabinoid receptors in our bodies, many researchers theorize that cannabis and humans co-evolved. Proof exists that humans used cannabis medicinally as early as 2800 BCE. Ancient ritual use is suggested by the finding of charred hemp seeds in a 5,000-year-old ritual object excavated in Romania (Russo et al., 2008). It was first grown agriculturally in China at least 6,000 years ago and was prized for its psychoactive properties in India as long ago as 2000 BCE. Arab traders brought cannabis to Africa while British colonists imported slaves from Africa and then workers from India who ensured the spread of cannabis use to Brazil and the Caribbean (Courtwright, 2001, pp. 39–41).

Functional uses of the cannabis plant have been known for thousands of years, and we are still discovering uses for hemp as a renewable resource. Hemp fibers from the plant have been used for making rope and cloth, while nutritious seeds and other parts of the plant have been used for oil and as feed for livestock. Biodegradable cellophane and compostable cellulose can be manufactured from the plant to replace the plastics and Styrofoam that are polluting our environment, and sustainable hempseed oil can be used as a biodiesel fuel (Holland, 2010a, pp. 6–8).

Early History in the United States

The colonists had many practical uses for hemp fiber, which is derived from the cannabis plant. They valued strong hemp fibers for rope and textiles, while they used oils and seeds from the plant in food. Cannabis was used as a medicinal ingredient in treatments for nausea, asthma, sleep disorders, stress, epilepsy, tumors, and glaucoma (Lusane, 1991, pp. 29–30). In Virginia, it was considered such an important crop in 1619 that the colony required every farmer to grow hemp. Use of hemp for rope and clothing decreased after the Civil War when the United States began to import more goods from abroad (Public Broadcasting System, 2019).

In nineteenth-century America, marijuana was a common ingredient in medicinal preparations. It is important to note that in the nineteenth century, the medical field had not yet professionalized. Doctors, pharmacists, and medicines were completely unregulated. Until the 1906 Pure Food and Drug Act, there was no federal oversight of ingredients, safety of food, or medicines. The 1906 Act required products meant for human consumption to list all ingredients on the label; however, it didn't restrict the kinds of ingredients that could be used.

Early Recreational Use and Regulation in the United States

Smoking cannabis for pleasure and relaxation, a practice introduced in the United States in the early 1900s by Mexican immigrants and sailors, exceeded its medicinal use. Ironically, the popularity of smoking marijuana recreationally coincided with the growth of the cigarette industry in America in the early 1900s. Tobacco had long been an important cash crop, and in the early 1900s pre-made cigarettes began to be available and a burgeoning advertising industry extolled tobacco use to a growing middle-class. Tobacco smoking increased and cleared a path for cannabis smoking.

Recreational cannabis use in a society that was more familiar with alcohol consumption than other recreational substances, coupled with the prejudice against nonwhites in the U.S. population, assured that racism tinged early attitudes about recreational use of marijuana. In 1911, the White South African government outlawed marijuana based on the fear that it was radicalizing Blacks and causing them to want equal rights. South Africa spearheaded an international campaign against the substance (Lusane, 1991, p. 34). Similar racist attitudes influenced views of cannabis in the United States: Almost a million Mexican workers came to the United States seeking work in the first three decades of the 1900s, while others came fleeing the Mexican Revolution of 1910. Some immigrants from Mexico brought marijuana with them. Their use of marijuana would probably have gone unnoticed, except that many Americans were leery of the immigrants, and anti-immigrant stories often linked Mexicans, cannabis, crime, and violence. The anti-immigrant, anti-drug stories often faulted marijuana use (calling it "The Marijuana Menace") as the cause of negative behavior (Public Broadcasting System, 2019).

In the early 1900s, the recreational use of marijuana filtered slowly into the American consciousness. Sailors from Latin America and dockworkers from Mexico, Cuba, and the Caribbean brought marijuana into port cities, especially port cities in the American South. Marijuana became popular in New Orleans, Louisiana after World War I. The association of marijuana with jazz and the underworld was born in Storyville, a district known for prostitution and crime (Lusane, 1991, p. 36). New Orleans (and Storyville specifically) was the birthplace of the nascent American art form of jazz, and many White and African American jazz musicians smoked cannabis, also called "tea," "weed," "muta," or "muggles" and wrote songs in homage to its psychoactive properties. Jazz musician Mezz Mezzrow, who published his autobiography in 1946, claimed that "tea puts a musician in a real masterly sphere, and that's why so many jazzmen have used it" (Mezzrow & Wolfe, 1946, p. 74). There is also evidence that U.S. troops stationed at the Panama Canal learned about the recreational use of marijuana from West Indian workers (Courtwright, 2001, p. 42).

The association of marijuana use with a demographic considered unsavory according to the racist norms of the times, prompted regulation (Lusane, 1991, p. 36). Local ordinances in some border cities began to outlaw marijuana, and by 1925, the state of Louisiana outlawed it. Many southern states were quick to follow suit. Enforcement of the laws often targeted African Americans and Mexicans (Lusane, 1991, p. 36). During the economic strife of the Great Depression (1929–1933) when unemployment rose, prejudice against immigrants and Mexican Americans increased. Accounts of crime prompted by marijuana use were an easy propaganda ploy to stir fear of these minority groups and create the idea that both nonwhite immigrants and marijuana were threats to society.

Federal regulation of marijuana in the United States began in the late 1930s, when a new federal agency, the Federal Bureau of Narcotics (FBN) was created. The federal government had started to regulate food and drugs in 1906 with the Pure Food and Drug Act, which required labels listing all ingredients on food and medicine products. The next major federal regulation of substances was the 1914 Harrison Act, which required that opiates be dispensed only upon the prescription of a physician. Alcohol was the next substance to be federally regulated during the period known as Prohibition (1920–1933). The FBN was founded during Prohibition to combat the use of narcotics (opiates and cocaine), and the first commissioner was ex-Prohibition agent Harry J. Anslinger, who launched an attack against cannabis after he was appointed head of the FBN in 1930. He remained at the post for more than three decades, and his racist attitudes infected propaganda stories he wrote for newspapers linking African Americans and Mexicans to violence and marijuana use. Notably, he shifted terminology toward the word marijuana instead of cannabis.

The FBN encouraged states to regulate marijuana, but by the late 1930s Anslinger decided on a different tactic that aimed for federal prohibition. He pursued a campaign characterizing marijuana as a "killer weed." He inflamed public opinion against marijuana by planting false news stories in the media about heinous crimes committed while under the influence of marijuana. His stories associated marijuana with Negroes maddened by its effects and Mexicans driven to violence after smoking the substance (Goode, 2005, p. 103). The stories exploited racist attitudes, and some scholars claim that Anslinger's propaganda was motivated by the desire to convince the federal government to increase the budget of the FBN. One of the most famous examples of anti-marijuana hype of the time is the 1937 movie, *Reefer Madness*. Clips of the movie can easily be found online, and it is worth watching for its portrayal of how marijuana drives its users to insanity and ruins their lives.

Newspaper magnate William Randolph Hearst happily colluded with Anslinger's propaganda and launched a news campaign against marijuana that linked it to Mexican immigrants with lurid stories of interracial sex and violence. Exercising a vendetta against Mexicans was one impetus for his attacks after Pancho Villa's army seized 800,000 acres of Hearst's land during the Mexican Revolution. Another motivation was the fear that high quality paper made from hemp would bite into profits from his lumber papermill industry (Lusane, 1991, p. 37). Hearst's newspapers published exaggerated stories of marijuana users becoming violent and rowdy, and by 1930, many states west of the Mississippi had outlawed the substance. In the public imagination it was clearly linked with Mexicans, African Americans, and criminals, and tinged with racial prejudice and distaste (Goode, 2005, p. 102).

For many decades in the United States, marijuana was associated primarily with lower- and working-class cultures and nonwhite minorities and therefore seen as a dangerous substance. Even though Hearst's stories were patently false, they stirred enough sentiment to pass the Marijuana Tax Act of 1937 (Lusane, 37–38; Goode, 102), the first federal regulation of marijuana. The Tax Act placed strict regulations on who could legally use or be in possession of marijuana. The Tax Act restricted possession, use, distribution, and sale of marijuana only to authorized individuals who registered and paid an excise tax. This law remained in effect until the 1970 Comprehensive Drug Abuse Prevention and Control Act supplanted it.

Marijuana and 1960s Counterculture

The popularity of marijuana exploded in the 1960s and 1970s, and simultaneously become more tightly regulated. To understand the regulation of substances introduced by the 1970 Comprehensive Drug Abuse Prevention and Control Act, it is essential to understand the social and political turmoil of the 1960s. Time and space constraints prevent a thorough analysis here, but the decade following World War II (1941–1945) was one of the major changes in the United States. Emerging as a victor from the war, the country experienced prosperity and a growing middle-class. The 1960s were also a time of controversy over Civil Rights, as African Americans and other minorities who had served in the military renewed their push for legal and social equality. Women, who had formed a backbone of the war industries domestically, also began to demand equal rights. At the same time, immigration reform in 1965 began to change the face of America as more people from Latin America and Asia entered the country. The nation was deeply divided over Civil Rights legislation and activism promoting equality for everyone regardless of race or ethnicity. By the end of the decade, several cities had seen urban riots sparked by issues of racial and economic inequality and a shift in the economy which saw stable, well-paid jobs leaving urban areas. The nation was traumatized by the assassination of President Kennedy in 1963, followed by the assassinations of Robert Kennedy and Civil Rights leaders Martin Luther King and Malcolm X in 1968.

Another major issue that wrought havoc on the fabric of American life was U.S. involvement in Vietnam. In 1947, President Harry S. Truman initiated the Cold War when he declared that the United States would do everything possible to stop the global spread of Communism. An entrenched Cold War fear of Communism prompted President John F. Kennedy to send advisors to South Vietnam to staunch the growing sentiment for Communism in North Vietnam. This hard stance was continued by President Lyndon B. Johnson, whose reaction to an alleged attack on an American ship in the Gulf of Tonkin was to send troops into Vietnam, enmeshing the United States in an expensive nine-year conflict. Aside from money, many lives were lost on both sides. American men between the ages of 18 and 26 were drafted to fight as the conflict escalated. The war was popular at first, but enthusiasm waned as it began to seem unwinnable and more American lives were lost. Anti-war protests spread and became more and more visible. Although political protest of U.S. involvement in Vietnam didn't necessarily go hand in hand with experimentation with psychoactive drug use, the anti-war movement ran parallel to the development of a counterculture in the nation.

A countercultural upheaval was undergirded by the existence of an American middle-class youth that was better-educated than ever before and had money to spend. Postwar prosperity in the United States made the development of youth culture possible. Teenagers and young adults began to relish their own creative fashions and a new music called rock and roll that spoke directly to them emotionally and to the social issues that concerned them. Even more importantly, disenchantment with democratic processes and government as well as social institutions meant many countercultural youths turned away from conventional, mainstream values. The blossoming counterculture dabbled in non-mainstream religions, alternative lifestyles, more open sexuality, and mind-altering drugs. While anti-war activism increased on college campuses, so did marijuana use.

Political and social movements overlapped at times, but the counterculture was specifically interested in rejecting the conservative social norms of family, gender, and sexuality that had been foundations for mainstream American values in the 1950s. Experimentation with psychoactive substances, including marijuana and psychedelics, was driven by a desire to change the individual self as a crucial step in transforming society. Although marijuana use was also recreational, for many users in the counterculture it went hand in hand with idealistic aspirations. Mind-expanding substances could enhance self-awareness, ease inhibitions, and facilitate liberating insights into new possibilities for individual growth and social structures. For members of the counterculture, often called hippies, using marijuana was not just rebellion or a fun way to get high; it was also often an idealistic journey seeking creativity and a new collective reality. The counterculture of the 1960s has been called naïve, radical, utopian, insightful, and self-conscious. The pursuit of self-knowledge was seen by some as self-indulgent, while others saw it as a necessary antidote to the disillusionment wrought by a mainstream society that fought in Vietnam without reason and valued superficial materialism and consumer culture. Marijuana was used as a tool to reorganize the individual psyche and "deepen insights into reality and human existence" (Bloom & Breines, 2003, pp. 227–229.) Often it went hand in hand with the music and fashions of youth culture. In Todd Gitlin's first-hand account of the 1960s, *The Sixties: Years of Hope, Days of Rage*, he accents how marijuana offered an initiation into the counterculture: "without it, you were an outsider looking in" and would never fully understand the social critique and insights of the protest music and popular culture of the hippies (Gitlin, 1987, p. 201). The counterculture, an indistinct mix of lifestyles rebelling against the mainstream, and sometimes political liberalism, is sometimes known by the vague catch-all phrase The New Left, even though there were many distinct amalgamations of culture and politics. Of course, not all Americans accepted liberal political or social attitudes, and during the 1960s a new conservativism, called The New Right, also grew.

By the 1970s, many trends of the counterculture had filtered into the mainstream. *Vogue* magazine featured spreads of models wearing hippie fashions like headbands, fringed vests, and paisley prints, and many films depicted youth culture and marijuana use. Youth culture had infiltrated mainstream culture, and just as the youth once mimicked cool jazz musicians who smoked pot, more and more adults mimicked the youth and imbibed in marijuana. During the 1970s, use of all illicit substances, including marijuana, increased, and peaked in 1979. By then, 55 million Americans had tried marijuana, and two-thirds of people aged between 18 and 25 had experimented with it (Courtwright, 2001, p. 44).

As the market for cannabis increased, so did sophisticated underground domestic cannabis agriculture and breeding. In the 1960s and 1970s, serious breeders sought a predictable, hardy crop with a high delta-1 tetrahydrocannabinol (THC) content, making it more potent. Breeders also wanted early maturing plants that were small in stature and less easily detected by observant neighbors or police (King, 2000, pp. 2–8). The sophistication of their breeding methods presaged the plethora of strains available today that are marketed for a variety of medical conditions.

The War on Drugs Officially Begins

The history of marijuana in the United States is a history of opposing movements and conflict over regulation. In the 1960s and 1970s, two conflicting attitudes about marijuana developed. One branch accepted the use of marijuana as a recreational and mind-expanding substance. The magazine *High Times* was founded in 1974, and casual use of marijuana increased, as did use of all illicit substances during the decade of the 1970s. Another branch viewed the new permissiveness with distaste, associated it with the decay of morals, and saw it as a threat to society, especially the youth.

As part of his 1968 presidential campaign platform, Nixon denounced increased crime rates in American urban areas, which had become increasingly segregated due to economic inequities and systemic racial discrimination. In 1970, he notched up his rhetoric to claim that America's crime problem could be solved by declaring a "War on Drugs." Although more Americans of college age were smoking marijuana and the use of heroin in urban areas was increasing, data did not show the "epidemic" of use among the youth that Nixon claimed. (Baum, 1996, pp. 26–27). A survey of a thousand college students showed that only a quarter of college students had even tried marijuana, and half of those did not try it a second time (Baum, 1996, p. 39). Politicians and the media, however, focused on "drug use" as a catch-all problem that lumped marijuana use with hard drug use (heroin and cocaine) and served as a code word for racial prejudice.

Nixon's War on Drugs instituted aggressive federal controls at a time when state-level and popular sentiment to legalize marijuana was increasing. In 1970, a benchmark in drug regulation was introduced by Nixon. Congress approved the Comprehensive Drug Abuse Prevention and Control Act, commonly called the Controlled Substances Act (CSA). Although it authorized funding for research, education, and treatment for problems caused by illicit substances, a major focus of the legislation was law enforcement. It created a federal schedule of substances that classified them according to a list of criteria, including potential for abuse and medical purposes. Marijuana was classified as a Schedule 1 substance, defined as having no medical use and a high potential for abuse, thus carrying the heaviest penalties for use, possession, or distribution. Heroin and LSD were also included as Schedule 1 controlled substances. The CSA also created the National Institute on Drug Abuse (NIDA), the first federal agency to address substance research, education, and prevention. Part of the research initiated by the CSA was a two-year study of the effects of marijuana. The multi-volume study was published in 1972–1973 as the findings of the National Commission on Marijuana and Drug Abuse. The study reported that marijuana use was not particularly harmful and recommended decriminalization of personal use. Although Nixon had eagerly pushed the CSA forward, he rejected the findings of the Commission as politically inconvenient and ignored its findings (Goode, 2005, 104). Cultivating favor with his conservative political constituency, Nixon used his newly created Bureau of Narcotics and Dangerous Drugs (BNDD) to pursue aggressive drug raids, especially in Northern California's Humboldt County, which had become a "hippie, agrarian pot culture" (Balko, 2013, p. 105). They had new tools, such as "no knock" raids, which meant law enforcement officials didn't have to announce themselves before breaking down the door to a place they suspected of drug activity. Local law enforcement often eagerly cooperated with federal agents due to their prejudice against the "longhairs" they felt had invaded their territory (Balko, 2013, p. 105). Nixon increased funding for anti-drug agencies and founded the Drug Enforcement Agency (DEA) in 1973.

Simultaneously, campaigns to decriminalize marijuana became more visible and experienced some success, even though Republican President Nixon had declared a War on Drugs. The National Organization for the Reform of Marijuana Laws (NORML) was founded in 1970. Oregon became the first state to decriminalize marijuana in 1973 by making possession of less than an ounce a civil offense that would incur only a small fine. Alaska followed suit two years later by eliminating all penalties for cultivation and possession of less than four ounces. In the late 1970s, while the Carter presidency waffled on liberal policies, the marijuana reform movement peaked. Although endorsing reduced penalties, Carter was unwilling to take a firm stand. The American Medical Association, the American Psychiatric Association, the American Bar Association, and the National Council on Churches supported decriminalization (making possession a civil offense), and by 1977 many states had demoted possession of a marijuana for personal use to a misdemeanor. By 1980, eleven states had decriminalized possession (Grinspoon, 2010: pp. xi–xxiv).

On the other hand, opposition to marijuana also became more pronounced in the late 1970s. Concerned parents formed organizations to combat what they saw as the corruption of youth provoked by widespread use of marijuana. Supported by the National Institutes on Drug Abuse (NIDA) and the DEA, these parents' groups became visible, powerful lobbies (Public Broadcasting System, 2019). One of the ideas they promoted which became most entrenched was the myth that marijuana was a "gateway drug" that led to the use of drugs like heroin and cocaine. No evidence for this theory exists. Although many individuals who use heroin and cocaine first use marijuana, very few individuals who try marijuana continue to other illicit drug use. These anti-drug lobbies became even more influential during the conservative Reagan Era of the 1980s (Baum, 1996, p. 53).

By the end of the 1960s, social and political controversies created turmoil in the United States. Urban areas were riddled with racial tensions, pockets of poverty, and crime. Anti-Vietnam sentiment had increased, and the streets of Chicago exploded with violence when protesters at the 1968 Democratic National Convention clashed with the Chicago police. President Johnson declined to run for President again and Richard Nixon, a conservative Republican, became president. In the 1970s, America experienced an economic recession, creating discontent. By the 1980s, a conservative backlash gained political power, the liberal trend toward marijuana declined, and a more conservative attitude influenced regulation.

The 1980s: The War on Drugs is Revived

Conservative Republican Ronald Reagan was elected U.S. president twice in the 1980s, and he and his wife Nancy Reagan ushered in a new era of anti-drug rhetoric and laws. Nancy Reagan coined the slogan "Just Say No," spoke at schools across the nation, and helped promote public service announcements designed to create an emotional response rather than educate the public. The Reagan administration supported stringent penalties for illicit drug use and instituted policies in opposition to harm reduction. For example, federal funding for needle exchange programs ended, even though such programs had been effective in reducing the incidence of HIV. The 1984 Comprehensive Crime Control Act created mandatory minimum prison sentences for illicit drug offenses, and as a result, the number of individuals in prison for drug offenses skyrocketed. Tools to fight the War on Drugs were implemented to their full capacity. No-knock warrants, which allowed police to break down doors when serving search warrants, and asset forfeiture, which allowed the seizure of any property related to a drug offense, were used frequently. Drug testing became mandatory for certain federal jobs and common for many jobs in the private sector. Students who had been convicted of a drug charge were made ineligible for financial aid. The publicity and media coverage was so convincing that by 1989 64% of Americans thought drug use was the number one problem in the country. Notably, many public service announcements and the "Just Say No" slogan failed to differentiate between marijuana and hard drugs that are addictive, like heroin.

One result of the rejuvenated War on Drugs in the 1980s was a soaring number of drug arrests. In 1988 almost 400,000 charges involved marijuana. Being found guilty of possessing one ounce of marijuana could result in a 15-year prison term (Lusane, 1991, p. 72). In general, approaches to the War on Drugs split over party lines. Republicans were more interested in funding interdiction and law enforcement, while Democrats pushed for equal funding for education, prevention, and treatment (Lusane, 1991, p. 73). Reagan created the White House Office of Drug Abuse Policy to supervise the War on Drugs, and in 1987 created the National Drug Policy Board. During the Reagan years budgets for federal anti-drug programs increased 39%, while funding for many other social programs was cut (Lusane, 1991, p. 78). In one of the ironies of drug policy, Reagan's efforts to curtail the flow of marijuana from Mexico resulted in a 25% increase in domestic production. When Reagan deployed federal law enforcement to crush marijuana production, especially in northern California, growers moved their crops indoors (Lusane, 1991, p. 78) and developed new strains to reduce the chance they would be detected (King, 2000, pp. 2–8). Indoor cultivation produced more potent marijuana than ever before, and the United States became the major marijuana producer in the world (Nadelmann, 1997, p. 291).

Racial Bias Persists in the War on Drugs

The War on Drugs had important consequences in communities of color. Between 1985 and 1989 the number of African Americans arrested on drug charges nationwide more than doubled, while the number of Whites arrested for drug charges increased by 27%, even though rates of drug use were the same in each racial group according to the National Institute of Drug Abuse. During the height of the drug war in 1989, the arrest rate on drug charges for African Americans was five times that of Whites. The rate of arrest, prosecution, conviction, and imprisonment for nonwhites exploded without any real world relation to rates of their drug use (Donzinger, 1996, p. 115).

Bowing to political pressure in the 1990s, President Bill Clinton continued many of Reagan's draconian anti-drug policies. California and Arizona led the nation in legalizing medical marijuana in the 1990s, but the DEA continued heavy-handed assaults on state-licensed medical cannabis facilities. Marijuana was still illegal at the federal level, and the Clinton administration wanted to send a political message (Balko, 2013, pp. 215–216). The first Bush administration continued to assault medical marijuana facilities, arresting owners and patients, and calling the suppliers "drug traffickers." The second Bush administration continued to ramp up funding for the War on Drugs and promoted military style policing tactics (Balko, 2013, p. 252). The Obama administration, despite lip service to more liberal policies, continued the assaults on medical marijuana dispensaries (Alexander, 2012, pp. 252–253; Balko, 2013, pp. 301).

Cannabis remains the most commonly used "illicit" substance in the United States, yet the lingering effects of past racially biased policies and institutional racism are still extant in the ways drug laws are enforced and the consequences of enforcement. Many police departments favor low-level possession arrests because they are easy, and in the early 2000s marijuana arrests were at an all-time high, accounting for approximately 40% of all drug arrests, or more than six million arrests between 2000 and 2010. Even though Whites imbibe in marijuana at equal or greater rates than nonwhites, young Blacks and Latinos are more commonly stopped and arrested for possession. Due to lingering laws from the 1980s, a drug conviction of any kind makes students ineligible for federal financial aid and may hinder someone from getting a job or housing (Levine, 2010, p. 205). A study of drug arrests between 2000 and 2008 in California pointedly noted that African Americans were disproportionately arrested on drug charges, revealing lingering effects of past racial bias and institutional racism still extant (White & Holman, 2012).

Drug war policies disproportionately affect communities of color and poor communities in which individuals have fewer resources that allow them to consume illicit substances in private, combat drug dependency problems, and retain legal counsel if they are arrested. Harsh drug laws have pummeled communities of color and sent disproportionate numbers of minorities and the lower class to prison for illicit drug offenses (Alexander, 2012), even though the members of those communities do not use illicit substances with any more frequency than the members of White, middle-class communities. The result is that the association between minorities and the lower classes and illicit drug use persists.

Prejudicial attitudes have influenced the ways in which government agencies have stifled cannabis research. While the National Institute of Drug Abuse has spent millions of dollars to study the harmful effects of marijuana, the research has failed to provide hard scientific evidence to support ineffective prohibitionist policies and penalties for cannabis use (Grinspoon, 2010, p. xii). The ways government agencies have inflated the harm of marijuana have kept it classified as a Schedule 1 substance, denying its medical benefit despite evidence to the contrary, as other chapters in this book discuss. Unbiased research is needed to discover the effects of cannabis use.

New Approaches

In the past 10 to 20 years, reform of drug regulation is gaining attention as the devastating consequences of the War on Drugs (especially in communities of color) become more obvious. Major ideas of the reform movement include the idea that social issues related to illicit drug use must be examined to determine the root cause of drug use rather than considering drug use itself the problem. When problems related to drug use exist, it should be addressed as public health issues rather than issues for law enforcement to curtail. Most importantly, policies should be grounded in scientific research rather than political popularity. As research and interest in psychoactive substances has gradually increased, scientists, intellectuals, and creative thinkers are discussing new and interesting ideas about the role marijuana may play within the ecosystem and especially as a plant that co-evolved with humans.

Michael Pollen, an influential journalist who writes about the intersection between nature and culture, theorizes some fascinating ideas that help us reorient our relationship with cannabis. He speculates that the marijuana plant may have evolved its psychoactive properties as a protection against being over-grazed or over-consumed. In turn, humans and other animals who developed biological receptors that interact with the psychoactive ingredients in marijuana may have co-evolved a beneficial relationship in which the plant helps them edit the immense amount of information and stimuli in their environment. Pollen postulates that the effects of marijuana can simultaneously help one focus intently on the present moment and the immediate task at hand, while temporarily forgetting (or editing out) less important things in short-term memory (Holland, 2010, pp. 373–382). Globally, many indigenous cultures still preserve traditions of plant medicines, including the use of plant medicines that induce non-ordinary states of consciousness, are used in the service of medicinal use, or for pragmatic enhancement of the senses.

Several countries have implemented new approaches to human use of psychoactive substances, including cannabis. In 1976, the Netherlands began to allow the sale and consumption of cannabis and hashish in coffee shops licensed specifically for cannabis use. In Amsterdam especially, coffee shops cater to tourists and locals who smoke marijuana or hashish. In the decades since 1976, the country has fine-tuned regulations that control the conditions of distribution and use of cannabis instead of blunt prohibition of these substances. For example, no one under the age of 18 can enter the coffee shops, the coffee shop must be a certain distance away from schools, and alcohol cannot be sold in the same establishments that sell cannabis products (Van der Veen, 2009). Despite the accessibility of cannabis, the percentage of the population using cannabis recreationally in the Netherlands has not increased, and its rate of use is half that of the United States (Moskas, 2008, pp. 191–192). Along with many countries like Canada, Ukraine, Germany, Denmark, and Switzerland, the Netherlands promotes education and harm reduction programs to reduce the harmful effects of substance use instead of jailing individuals who use a variety of psychoactive substances. In 2001, Portugal removed all criminal penalties for possession of drugs and replaced punishment with an approach that focused on promoting health and reducing harm caused by certain kinds of use. Several other countries, including the Czech Republic, New Zealand, and Ecuador have decriminalized drug use. These approaches allow for legal, regulated markets to develop, while addressing possible health problems that some individuals may develop.

Today (in 2020) almost half of the states in the United States have made medical marijuana legal, although regulations vary widely among states and are in constant flux. For example, in New York State, medical marijuana became legal in January 2016 under tight controls. Originally, only doctors who had special training were allowed to prescribe medical marijuana, and only five licensed dispensaries were allowed to distribute it. The marijuana could not be smoked, and medical marijuana was only allowed for a tiny handful of very serious medical conditions (for example, life-threatening cancer) for individuals who registered with the state to get a prescription. However, within a few years, more conditions were added to the list of conditions for which marijuana could be prescribed, and legislation in New York proposed making marijuana legal for recreational use. While as of 2019, recreational cannabis hasn't been made legal, it has been further decriminalized, which means penalties have been reduced to a non-criminal, misdemeanor offense. Scientific research is calling attention to the pragmatic and medicinal uses of cannabis, and the cultural history of marijuana that has associated marijuana use with minorities and the lower class is beginning to fade. Legislation is only part of social change, however, and public attitudes must also rest on data and information rather than political or racially charged propaganda or stereotypes. Although many jokes have been made about "stoners" who smoke marijuana daily and do nothing but sit on the couch, watch television, and snack, evidence exists that daily marijuana use can be compatible with professional jobs and successful careers. Clearly other factors are more influential on the "amotivational syndrome" that is the butt of jokes. As well, we need to continue to investigate what stereotypes are embedded in the inchoate medical marijuana industry and the marijuana businesses that are forming. Wendy Chapkis, a scholar of gender and sexuality, calls attention to the sexualized images of women used in marijuana advertising. Additionally, medical marijuana is disproportionately the domain of women, which coincides with a stereotype of women as caregivers, while the for-profit legal marijuana business, as well as legislative reform efforts, is dominated by men (Chapkis, 2013).

Cannabis products stripped of THC but retaining cannabinoid (CBD) are legal and popular as an over-the-counter panacea for many ailments. Special stores sell CBD in various forms such as oils, tinctures, drops, salves, or lozenges. Although many people buy these products without medical advice, they claim relief from aches and pains, insomnia, depression, and anxiety. While evidence exists that cannabis has medicinal use, studies assessing the long-term effects of cannabis use have been inconclusive due to complicating variables of onset of use and duration of use (Filbey, et al., 2014). One area of interest is the potential of medical cannabis to manage pain and prevent or mitigate opiate use (Peters, 2013). More research is clearly needed to develop a clearer picture of the risks and benefits of medical cannabis.

As the racist context for marijuana use and the association of cannabis with underground subcultures, crime, minorities, and hippies slowly diminish, reform movements are gaining ground. American social norms and laws are changing to accommodate medical use, state by state. At the time of this publication several states, including Washington, Colorado, and Vermont have made recreational use of marijuana legal. Other frontiers remain, namely decriminalization or legalization at the federal level. There is also an inchoate discussion of cannabis for spiritual purposes and personal growth, called the "conscious cannabis" movement. These uses hark back to the 1960s counterculture as well as ancient cultures and indigenous traditions. Now that laws are changing, perhaps that discussion will enter the public sphere. Writer Chris Bennett proposes that "humanity has a natural indigenous right to all of the plants of the Earth ... Any law that stands in the way of that relationship is an abomination to both God and nature" (Bennett, 2010, p. 26). The past three decades have culminated in major changes for the role of cannabis in U.S. culture; the next decades present new opportunities to explore new functional, legal, medical, and spiritual relationships with cannabis.

References

Alexander, M. (2012). *The new Jim Crow: Mass incarceration in the age of colorblindness.* New York: The New Press.

Balko, R. (2013). *The rise of the warrior Cop: The militarization of America's police forces.* New York: Public Affairs/Perseus Books.

Baum, D. (1996). *Smoke and mirrors: The war on drugs and the politics of failure.* New York: Little, Brown and Co.

Bennett, C. (2010). Early/ancient history. In J. Holland (Ed.), *The pot book: A complete guide to cannabis: Its role in medicine, politics, science and culture* (pp. 17–26). Rochester, VT: Park Street Press.

Bloom, A., & Breines, W. (Eds.) (2003). *Taking it to the streets: A sixties reader* (2nd ed.). New York: Oxford University Press.

Chapkis, W. (2013). The trouble with Mary Jane's gender. *Humbolt Journal of Social Relations, 35,* 71–88.

Courtwright, D. T. (2001). *Forces of habit: Drugs and the making of the modern world.* Cambridge, MA: Harvard University Press.

Donzinger, S. R. (Ed.) (1996). *The real war on crime: The report of the national criminal justice commission.* New York: National Center on Institutions and Alternatives.

Drug Policy Alliance, A Brief History of the Drug War. Retrieved from http://www .drugpolicy.org/issues/brief-history-drug-war

Filbey, F., Aslan, S., Calhoun, V., Spence, J., Damaraju, E., Caprihan, A., & Segall, J. (2014). Long-term effects of marijuana use on the brain. *Proceedings of the National Academy of Sciences of the United States of America, 111*(47), 16913–16918. Retrieved from http://www.jstor.org.library.esc.edu/stable/43279411

Gitlin, T. (1987). *The sixties: Years of hope, days of rage.* New York: Bantam Press Books.

Goode, E. (2005). *Drugs in American society.* New York: McGraw Hill.

Grinspoon, L. (2010). Foreword. In J. Holland (Ed.), *The pot book: The complete guide to cannabis: Its role in medicine, politics, science and culture* (pp. xi–xxiv). Rochester, VT: Park Street Press.

Holland, J. (Ed.) (2010a). *The pot book: A complete guide to cannabis: Its role in medicine, politics, science and culture* (pp. 6–8). Rochester, VT: Park Street Press.

Holland, J. (Ed.) (2010b). Gardeners rights, forgetting and co-evolution: An interview with Michael Pollen. In Holland, J. (Ed.), *The pot book: A complete guide to cannabis: Its role in medicine, politics, science and culture* (pp. 373–382). Rochester, VT: Park Street Press.

King, J. (2000). *The cannabible* (pp. 2–8). Berkeley, CA: Ten Speed Press.

Levine, H. G. (2010). Arrest statistics and racism. In J. Holland (Ed.), *The pot book: A complete guide to cannabis: Its role in medicine, politics, science and culture.* Rochester, VT: Park Street Press.

Lusane, C. (1991). *Pipe dream blues: Racism and the war on drugs.* Boston, MA: South End Press.

Mezzrow, M., & Wolfe, B. (1946). *Really the blues.* New York: Citadel Press.

Moskas, P. (2008). *Cop in the hood: My year policing Baltimore's Eastern district.* Princeton, NJ: Princeton University Press.

Nadelmann, E. A. (1997). Drug prohibition in the US: Costs, consequences and alternatives. In C. Reinarman & H. Levine (Eds.), *Crack in America: Demon drugs and social justice* (pp. 288-316). Berkeley, CA: University of California Press. 288–316.

Public Broadcasting System, Marijuana Timeline. (2019). Retrieved from http:// www.pbs.org/wgbh/pages/frontline/shows/dope/etc/cron.html

Peters II, D. C. (2013). Patients and caregivers report using medical marijuana to decrease prescription narcotics use. *Humboldt Journal of Social Relations, 35,* 24–40. Retrieved from http://www.jstor.org.library.esc.edu/stable/humjsocrel.35.24

Russo, E. B., Jiang, H. E., Li, X., Sutton, A., Carboni, A., del Bianco, F., ... Li, C. S. (2008). Phytochemical and genetic analyses of ancient cannabis from Central Asia. *Journal of Experimental Botany*, *59*(15), 4171–4182.

Van der Veen, H. (2009). Regulation in spite of prohibition: The control of cannabis distribution in Amsterdam. *Cultural Critique*, *71*(1), 129–147. Retrieved from http://www.jstor.org.library.esc.edu/stable/25475504

White, K., & Holman, M. (2012). Marijuana prohibition in California: Racial prejudice and selective-arrests. *Race, Gender and Class*, *19*(3/4), 75–92. Retrieved from http://www.jstor.org.library.esc.edu/stable/43497489

Chapter 3

Clash of Laws

How States are Legalizing Marijuana[1] in the Shadow of a Federal Prohibition

Heather Trela

Until the early twentieth century, marijuana was used in the United States in a variety of ways and was mostly unregulated. Britain encouraged early colonists to grow hemp, and the crop was used in the production of rope, paper, and cloth. Marijuana was also an ingredient in mainstream medicines as a treatment for a variety of ailments, including cholera, dysentery, alcoholism, opiate addiction, epilepsy, and asthma. The recreational smoking of marijuana was also introduced, though it was not widespread or widely accepted.

The first federal regulation of marijuana occurred with the 1906 Pure Food and Drug Act, which required that over-the-counter drugs and foods containing certain narcotics, including "cannabis," had to be clearly labeled. Misbranding of these items was a misdemeanor offense, carrying a maximum penalty of a $500 fine and a year in prison. (Pure Food and Drug Act, 1906). The Act had less to do with criminalizing marijuana or the other narcotics used in these products than it was to ensure transparency in the contents of the products consumers were purchasing and avoid adulterated or poisonous products from hitting the market. While the Act required accuracy in the content of the products, it did not require that products were effective or lived up to medical claims made about the product.

Beginning in 1910, the Mexican Revolution resulted in a large influx of Mexican immigrants to the United States looking to escape the violence and unrest in their country. Xenophobic fears of these new arrivals spread across the United States, and Mexican immigrants were blamed for many of society's ills, including increased crime and economic downturns. The fact that the immigrants brought their cultures and practices with them to the United States and didn't immediately assimilate was also threatening to many people. This included the use of marijuana for both medical and recreational purposes. While Americans were familiar with "cannabis" and its usages at their local pharmacies, they were suspicious of the "marihuana" (later marijuana)

---

1 In this chapter, I primarily use the term marijuana, rather than cannabis, to reflect the terminology used in many of the policies discussed.

associated with these new residents. That simple name change stoked many fears, and the recreational use of marijuana by the immigrants was believed to fuel some of their "dangerous" behavior. As a way to target the immigrants, states began to ban marijuana, beginning with the Commonwealth of Massachusetts in 1911 (2011). Cities would follow, with El Paso, Texas banning marijuana in 1915 after a person of Mexican descent killed a police officer and wounded others while he claimed to be high on marijuana (Long, 2019). By 1931, twenty-nine states had passed marijuana prohibitions.

In 1937, Congress passed the Marihuana Tax Act to "impose an occupational excise tax upon certain dealers in marihuana, to pose a transfer tax upon certain dealings in marihuana, and to safeguard the revenue therefrom by registry and recording." (Marihuana Tax Act, 1937). The act did not criminalize the drug per se, but failure to pay said taxes or follow regulations was punishable by fines up to $2,000, up to five years in jail, or both. This applied to physicians, dentists, surgeons, and other healthcare providers who would proscribe any form of medication containing marijuana. The Marihuana Tax Act stayed on the books until 1969 when the Supreme Court struck it down as a violation of the Fifth Amendment protection against self-incrimination in *Leary v. United States* (1969).

After the Marihuana Tax Act was deemed unconstitutional, the Nixon administration encouraged Congress to create a new system for classifying drugs based on their medical utility and addictive potential. The result was the 1970 Controlled Substances Act (CSA), which established federal drug policy. Marijuana—like heroin and LSD—was classified as Schedule I, meaning it has no currently accepted medical use and has a high potential for abuse. President Richard Nixon, an opponent of marijuana and its associated use by the counterculture, personally lobbied Congress to make marijuana a Schedule 1 drug. With this classification, marijuana became illegal under federal law (Table 3.1).

However, the CSA left open the possibility for states to also make laws related to controlled substances, as long as state and federal law could coexist. Section 903 stated:

> No provision of this subchapter shall be construed as indicating an intent on the part of the Congress to occupy the field in which that provision operates, including criminal penalties, to the exclusion of any State law on the same subject matter which would otherwise be within the authority of the State, unless there is a positive conflict between that provision of this subchapter and that State law so that the two cannot consistently stand together (Controlled Substances Act, 1970).

In 1996, California became the first state to take advantage of this provision, enacting legal medical marijuana with the passage of Proposition 215, otherwise known as the Compassionate Use Act. In the next four years, Oregon,

Table 3.1 Clash of laws

Schedule I	No currently accepted medical use and a high potential for abuse.	Heroin, LSD, marijuana, peyote, Quaaludes, and MDMA.
Schedule II	A high potential for abuse which may lead to severe psychological or physical dependence.	Cocaine, hydromorphone, methadone, oxycodone, fentanyl, morphine, opium, codeine, hydrocodone, amphetamine.
Schedule III	A moderate to low potential for physical and psychological dependence.	Products containing less than 90 milligrams of codeine per dosage unit (Tylenol with codeine), ketamine, anabolic steroids, testosterone.
Schedule IV	A low potential for abuse and low risk of dependence.	Xanax, Soma, Darvon, Darvocet, Valium, Ativan, Talwin, Ambien, Tramadol.
Schedule V	Drugs with lower potential for abuse than Schedule IV and consist of preparations containing limited quantities of certain narcotics.	Lomotil, Motofen, Lyrica, Parepectolin, cough preparations with less than 200 milligrams of codeine or per 100 milliliters.

Alaska, Washington, Maine, Hawaii, Nevada, and Colorado followed suit. Colorado became the first state to legalize adult-use/recreational marijuana in 2014 with Amendment 64. As of January 2020, eleven states and the District of Columbia have passed legislation permitting adult-use marijuana, and 33 states and the District of Columbia have medical marijuana laws on the books (Figure 3.1).

What caused this proliferation of state legalization of marijuana despite the federal prohibition? The federal government was initially hostile to states implementing marijuana policy, often threatening action. After California passed the Compassionate Use Act of 1996, then Attorney General Janet Reno indicated that physicians that followed state law would be the target of federal law enforcement and could lose their prescription licenses from the Drug Enforcement Agency and be banned from participating in Medicare and Medicaid programs (Annas, 1997).

California physicians sued on First Amendment grounds, arguing that such ultimatums by the United States Department of Justice have a chilling effect on patient-physician communication. A Federal district judge issued a temporary restraining order against federal action (Golden, 1997).

The federal government, however, scored a subsequent victory in the 2005 Supreme Court case *Gonzalez v. Raich* (2005). At issue was whether the federal Drug Enforcement Agency (DEA) could seize and destroy home-grown marijuana plants from a California resident, despite the fact that the marijuana was recommended to be used by a doctor under the state's

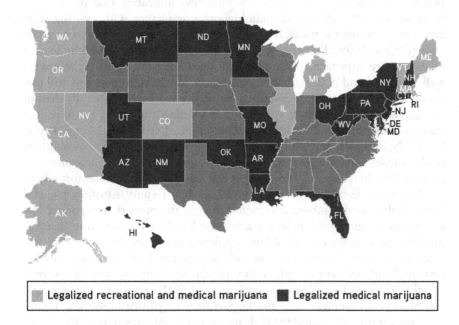

Legalized recreational and medical marijuana   **Legalized medical marijuana**

Figure 3.1 Map of states where cannabis is legal

Compassionate Use Act. The California residents argued that the CSA was an unconstitutional overreach of Congress's Commerce Clause power. The federal government argued that the Controlled Substances Act preempted, or overrode, state law and that making an exception for California's Compassionate Use Act would essentially make the CSA unenforceable. The Supreme Court ruled in favor of the federal government and their ability to prohibit the local cultivation of marijuana, regardless of state legality:

> Given the enforcement difficulties that attend distinguishing between marijuana cultivated locally and marijuana grown elsewhere, and concerns about diversion into illicit channels, we have no difficulty concluding that Congress had a rational basis for believing that failure to regulate the intrastate manufacture and possession of marijuana would leave a gaping hole in the CSA .

The decision in *Gonzalez v. Raich* reaffirmed that though state legalization was to the contrary, the federal government had the right to enforce the Controlled Substances Act and marijuana's Schedule I status.

However, during the Obama Administration, federal attitudes toward state marijuana laws began to soften. In 2009 then Deputy Attorney General

David Ogden wrote a memo to U.S. attorneys indicating that prosecuting those who are "in clear and unambiguous compliance with existing state laws providing for the medical use of marijuana" was not going to be a priority (Ogden, 2009). Essentially, the Department of Justice was going to take a laissez-faire approach to state medical marijuana programs if these were well-regulated and didn't cause any problems. While marijuana was still illegal under federal law, the Department of Justice would generally disrupt the implementation of state marijuana law unless there was a compelling reason. This signaled to states that the threat of federal prosecution was less likely, and after the Ogden memo, more than twenty states passed new medical marijuana laws or expanded their current medical marijuana program. After the passage of legislation in Colorado and Washington allowing for adult-use marijuana usage in 2013, then Deputy Attorney General James Cole issued a subsequent memo to U.S. attorneys that expanded the Ogden memo guidelines to cover adult-use legislation, reiterating that "in jurisdictions that have enacted laws legalizing marijuana in some form and that have also implemented strong and effective regulatory and enforcement systems," enforcement of federal law related to marijuana would not be a priority (Cole, 2013) . However, on January 4, 2018, then Attorney General Jeff Sessions announced that the Department of Justice under the Trump Administration will rescind the Cole memo guidance, thus putting the power in the hands of U.S. attorneys, who will ultimately have the discretion on whether to seek prosecution of those who violate federal drug law (Guzman, 2018). The decision by Attorney General Sessions to abandon the strategy outlined in the Cole memo did not come as a surprise because Sessions is a longtime opponent of marijuana, famously saying in 2016 that "good people don't smoke marijuana."

Congress also took action to give state marijuana programs some protection. In 2014, the Rohrabacher-Farr amendment was added to federal budget bills, prohibiting the Department of Justice from using federal funds to interfere with the implementation of state laws that legalize medical marijuana, while not altering the legality of marijuana at the federal level. Some versions of the amendment have been included in every federal budget bill since, but must be renewed with every new budget bill. The coverage lapses in the event of a government shutdown. The bill does not offer any protection for states that have adult-use marijuana programs.

In June 2019, the U.S. House of Representatives passed the Blumenauer-McClintock-Norton amendment that would have also prohibited the Department of Justice from using federal funds to interfere with state adult-use marijuana programs, but it did not gain enough support in the Senate. In 2017, then Attorney General Jeff Sessions personally asked Congress to undo the protection granted by the Rohrabacher-Farr amendment, stating that it inhibits the Department's authority to enforce the Controlled

Substances Act (Ingraham, 2017). In his 2017 letter to congressional leadership, Sessions said:

> I believe it would be unwise for Congress to restrict the discretion of the Department to fund particular prosecutions, particularly in the midst of an historic drug epidemic and potentially long-term uptick in violent crime. The Department must be in a position to use all laws available to combat the transnational drug organizations and dangerous drug traffickers who threaten American lives (Sessions, 2017).

Tensions have somewhat cooled under the tenure of Attorney General William Barr. Though Barr is not a proponent of legalized marijuana, his approach is less combative than his predecessor. Barr has chosen to view marijuana legalization through the lens of a state's rights issue. During his Senate confirmation hearing he stated that, while he personally "would still favor one uniform federal rule against marijuana," he recognized that "if there is not sufficient consensus to obtain that, then I think the way to go is to permit a more federal approach so states can, you know, make their own decisions within the framework of the federal law" (Godlewski, 2019). To date, prosecution of state-legalized marijuana sales has not been a priority of the Department of Justice under Attorney General Barr's tenure.

While the pendulum of federal action under the Obama Administration swung toward, allowing for the proliferation of state marijuana laws despite the federal prohibition, some action under the Trump Administration has created additional uncertainty for those same state programs. While the federal government to date has not increased enforcement of federal law, state marijuana programs are operating under much less clear guidance then when many of those programs were implemented. Still, state marijuana programs do not appear to be going anywhere, with a number of states slated to implement new marijuana policy in the 2020 election.

Clash of Laws

States, however, do not only have to be concerned with Department of Justice enforcement when it comes to their marijuana programs. The federal prohibition of marijuana casts a shadow over much of the structure and operation of state marijuana industries and presents numerous challenges that states must consider when implementing their medical or adult-use marijuana legislation.

Access to Financial Institutions

The majority of banks and credit unions in the United States are regulated by a number of federal agencies, including the Federal Deposit Insurance

Corporation (FDIC), Federal Reserve System (FRS), Office of the Comptroller of the Currency (OCC), and the National Credit Union Administration (NCUA). As a result, the majority of United States financial institutions are hesitant to provide any access to those in the marijuana industry for fear of running afoul of federal law and incurring potential fines. When the Department of Justice abandoned the guidance of the Cole memo, it also upended the regulations that gave banks and credit unions some coverage to work with marijuana businesses. The foundation for the Department of the Treasury's Financial Crimes Enforcement Network guidelines for financial institutions was based on the Cole memo, and no new guidelines have been issued to offer clarification (United States Department of the Treasury, 2014). This has forced the bulk of companies operating state-legal marijuana activities to operate primarily as a cash-only business. This also extends to customers who patronize these companies—dispensaries are unable to accept payment via debit card, credit card, or check. The marijuana businesses that have been able to find financial institutions that are willing to take their business often wind up paying higher fees for the privilege. For example, the only bank in Massachusetts that served the medical marijuana industry levied a $5,000 a month charge to have a checking account (Bartlett, 2018).

Being an unbanked industry creates a number of additional hurdles for marijuana-related businesses. Marijuana businesses are unable to take out loans, preventing future expansion or investment in equipment. Since they have no other option to pay their employees and expenses, this necessitates having large sums of cash on hand at any given time which can create a public safety issue because it makes these businesses a target for theft. In 2015, 50% of cannabis dispensaries were robbed or burglarized, and thieves walked away with an average of $20,000–$50,000 in a single act (Wharton Public Policy Initiative, 2017).

An excessive amount of cash on hand also provides another kind of threat to marijuana dispensaries—civil asset forfeiture. Civil asset forfeiture allows law enforcement officers to seize assets they suspect, by a "preponderance of the evidence," were involved in a crime. Unlike criminal forfeiture, where assets cannot be seized without a conviction, in civil forfeiture the person whose property is confiscated does not have to be convicted or even charged with a crime. The property, not the owner, is considered the defendant. Law enforcement is able to keep what is seized or keeps the profits if assets are sold off. Once property is seized through civil asset forfeiture, the burden of proof is on the owner to prove the property's innocence by going to court. Unlike the more familiar judicial standard of innocent until proven guilty, assets seized though civil asset forfeiture are guilty until proven innocent. Civil asset forfeiture has always been somewhat controversial, and several states have passed legislation to put limitations on its practice.

In July 2017, then Attorney General Jeff Sessions announced that the Justice Department would allow federal agency forfeiture, also known as "federal adoptions," of assets seized by state and local law enforcement agencies. The practice, an expansion of civil asset forfeiture, was curtailed by the Obama Administration in 2015 by then Attorney General Eric Holder (United States Department of Justice, 2015). The federal adoptions provision that the Department of Justice reinstated provides a loophole for law enforcement to get around any restrictions on civil asset forfeiture in their state. Under federal adoptions, state and local agencies can circumvent state laws on civil asset forfeiture by partnering with a federal agency to seize property that is believed to violate federal law. Up to 80% of the proceeds from equitable sharing are then returned to the state or local agency. Through federal adoptions, state and local law enforcement agencies are able to use the potentially more lenient federal standard of proof ("preponderance of evidence") to seize assets that otherwise may be restricted by state statute. Marijuana dispensaries could be particularly vulnerable to being targeted through federal adoption, given marijuana's status as a Schedule I drug that is illegal in the eyes of the federal government.

Limited access to financial institutions also complicates the ability of states to collect the revenue they anticipated from the taxation of the marijuana industry. States not only have to make accommodations for large cash payments of tax receipts, it is more difficult for the state to track marijuana industry revenue to tax accurately without banking records or credit card statements for sales. Furthermore, despite the federal ban and the fact that marijuana companies are not eligible to take many federal business tax deductions available to other industries, they still have to pay federal taxes. The Internal Revenue Service has had to make special arrangements to process these large cash payments.

Congress has taken initial steps to provide some guidance for financial institutions that would be open to working with the marijuana industry if there was no fear of violating federal policy. In September of 2019, the U.S. House of Representatives passed the Secure and Fair Enforcement (SAFE) Banking Act which would prohibit "a federal banking regulator from penalizing a depository institution for providing banking services to a legitimate marijuana-related business." (Secure and Fair Enforcement Banking Act, 2019). At this time, the bill has yet to be voted on by the Senate.

Taxation

The ability to generate tax revenue of the sale of marijuana is one of the driving forces behind continued legalization. Many states are still recovering from the economic downturn of 2008 and see great potential to refill state coffers with the revenue from state marijuana sales. States that have implemented marijuana programs, however, have had to create their taxation structure without any guidance from the federal government and often with imperfect information about the market. This has led to a wide variation in how states tax marijuana sales and imperfect forecasting models.

While prescribed medicines are generally exempt from taxation, marijuana's Schedule I status and lack of Food and Drug Administration (FDA) approval means that it cannot actually be prescribed; doctors can suggest marijuana for several medical issues as outlined by the individual state, but they do not write a script that patients fill at a dispensary. As a result, the purchase of medical marijuana could be subject to the same general sales tax as other products purchased in the state, though several states have decided to grant medical marijuana an exemption or charge a slightly lower rate.

The bulk of revenue that states anticipate levying via taxation is on adult-use marijuana. When setting the taxation rate as part of their adult-use marijuana policy, states are striving to find a sweet spot—a taxation rate that is high enough to bring in as much revenue to the state as possible, but a rate that is not so high that it results in pricing out legal adult-use marijuana for consumers, thereby making black market sales more financially attractive. People are likely to be willing to pay some premium for being able to legally buy marijuana: There is a value to not having to worry about being arrested or about the quality and composition of what they are buying. However, if the state charges too much, that alters the cost-benefit analysis of consumers and may allow the illicit marijuana market to continue to flourish despite legalization.

State taxation policies for adult-use marijuana vary widely by state, both in rate and type of taxes. States impose an excise tax, a sales tax, or a combination of both. Excise taxes vary in how these are accessed. California and Alaska tax marijuana by weight, while other states access taxation based on the price of marijuana sales at the wholesale transaction, the consumer purchase, or both. California is the currently the only state that levies both types of excise taxes. The rate of retail excise taxes charged by states range from a low of 10.75% in Massachusetts to a high of 37% in Washington. California, Massachusetts, Nevada, and Washington, and all charge a general sales tax in addition to marijuana-specific taxation. Illinois, the latest state to legalize adult-use marijuana, has implemented a three-tiered excise tax system, depending on the level of Tetrahydrocannabinol (THC) in the product, as well as a wholesale tax (Berg, 2020). Additionally, most states with adult-use marijuana also allow local governments to add another layer of taxation. In Alaska, California, Massachusetts, and Oregon local governments can collect their own marijuana taxes, and localities in Alaska, California, Colorado, Nevada, and Washington can charge local sales tax on adult-use marijuana sales (Dadayan, 2019). Cook County in Illinois, home of Chicago, is expected to implement a marijuana sales tax later in 2020.

There are several inherent challenges for states that are trying to forecast how much revenue adult-use marijuana will generate and what the proper rate of taxation should be. Because the legalization of adult-use marijuana is relatively new and has only been rolled out in a handful of states, there is still uncertainty about the demand, supply, and long-term growth of the industry.

While the legalization of marijuana is politically popular—a September 2019 Pew Research Center survey found that 67% of Americans favored marijuana legalization (Daniller, 2019)—that does not necessarily correlate to actual consumption. Information on marijuana usage is often unreliable: It relies on self-reporting on surveys, which may not present an accurate data because people may be leery of reporting a violation of federal law (especially if they are a recipient of benefits from any federal programs), or may simply downplay their drug usage out of judgment or embarrassment. The pattern of consumption also has to be considered. States that implement adult-use marijuana programs may see an initial surge of consumption after legalization, but the numbers may level off over time as the novelty wears off or the market stabilizes. Colorado and Washington have the most mature adult-use markets, having been the first two states to legalize, and while they continue to bring in tax revenues from marijuana, the growth in revenues has slowed considerably or has decreased from peak numbers (Chapman et al., 2019). For states that have excise taxes tied to price, fluctuations in the cost of adult-use marijuana will also have ramifications: If the licensed dispensaries produce more marijuana than expected, there is no way to sell off the surplus outside of the state. The federal prohibition on marijuana means that states that have legalized marijuana cannot send any excess product to other states that may have scarcity or that could absorb more product. Legal marijuana is an intra-state model—if marijuana that is legally grown crosses state lines, it would invite federal intervention. If the state marijuana market is flooded with supply, the price will drop and predicted tax revenue would drop unless accompanied by an increase in demand to offset the losses. This has been an issue in Oregon, where overproduction led marijuana prices to drop by 50% from 2016 to 2018 (Hussain, 2019). States also must try to predict the rate at which people will abandon the black market for the legal market as well as the percentage of those people who will stick with the legal market. Since black market consumption in and of itself is not easy to measure accurately, this introduces yet another variable that clouds tax revenue forecasting. Without a clear picture of what the expected market for adult-use marijuana is going to be, setting the appropriate tax rate and predicting revenue becomes more complex.

Economic Development

Another benefit states expect to see with the legalization of marijuana is the creation of jobs and increased economic development. Once marijuana policy is enacted, a state economy must establish a complete industry infrastructure and supply chain in a very short period of time. Legal state marijuana industries are highly regulated, necessitating state licensing for jobs like cultivators, processors, distributors, retailers, and testing facilities. This all has to be contained within state borders because of federal restrictions; states cannot outsource any of these services to out-of-state or international providers. States also differ in the degree that they allow vertical integration—the ability of firms to control different aspects of the supply chain—of their marijuana industry. Arizona, New Mexico, Hawaii, Minnesota, Florida, New York, Vermont, New Hampshire, Massachusetts, New Jersey, and Delaware require vertical integration for medical marijuana markets, and firms must hold licenses for cultivation, product manufacturing, and retail. No states currently require vertical integration for the adult-use market, though some states do allow it. Washington has prohibited vertical integration for both adult-use and medical marijuana markets (Peña, 2019). Those states in favor of a vertically disintegrated market believe it is more likely to expand economic opportunity to more vendors and spread the wealth.

Because of the federal marijuana prohibition, the growth of the marijuana industry is not reflected in traditional data sets and muddies the waters for states that are trying to predict the potential economic development of marijuana legalization. The Census Bureau, Bureau of Economic Analysis, Internal Revenue Service, and Bureau of Labor Statistics rely on a firm's North American Industry Classification System (NAICS) code. The NAICS system does not currently have a category for the marijuana industry, despite the fact that these firms are required to respond to surveys and submit tax returns using NAICS codes. Therefore, dispensaries, manufacturers, and cultivators must choose other categories, such as Other Food Crops Grown Under Cover, Medicinal and Botanical Manufacturing, Miscellaneous Store Retailers, and Pharmacies and Drug Stores, which do not accurately capture their industry (Schultz, 2019). The NAICS system is scheduled to be reevaluated and revised in 2022 and could perhaps be updated to reflect the growth and prevalence of the marijuana industry in America. In the interim, states that have legalized marijuana have begun keeping their own statistics. This data is preferable to national estimates, but there is not one universal methodology states are using, which can complicate comparisons across states. Many states that have adult-use marijuana programs are still in their infancy, so economic impact and job creation data is not yet available.

There are some additional special considerations that state economic impact calculations for the marijuana industry must also take into account. So far, every state that has legalized adult-use marijuana has permitted local governments to opt out of the industry. The threshold depends on the state, but usually counties or large cities are given the option to prohibit marijuana-related businesses from their jurisdiction. Possession and consumption of marijuana remains permissible in these areas, but dispensaries, grow facilities, processing plants, and other related industries could be prevented from operating. When Washington legalized adult-use marijuana in 2014, approximately 25% of cities opted out. Nearly half of municipalities prohibited sales in Nevada when they legalized in 2017, and California, saw 300 of 482 municipalities ban marijuana operations upon legalization in 2016

(Kapos, 2019). Depending on how many municipalities opt out, the scope of the economic gains from legalizing marijuana could be muted. If state residents cannot easily access legal marijuana because dispensaries are banned from their county or city, demand will be diminished and job creation may be thwarted. The cost to municipalities for choosing to prohibit marijuana industries in their jurisdiction is exclusion from receiving any cut of the revenue from marijuana sales in the state.

Job creation numbers may also be tempered by jobs that are lost because of the legalization of marijuana because the federal government requires many employers to implement drug-free workforce policies or carry out regular drug testing:

> The Drug-Free Workplace Act of 1988 required all federal contractors to implement a drug-free workplace policy statement that prohibits the manufacture, use, and distribution of controlled substances in the workplace. While the Act does not require drug testing, employees are subject to action if evidence of marijuana use is found. Executive Order 12564 requires all federal employees to refrain from the use of illegal drugs and requires mandatory drug testing for all employees in law enforcement, national security, protection of life and property, and public health and safety. Many states and local law enforcement and emergency service providers also undergo regular testing. The Omnibus Transportation Employee Testing Act of 1991 requires drug and alcohol testing of safety-sensitive employees in aviation, trucking, railroads, mass transit, pipelines, and other transportation industries. (Schultz, 2019)

Private companies can also set their own drug-screening policies for employment, and while some are changing standards as more states legalize marijuana, many have not. The prolonged period that marijuana stays in a person's system—potentially up to 30 days—means that employees who may enjoy legalized marijuana in their off-hours would test positive in a drug screening, and employees who consume marijuana during work hours would be impaired in their job performance.

Environmental Concerns

States must also consider other costs that arise from embracing the marijuana industry. Marijuana cultivation is not necessarily an environmentally friendly procedure because "Marijuana is a water- and nutrient-intensive crop. Its cultivation is associated with land clearing, the diversion of surface water, agrochemical pollution, and the poaching of wildlife in the United States and internationally. Where grown indoors, it can require extensive energy inputs with potentially negative effects on climate." (Carah et al., 2015)

Marijuana plants are thirsty creatures: A single mature weed plant can consume almost 23 liters of water per day (for context, wine grape plants consume approximately 13 liters) (Oregon Cannabis Environmental Best Practices Task Force, 2016). Where marijuana plants are grown creates different additional environmental impacts. Indoor cultivation is an attractive option for many businesses: The product is more secure, the consistency of the grow conditions are controlled, multiple harvests can occur a year, and it opens up cultivation options for areas of the country that do not have the climate for outdoor marijuana cultivation. Reliance on indoor cultivation, however, necessitates grow lights, ventilation systems, and climate control. These all can consume a lot of electricity, especially lighting, which may have brightness that rivals what is found in a hospital operating room. Many indoor grow facilities operate 24 hours a day, resulting in round-the-clock energy consumption. The total electricity intensity for an indoor marijuana facility has been estimated to be approximately 200 watts per square foot (Mills, 2012). Moving marijuana cultivation outside may be less energy-intensive, but it introduces other equally damaging environmental concerns such as deforestation, destruction of wildlife, and the use of pesticides (Warren, 2015). To prevent losing marijuana crops to mold or mites, many outdoor growers rely on pesticides to keep the plants protected. However, since the U.S. Environmental Protection Agency (EPA) doesn't regulate or provide guidance on what pesticides should be used because of the federal ban on marijuana, this leaves it up to individual states to make these determinations. The states, however, do not have the data or research of the EPA in making these decisions, resulting in a patchwork quilt of regulations in states that have legal marijuana:

> Beyond California's northern border, for example, Oregon requires testing for a different set of pesticides and enforces different limits for residue levels on cannabis products. In some cases, Oregon's limits are tighter than California's; in others, they are more lenient. Cross another border into Washington, where recreational cannabis sales began in 2014, and pesticide testing is not required at all (Seltenrich, 2019).

Environmental issues were not addressed in much of the early legalization of marijuana, but as the industry continues to flourish and the potential toll that cultivation takes on the environment is becoming more apparent, states are beginning to take more concrete measures to address the issue. Illinois, which legalized adult-use marijuana in 2019, has limits on the amount of water and electricity that growers can use (Illinois Public Act 101-0027, 2019). In California, legal marijuana industries must comply with the state's California Environmental Quality Act (CEQA), which requires environmental impact assessments for construction or projects that will change the physical environment of the state (Britschgi, 2019). While these regulations are aimed at protecting the environment, there is the side-effect of increasing the cost of operating in the state's legal marijuana industry, inadvertently making the black market a more fiscally attractive alternative. More research also has to be done on the long-term impacts of legal marijuana to provide states with the best data for formulating their policies.

Social Justice

Historically, while marijuana usage is similar among different racial and socio-economic backgrounds, arrests for marijuana possession are concentrated among people of color, particularly Blacks and Hispanics (Vitiello, 2019). As more and more states legalize recreational marijuana, many are also considering how to address social justice concerns to make sure that individuals who disproportionally paid the price for marijuana prohibition are not excluded from reaping the rewards of state legalization. This has taken different forms in different states. Some states that have not made the leap to full legalization of adult-use marijuana have decriminalized possession, making small amounts of marijuana either a civil infraction or a low-level misdemeanor that carries no jail time; however, violators can still be punished by a fine. While decriminalization doesn't eliminate the burden of punishment for marijuana possession completely or remedy patterns of enforcement, it does remove the threat of jail time from the equation.

States and localities have also started to implement the expungement or sealing of certain prior marijuana arrests and convictions from a person's record, so that in the eyes of the law the infraction never happened. Expungement is traditionally available for nonviolent offenders and primarily for low-level possession convictions. The expungement process can be automatic (Illinois), though the vast majority of states handle expungement via a petition process initiated by the individual with the criminal record. The petition process can be cumbersome, time consuming, expensive, and relies on the individual knowing how to maneuver through the judicial system, which creates some barriers to individuals who qualify for their records to be expunged from actually doing so. "Of 78,000 cannabis-related convictions that could be set aside in Oregon, for example, only several hundred requests for set-asides were received in 2015 and 2016. And whereas nearly half a million people were arrested for cannabis-related offenses over the past decade in California, less than 5,200 applications were received (through March 2018) to reclassify these offenses" (Adinoff and Reiman, 2019).

States are also taking steps to encourage diversity in the legal marijuana industry. Participating in many aspects of the legal market requires a license from the state, which can be expensive. License fees for a retailer in California, for example, range from $10,000 for a small business to $300,000 for a larger business with the size of the business based on revenue (Adinoff and

Reiman, 2019). Additionally, states have requirements for testing, security, and environmental protections that can add several hundreds of thousands of dollars to start-up expenses. In addition to federal prohibition on marijuana diminishing the chance of getting a loan to cover these costs, people of color historically have had difficulties in accessing the capital needed to gain entry to the legal marijuana market (Fairlie et al., 2016). To try and eliminate some of these barriers, states have implemented a variety of programs. In California, there is grant funding available to assist minority-owned businesses in the adult-use marijuana industry (California Cannabis: State and Local Equity Programs, 2018). Illinois, which uses a scoring system for license determinations, grants additional points on applications for qualified social equity applicants (Illinois Department of Commerce & Economic Opportunity, n.d.), while Massachusetts gives qualified social equity applicants training and technical assistance in areas such as accounting and sales forecasting, legal compliance, farming best practices, and navigating the municipal process (Commonwealth of Massachusetts Cannabis Control Commission, 2019). Michigan offers reduced licensing fees for business owners with a prior marijuana-related conviction or who reside in one of the identified communities that have been disproportionately impacted by previous marijuana prohibition (Michigan Department of Licensing and Regulatory Affairs, n.d.).

Legislative Process

Even the passage of marijuana laws is complicated by the federal prohibition. The early adopters of medical marijuana programs, and almost all adult-use programs, have been enacted by the initiative process rather than by state legislative action. The initiative process takes the legislature out of the lawmaking process, allowing citizens to decide directly whether a statute should be approved. The initiative process varies from state to state in the requirements but, generally, citizens are able to get proposed legislation or a constitutional amendment on the ballot if they meet the state's predetermined signatory requirements. In theory, once an initiative passes, lawmakers are forced to then implement the will of the voters; it's a way to force an issue on the agenda that lawmakers are either ignoring or are unable to come to a consensus on for legislation.

However, adult-use marijuana has struggled to be passed though state legislative action. Of the 11 states that permit adult-use marijuana, only Vermont (2018) and Illinois (2019) did so through acts of the legislature. Vermont is a bit of an outlier in that, while adult-use marijuana is legal, the legislation enacted only permitted home cultivation of a small number of marijuana plants and failed to tackle the more complex issue of creating a commercial market for retail sales. One reason the legislative avenue for adult-use marijuana tends to be more difficult is that it forces elected officials to take responsibility for their vote, which may be daunting given that there are so many unknowns associated with the impact of marijuana. Because federal prohibition has made marijuana difficult to study, there is not a clear body of evidence on how long-term marijuana usage affects the body. The data from states that have legalized adult use on societal concerns, like marijuana-related traffic accidents and youth consumption, have been somewhat anecdotal and hard to draw conclusions from given the limited timeframe of implementation. This lack of information may contribute to some legislators being hesitant to provide an affirmative vote on adult-use marijuana: Without a clear picture of the consequences of legalization, the risk may outweigh the reward.

Creating a state adult-use program in the shadow of federal constraints and a potential crackdown may also contribute to the legislative gridlock. There are extra hurdles and complexities associated with implementing marijuana policy, discussed previously, that other legislation doesn't have to address. Additionally, while marijuana legalization enjoys popular support, it is not clear that implementing marijuana policy is an important factor in determining a candidate's reelection success. In fact, with many counties and cities leaning toward opting out of a statewide adult-use marijuana program, some legislators have an incentive to not support a bill.

The federal prohibition on marijuana hasn't stopped states from implementing medical and adult-use marijuana programs, but it has made doing so substantially more difficult and manifests itself in almost every decision-making process for the industry. As a result, marijuana policy in America has been created mostly by trial and error, with the experiences of early adapters in implementing marijuana laws serving as a potential roadmap for other states considering legalization. To paraphrase U.S. Supreme Court Justice Louis Brandeis, states can serve as "laboratories of democracy" that can inform legislation in other states. California and Colorado helped pave the way for other states to create medical and adult-use programs. Even so, the marijuana industry remains in a constant state of flux; given the uncertainty that a new President, Congress, or Attorney General can bring, threat of federal enforcement always exists. Federal and state laws have generally been able to coexist, but a showdown is always around the corner. Until federal marijuana policy changes, that tension will continue to exist.

References

Adinoff, B., & Reiman, A. (2019). Implementing social justice in the transition from illicit to legal cannabis. *The American Journal of Drug and Alcohol Abuse, 45*(6), 673–688

Annas, G. J. (1997). Reefer madness – the federal response to California's medical marijuana law. *New England Journal of Medicine, 337*(6), 435–439. Retrieved from https://www.nejm.org/doi/full/10.1056/NEJM199708073370621?url_ver=Z39. 88-2003&rfr_id=ori%3Arid%3Acrossref.org&rfr_dat=cr_pub%3Dpubmed

Bartlett, J. (2018, June 27). 'Cannabis premium': If you want to bank marijuana money, it will cost you. *Boston Business Journal.* Retrieved from https://www.biz journals.com/boston/news/2018/06/27/cannabis-premium-if-you-want-to-ba nk-marijuana.html

Berg, A. (2020, January 9). Illinois cannabis taxes among nation's highest, could keep black market thriving, Illinois policy. Retrieved from https://www.illinois policy.org/illinois-cannabis-taxes-among-nations-highest-could-keep-black-m arket-thriving/

Britschgi, C. (2019, April 18). Could this California environmental law be the cannabis industry's "silent killer"? *Reason.* Retrieved from https://reason.com/2 019/04/18/could-this-california-environmental-law-be-the-cannabis-industrys -silent-killer/

California Cannabis: State and Local Equity Programs, SB 1294, Chapter 794 (2018).

Carah, J., Howard, J., Thompson, S., Short Gianotti, A., Bauer, S., Carlson, S., ... Power, M. (2015, August). High time for conservation: Adding the environment to the debate on marijuana legalization. *BioScience, 65*(8), 822–829.

Chapman, J., Levin, A., Murphy, M., & Zhang, A. (2019, August). *Forecasts hazy for state marijuana revenue.* The Pew Charitable Trusts. Retrieved from https:// www.pewtrusts.org/en/research-and-analysis/issue-briefs/2019/08/forecasts-haz y-for-state-marijuana-revenue

Cole, J. M. (2013, August 29). *Guidance regarding marijuana enforcement (official memorandum).* Washington, DC: U.S. Department of Justice, Office of the Deputy Attorney General. Retrieved from https://www.justice.gov/iso/opa/resources/305 2013829132756857467.pdf

Colorado Constitution art, XVIII, § 16.

Commonwealth of Massachusetts (2011). *Acts and resolves passed by the General Court of Massachusetts.* Boston, MA: Secretary of the Commonwealth

Commonwealth of Massachusetts Cannabis Control Commission (2019, June 3). *Social equity program participants receive introductory training for entering the adult-use cannabis industry in Massachusetts.* Retrieved from https://mass-ca nnabis-control.com/social-equity-program-participants-receive-introductory-training-for-entering-the-adult-use-cannabis-industry-in-massachusetts/

Controlled Substances Act (1970). Pub, L, 91-513, 84 Stat. 1236.

Dadayan, L. (2019, October). Are states betting on sin? The murky future of state taxation, tax policy center. Retrieved from https://www.urban.org/sites/default /files/publication/101132/are_states_betting_on_sin_the_murky_future_of_sta te_taxation_1.pdf

Daniller, A. (2019, November 14). *Two-thirds of Americans support marijuana legalization.* Pew Research Center. Retrieved from https://www.pewresearch.org/ fact-tank/2019/11/14/americans-support-marijuana-legalization/

Fairlie, R., Robb, A., & Robinson, D. (2016, December 15). Black and White: Access to capital among minority-owned startups, Stanford institute for economic policy research. Retrieved from https://siepr.stanford.edu/sites/default/files/publications/ 17-003.pdf

Godlewski, N. (2019, April 10). Attorney General Barr Says he would favor making marijuana illegal across the United States. *Newsweek.* Retrieved from https://ww w.newsweek.com/attorney-general-barr-marijuana-law-1392561

Golden, T. (1997, April 12). Federal judge supports California doctors on marijuana issue. *New York Times*. Retrieved from https://www.nytimes.com/1997/04/12/us/federal-judge-supports-california-doctors-on-marijuana-issue.html

Gonzalez v. Raich, 545 US 1 (2005).

Guzman, S. (2018, January 4). *Sessions terminates US policy that let legal pot flourish*. Associated Press. Retrieved from https://apnews.com/19f6bfec15a74733 b40eaf0ff9162bfa

Hussain, S. (2019, June 24). Oregon has too much cannabis. Two laws may help the state manage its surplus. *Los Angeles Times*. Retrieved from https://www.latimes.com/nation/la-na-oregon-legislature-tackles-supply-marijuana-20190624-story .html

Illinois Department of Commerce & Economic Opportunity (n.d.). Illinois adult-use cannabis social equity program. Retrieved from https://www2.illinois.gov/dceo/CannabisEquity/Pages/default.aspx

Ingraham, C. (2017, June 13). Jeff sessions personally asked congress to let him prosecute medical marijuana providers. *Washington Post*. Retrieved from https://www.washingtonpost.com/news/wonk/wp/2017/06/13/jeff-sessions-personally-asked-congress-to-let-him-prosecute-medical-marijuana-providers/

Kapos, S. (2019, September 23). Illinois cities turn their backs on pot as legalization approaches. *Politico*. Retrieved from https://www.politico.com/story/2019/09/2 3/illinois-marijuana-legalization-city-ban-1506494

Leary v. United States, 39 US 6 (1969).

Long, T. (2019, November 14). 1915: El Paso becomes first city in United States to outlaw marijuana. *El Paso Times*. Retrieved from https://www.elpasotimes.com/story/news/2019/11/14/el-paso-history-pot-possession-first-city-outlaw-weed-t bt/2579079001/

The Marihuana Tax Act of 1937, Pub.L. 75–238, 50 Stat. 551.

Michigan Department of Licensing and Regulatory Affairs (n.d.). Social equity (adult-use marijuana). Retrieved from https://www.michigan.gov/lara/0,4601,7-1 54-89334_79571_93535---,00.html

Mills, E. (2012, July). The Carbon footprint of indoor cannabis production. *Energy Policy*, 46, 58–67.

Ogden, D. W. (2009, October 19). "Investigations and prosecutions in states authorizing the medical use of marijuana" (official memorandum). Washington, DC: United States Department of Justice, Office of the Deputy Attorney General. Retrieved from https://www.justice.gov/sites/default/files/opa/legacy/2009/10/19/medical-marijuana.pdf.

Oregon Cannabis Environmental Best Practices Task Force (2016, August 16). *Working Document*. Retrieved from https://www.oregon.gov/olcc/marijuana/Documents/CEBP/WorkingDocument_CEBP_08162016.pdf

Peña, J. (2019 March). Jack of all trades or master of one? Marijuana *Business Magazine*. Retrieved from https://mjbizmagazine.com/vertical-integration/

Pure Food and Drug Act of June 30, 1906. 34 Stat. 768. Ch. 3915. Public Law 384.

Schultz, L. (2019, April 25). The economic impact of developing the adult-use cannabis industry in New York, Rockefeller institute of government. Retrieved from https://rockinst.org/issue-area/the-economic-impact-of-developing-the-adult -use-cannabis-industry-in-new-york/

Secure and Fair Enforcement Banking Act of 2019, H.R.1595, 116th Congress (2019).

Seltenrich, N. (2019, April 25). Into the weeds: Regulating pesticides in cannabis. *Environmental Health Perspectives*, 127(4), 1–8.

Sessions III, J. B. (2017, May 1). "Department of justice appropriations" (letter to the congressional leadership, U.S. Department of Justice, office of the Attorney General). Retrieved from https://www.scribd.com/document/351079834/Sessions -Asks-Congress-To-Undo-Medical-Marijuana-Protections

United States Department of Justice (2015, January 16). "Attorney general prohibits federal agency adoptions of assets seized by state and local law enforcement agencies except where needed to protect public safety" (news release, U.S. Department of Justice). Retrieved from https://www.justice.gov/opa/pr/attorney-general-prohibits-federal-agency-adoptions-assets-seized-state-and-local-law

United States Department of the Treasury (2014, February 14). "BSA expectations regarding marijuana-related businesses," Guidance FIN-2014-G001, U.S. Department of the Treasury, financial crimes enforcement network. Retrieved from https://www.fincen.gov/sites/default/ files/shared/FIN-2014-G001.pdf

Vitiello, M. (2019, July 27). Marijuana legalization, racial disparity, and the hope for reform. *Lewis and Clark Law Review*, 23(3), 789–821.

Warren, G. S. (2015). Regulating pot to save the polar bear: Energy and climate impacts of the marijuana industry. *Columbia Journal of Environmental Law*, 40(3), 385–432.

Wharton Public Policy Initiative (2017, November 20). *Cash, crime, and cannabis: Banking regulations in an illegal market*. Retrieved from https://publicpolicy .wharton.upenn.edu/live/news/2214-cash-crime-and-cannabis-banking-regulatio ns-in-an/for-students/blog/news.php#_edn2

Chapter 4

The Business of Cannabis

Paul Seaborn

Introduction

The business landscape for cannabis is unlike that of any other industry due to the unique nature of the cannabis plant, its complex history and current legal status, and the wide range of regulations in jurisdictions where cannabis has recently been legalized. The recent trend of cannabis legalization in various U.S. states and in countries such as Uruguay and Canada has resulted in the creation of a wide variety of cannabis businesses. These include "plant-touching" businesses ranging from cultivators, processors, and manufacturers to retailers and testing facilities, as well as ancillary business such as technology companies and professional services firms that have a cannabis focus. The business landscape has changed significantly in recent years, and the pace of change is unlikely to slow in the years to come.

The range of cannabis products available for purchase is already quite broad and continues to increase as new jurisdictions legalize and new companies enter the market with innovative products. A wide variety of cannabis strains have emerged that vary in name, potency, and cannabinoid profile, and cannabis is increasingly being processed into a wide variety of new product forms which differ dramatically in physical form, concentration, and consumption experience.

The purchase process for cannabis products is also quite different from the purchase process for traditional prescription drugs or over-the-counter medicine. In legal jurisdictions, two primary channels for purchasing legal cannabis have emerged—a commercial medical cannabis market and a commercial "adult-use" or "recreational" cannabis market. The majority of purchases in these markets take place in physical stores that have been granted specific cannabis retail licenses, but a few other purchase methods exist in jurisdictions such as Canada and for certain products such as industrial hemp-derived CBD products. Traditional medical professionals have a formal role in the medical cannabis channel but little to no role in other channels. Traditional health care plans offered through Medicare, Medicaid, and private insurance typically provide no coverage for cannabis purchases even in states where cannabis has been legalized and where individuals meet state qualifications for medical access. Legal, non-commercial options for obtaining cannabis include personal home growing and/or assistance from a designated caregiver.

With cannabis legalization still in its early stages, predicting the future for cannabis businesses is a challenging task. However, among the likely developments in upcoming years are expanded U.S. federal legal protections, the growth of national and international organizations and brands as existing barriers are reduced, and both greater understanding and greater scrutiny of the impacts of cannabis consumption and legalization.

In the sections below, this chapter first provides an overview of the unique environment in which cannabis businesses operate and then describes the several types of cannabis businesses that exist. Next, it describes the various channels and locations through which eligible individuals can purchase cannabis and the unique characteristics and available products for each. Finally, thoughts on the future outlook for the cannabis industry are provided.

Business Landscape

The business landscape for cannabis is unlike that of any other industry due to the unique nature of the cannabis plant, its complex history and current legal status, and the wide range of regulations in jurisdictions where cannabis has recently been legalized. While there are some similarities between the emerging legal cannabis industry and well-established industries such as alcohol, tobacco, and pharmaceuticals, the extent of these similarities is quite limited.

For the majority of the 20th century, cannabis was illegal throughout the United States and in most of the world.[1] Although these restrictions eliminated the legal market for cannabis, cannabis continued to be available to some extent through illegal means. More recently, individual U.S. states and various countries have begun to legalize cannabis for medical and/or other purposes.

California became the first state to legalize medical marijuana with the passage of Proposition 215 in 1996, followed by Alaska, Oregon, and Washington in 1998. In November 2012, Colorado and Washington became the first U.S. states and the first jurisdictions in the world to legalize non-medical adult use of cannabis. At the state level, 11 states have legalized

---

1 In the United States, the Marihuana Tax Act of 1937 effectively made all forms of the cannabis plant illegal at the federal level. Cannabis of any kind was formally made illegal under federal law in 1970 under the Controlled Substances Act, in which Congress classified cannabis as a Schedule I drug. Schedule I has the highest level of control, designating a substance as having no safe medical use and a high risk of abuse or misuse.

both medical and adult-use marijuana, and 33 have legalized some form of medical marijuana.[2] Another 14 states allow products containing cannabidiol (CBD) with minimal THC content. In many states, including Colorado, Washington, California, and Nevada, these cannabis programs have originated from ballot initiatives with a variety of sponsors and varying levels of detail. In other states, such as Vermont, legalization has originated in the state legislature. In each legalized U.S. jurisdiction, except Vermont and the District of Columbia, some provision has been made for the commercial production and sale of cannabis rather than just allowing for personal cultivation and consumption.

Countries that have legalized the medical use of cannabis in some form include Argentina, Australia, Canada, Chile, Colombia, Croatia, Germany, Greece, Israel, Italy, Jamaica, Lithuania, Luxembourg, Norway, the Netherlands, New Zealand, Peru, Portugal, Poland, Switzerland, and Thailand. However, many of these countries have yet to establish a legal commercial medical cannabis industry. Only two countries have legalized non-medical adult use. Uruguay became the first country to do so in December 2013, although sales did not begin until July 2017. Canada, where medical cannabis was legalized in 2001, expanded legalization to include adult use in June 2018 with sales beginning in October of the same year.

In the United States, law and regulation affecting cannabis is not restricted to a single level of government, piece of legislation, or regulatory body with consistent views. Instead, the legal landscape involves a myriad of federal, state and local legislation, regulation, and regulatory and enforcement bodies with often conflicting or contradictory views.

At the U.S. federal level, the Drug Enforcement Agency (DEA) continues to classify marijuana as a Schedule 1 drug, making it illegal for possession, research, commerce, or interstate transport or sale. Among the many impacts of this federal status are limited access to banking and capital for state-licensed and compliant marijuana businesses. While some national and state-chartered banks and credit unions such as GRN Funds in Washington and Safe Harbor Private Banking in Colorado have publicly welcomed cannabis accounts, the majority have not. Similarly, the federal status of cannabis has meant that cannabis businesses have limited access to intellectual property protections such as trademarks and patents (Landau and Wright, 2019; Schuster and Wroldsen, 2018).

Implementation of a state cannabis program involves a myriad of regulatory considerations regarding access, safety, degree of oversight, protection of youth, taxation, and other details. Some U.S states such as Nevada, Illinois, and Massachusetts have enacted a limited licensing model where a fixed number of cannabis business licenses are made available through

2 These state totals are current as of February 2020.

either a lottery or merit-based application process. In the case of Illinois, for example, a maximum of 60 medical dispensing organizations are permitted.[3] Other states such as Colorado have an open licensing model in which a comprehensive set of requirements for obtaining a cannabis business license has been established but with no fixed cap on the total number of licenses that can be issued at the state level.

Another point of differentiation among states is their approach to *vertical integration*, a business strategy by which one company participates in multiple (or all) stages of a product's supply chain. Vertical integration requires a wider range of skills and resources but also provides greater control over the full production process. In cannabis, vertical integration can encompass stages such as cultivation, processing or manufacturing, and sales. When Washington voters passed Initiative 502 (I-502) in 2012, the referendum language mirrored post-prohibition alcohol laws prohibiting vertical integration. This had the result of slowing the initial flow of cannabis products to customers following legalization (Van Leynseele, 2019). Other states, such as Colorado and Massachusetts, initially required at least some degree of vertical integration, with cultivators also required to sell to patients or customers, and retailers required to cultivate their own cannabis products. Required vertical integration has been thought to simplify the oversight responsibilities for the state by reducing the total number of license-holders and reducing transfers of cannabis between them.

States have also typically imposed a wide variety of *security requirements* on cannabis businesses, including background checks on all participating individuals, requirements for "seed to sale" physical tracking of cannabis, video surveillance of licensed facilities, careful disposal of any waste plant material, and child-proof packaging of finished products. Penalties for non-compliance can include the revocation of individual and business licenses and fines. For example, in Illinois Section 1290.510 of the Administrative Code, Grounds for Discipline, provides 30 different grounds on which the Department of Financial and Professional Regulation-Division of Professional Regulation "may refuse to issue or renew, place on probation, temporarily suspend, suspend, or revoke a dispensing organization registration or agent identification card." It also states: "If the Division determines that the dispensing organization committed a violation, the Division may take any disciplinary or non-disciplinary action as the Division may deem proper, including fines not to exceed $10,000 for each violation."[4]

Across legal jurisdictions, cannabis businesses consistently face significant restrictions on advertising (Seaborn and Miller, 2014). For example, in Illinois no registered dispensing organization can:

3 410 Ill. Comp. Stat. 130/115 (a)
4 68 Ill. Admin. Code § 1290.510.

place or maintain, or cause to be placed or maintained, an advertisement of cannabis or a cannabis-infused product in any form or through any medium:

1. Within 1,000 feet of the perimeter of a school grounds, playground, recreation center or facility, child care center, public park or library, or any game arcade admission to which is not restricted to persons age 21 years or older;
2. On or in a public transit vehicle or public transit shelter; or
3. On or in a publicly owned or -operated property.

Despite similar restrictions in Oregon, research in that state demonstrated that more than half of adults reported exposure to cannabis advertising after legalization and people who did not use marijuana and those aged 18 to 24 years were as exposed to advertising as other groups (Fiala, Dilley, Firth & Maher, 2018). Debate is ongoing as to whether existing advertising restrictions in various jurisdictions are excessive or perhaps not extensive enough (Caulkins, 2018).

Cannabis businesses also face further sources of regulatory variation. Many states have also allowed counties and municipalities to implement their own regulations for cannabis businesses, giving those bodies the choice to implement additional restrictions on cannabis businesses above and beyond those imposed by the state or ban commercial cannabis activities altogether. For example, even though Colorado voters passed Amendment 64 in November 2012, legalizing adult use of cannabis, the state's second-largest city, Colorado Springs, banned retail marijuana sales within its boundaries. In contrast, the state's largest city, Denver, allowed retail sales but later placed a cap on the number of retail marijuana store licenses due to concerns about the concentration of cannabis stores in certain areas of the city.

Industrial hemp has also been increasingly treated differently than marijuana, both at the federal level through the 2014 and 2018 Farm Bills and at the state level where some states have implemented industrial hemp programs. Some of these state programs have explicitly allowed for the commercial sale of hemp-derived products, including CBD products, while others have restricted commercial sale or not taken any position on the matter.

As a result of this complex web of legality and regulation, activities that are straightforward or taken for granted in other industries are often impossible or much more challenging for cannabis businesses. The ability of U.S. dispensaries to accept credit card payments has been and continues to be rare due to an unwillingness of national credit card processors to handle transactions that are considered in violation of U.S. federal law. The lack of credit card processing results in an increase in cash transactions that puts dispensaries, their employees, and their commercial partners in a position of having to handle significant amounts of cash. Cannabis businesses are also ineligible for typical federal bankruptcy protections due to marijuana being federally illegal.

Because the listing requirements for stock exchanges such as the New York Stock Exchange and NASDAQ include businesses being in full compliance with the laws in their home country, "plant-touching" U.S. cannabis companies have been unable to list their stock on these exchanges, whereas ancillary cannabis companies and "plant-touching" Canadian cannabis companies have done so. Similarly, many institutional investors such as state pension funds and private investment funds are either prohibited or reluctant to invest in cannabis businesses in the current legal environment.

As with alcohol and tobacco, states have allowed for a wide range of taxes to be applied to cannabis at both the state and local levels. Indeed, the generation of substantial tax revenue has been one of the arguments used in favor of cannabis legalization. However, there are significant complexities in generating tax revenue from a federally illegal substance and ongoing debates as to whether taxation levels are sufficient relative to regulatory costs and societal impacts.[5] Oregon, which does not have a general sales tax, levies a 17 percent sales tax on marijuana.[6] In Colorado, taxes for medical cannabis are lower than those for recreational cannabis, with a 15 percent excise tax on the sale of marijuana from a cultivator to a retailer as well as a 15 percent sales tax on recreational sales.[7] A portion of Colorado state tax revenue is specifically directed to K-12 education and exceeded 90 million dollars in 2017–18.[8] Counties and municipalities also may apply specific cannabis taxes. Higher cannabis taxes can be appealing to jurisdictions looking to cover the cost of industry oversight and generate additional revenues that can support other government programs. However, higher taxes also make illegal options more attractive to cost-conscious consumers.

Cannabis businesses are the target of significant criticisms, many of which stem from their operations but also from factors not fully within their control. Unlawful diversion of cannabis from legal jurisdictions to other jurisdictions that have yet to legalize continues to be a societal issue problematic for many stakeholders. Yet even cannabis businesses in full compliance with U.S. state law have little ability to prevent such diversion. Similarly, the lack of clear and consistent standards for both cannabis-impaired driving and the public or social consumption of cannabis is a focus of concern

5   Mikos, R.A., 2010. State Taxation of Marijuana Distribution and Other Federal Crimes. U. Chi. Legal F., p. 223.
6   How High Are Recreational Marijuana Taxes in Your State? Tax Foundation. https://taxfoundation.org/state-marijuana-taxes-2018/
7   Retail Marijuana Sales Tax Changes Fact Sheet. Colorado Department of Revenue, Taxation Division. https://www.colorado.gov/pacific/sites/default/files/2017JulySB267.pdf
8   Marijuana Tax Revenue and Education. Colorado Department of Education. https://www.cde.state.co.us/communications/2019marijuanarevenue

that also requires the broader involvement of a variety of stakeholders to be addressed. Cannabis businesses have also been criticized for a lack of diversity in ownership and employment in terms of race, gender, and socioeconomic status—a particular disappointment to those who had hoped legalization would provide increased opportunity to disadvantaged groups. In some cases, well-intended regulations setting the required qualifications for industry participation, such as proof of significant investment capital, have contributed to the lack of diversity. Increasingly, there are calls for intentional programs of inclusion in the industry (Rahwanji, 2019).

The cannabis industry operates in a very unusual business landscape with no two states or countries adopting the same cannabis regulatory approaches. Frequent changes in the legal status and regulation of cannabis at all levels result in a very dynamic business environment, requiring modifications in practices that affect both businesses and their customers.

Types of Cannabis Businesses

Legalization of cannabis in its various forms has resulted in the creation of a wide variety of cannabis businesses. These businesses can be divided into two primary categories—"plant-touching" businesses that directly handle the cannabis plant and "ancillary" or supporting businesses— that play a role in the industry but do not directly handle cannabis. Cultivators and dispensaries are two of the most common and visible types of plant-touching businesses, but additional businesses include processors and manufacturers as well as testing and transportation services. Typically, all of these businesses must obtain and maintain a specific state or national license to operate legally. The range of ancillary cannabis businesses is immense and includes technology companies, packaging and equipment manufacturers, and professional services firms with a cannabis focus, to name a few. Since these businesses do not directly handle cannabis, they are typically not required to obtain a specific cannabis business license and are able to operate in a manner more similar to non-cannabis businesses. More detail on specific types of cannabis businesses is provided below.

Licensed "Plant-touching" Cannabis Businesses

Cultivators

Cultivation businesses grow cannabis for consumption in flower form or for subsequent processing into a variety of other product forms. Cultivation takes place in one of three environments—indoors, in greenhouses, and outdoors. Indoor cultivation relies heavily on lighting and air conditioning equipment that provides maximum control over growing conditions regardless of the outside climate. This has allowed cannabis production to flourish in each legalized U.S. state but requires significant electricity and equipment. Greenhouse cultivation takes advantage of available natural light but also allows for significant control over growing conditions. Outdoor cultivation has the greatest reliance on natural conditions but, as a result, also offers the lowest production costs. Successful cultivation in all three of these environments requires obtaining suitable strains of cannabis strains from seeds or by cloning, maintaining suitable conditions for growing in an efficient manner, and avoiding crop losses due to pests or equipment problems. Due to a lack of federal legality in the United States, it has fallen to individual states to develop regulations regarding the use of pesticides and other chemicals during the cultivation process and to establish other requirements for cultivation safety and security, such as perimeter fencing. Most cultivators are also involved in at least some basic processing of cannabis plants after harvest, typically curing and trimming. Both of these processes are labor-intensive tasks in a business where automation is still in its infancy. In many legal states, multiple tiers of cultivation licenses have been issued based on the permitted size of the licensed cultivation facility.[9] In U.S. states where both medical and recreational cannabis has been legalized, cultivation licenses are usually specific to either the medical or recreational market, and each cannabis plant must be designated for one of these markets.

Processors and Manufacturers

While some cannabis is sold to customers in its natural form as "flower," processors and manufacturers are increasingly in the business of extracting cannabinoids and other cannabis compounds and creating concentrates that can be consumed in isolation or infused into a wide variety of end products. Extraction of cannabinoids is a highly technical process that can involve the use of butane hash oil, CO_2, and other methods in conjunction with specialized equipment. The resulting concentrate can take a variety of physical forms, including wax, oil, or shatter that can be smoked or vaporized on its own. Cannabis distillate is a particular form of oil where impurities, waxes, terpenes, and other plant matter have been removed. Distillate can be vaporized or dabbed, added to flower and smoked, or infused into a variety of cannabis edibles including gummies, beverages, baked goods, and candies. Cannabis is also processed and manufactured into topical products such as creams, lotions, and bath soaks. In addition to products intended for humans, there has been an increase in the development of cannabis-derived pet products. The range of cannabis products now legally available continues to increase as new jurisdictions legalize, new companies enter the market, and consumer demand and sophistication increases. Because cannabis is

---

9 For example, Washington has three tiers of cultivation licenses and Colorado has five tiers.

an agricultural product that currently cannot be transported widely across state and national borders, there is considerable variation in the strain, potency, and condition of cannabis products. Even products sold under the same name can vary significantly from state to state or over time.

Retailers/Dispensaries

Facilities that sell cannabis to end customers are the most visible to the public and to cannabis consumers. Like cultivators and processors, these businesses are subject to a variety of specific regulations relating to permissible products, transaction content, and physical access to their facility and products. The location and operating practices of these businesses is the subject of both standard zoning and safety regulation as well as cannabis-specific policy. Much debate has ensued over the effects of physical cannabis stores on neighborhood safety, property values, traffic, and cannabis usage. In a study of Washington state both before and after legalization, increasing cannabis retail access was associated with increased current and frequent cannabis use among adults (Everson, Dilley, Maher & Mack, 2019). Some jurisdictions limit the number of retail dispensary locations that one business can own or control, while in other states, such as Colorado, there are no such state limits, and some individual businesses operate a large number of different retail locations.

Among licensed cannabis businesses, medical dispensaries are the most connected to traditional medical practitioners and organizations. This is because of the responsibility that state medical marijuana programs have assigned physicians to evaluate whether individuals have a qualifying medical condition warranting the issuance of a medical marijuana card. In Illinois, for example, more than 4,500 doctors certified patients for medical marijuana between July 1, 2018 and June 30, 2019 (Schencker, 2019). The number of eligible patients for medical dispensaries in a given state is significantly affected by the availability of doctors willing to evaluate these individuals and issue medical cards, the breadth of qualifying conditions, and the overall simplicity or complexity of the state's medical card application process.

Testing Services

Testing of the contents and safety of products is common in cannabis, as it is for a wide variety of other agricultural and commercial products. Additional challenges in the U.S. cannabis industry include an absence of national standards or testing services. This has led individual states such as Colorado to develop their own standards for cannabis production and to issue licenses to commercial testing companies who are responsible for testing products in the state. The reliability and interpretation of testing results is an ongoing challenge for two primary reasons. First, cannabis crops, like all other agricultural products, naturally vary in composition even when cloned from the same plant or originating from the same set of seeds. Second, testing standards and technologies are still in their infancy, and the standards against which cannabis products are measured are frequently revised by regulators.

Transportation/Delivery Companies

A number of states and countries that have legalized cannabis have also chosen to issue licenses to companies that specialize in transporting cannabis between other licensed businesses, or in some cases such as California, delivering cannabis to the homes of end customers who have placed orders with licensed dispensaries remotely. Because marijuana remains illegal at the U.S. federal level, any such transportation must not cross U.S. state lines.

Social Consumption Venues

There are only a few jurisdictions that have allowed for the legal public consumption of cannabis in a commercial establishment. The lack of legal public consumption venues is significantly different from alcohol and more similar to tobacco in recent years. Even in states such as Colorado where the legalized adult use of cannabis took effect in 2014, state and local approval for such businesses has been slow to occur due to the newness of the legalization concept and concerns about public visibility, secondhand smoke, youth exposure, and impacts on surrounding areas. California, and in particular the San Francisco Bay Area, has been an early leader in the approval of social consumption businesses.

Multi-state Operators (MSOs)

The emergence of national brands and producers has so far been held back by a variety of legal and logistical obstacles—prohibition of interstate commerce, limited access to capital and traditional banking, and limited state licenses in some state markets. Nonetheless, a few companies have successfully navigated these challenges to create organizations that legally operate in more than one U.S. state, typically referred to as Multi-State Operators (MSOs). Such businesses can share operating procedures, product specifications, and human resources. Since MSOs cannot transport cannabis between U.S. states, they must create separate supply chains in every state in which they operate.

Ancillary Cannabis Businesses

Professional Services Firms

For almost every type of professional services, businesses have emerged that specialize in serving cannabis clients. Services provided by such firms include legal services, consulting services, marketing/branding/public relations services, accounting services, financial services, human resources, and real estate and construction services. The emergence of cannabis-specific services firms can be attributed to two primary factors—reluctance by existing professional services businesses to serve cannabis clients, as well as the unique needs and challenges of the cannabis industry that require special expertise and experience.

Technology Providers

The specialized nature of cannabis businesses has spurred the emergence of a variety of technology companies to serve them, including seed to sale tracking systems that connect licensed businesses and regulatory authorities, point of sale systems that support and track dispensary purchases, and analytics tools that provide insight into industry trends. For cannabis consumers, technology companies have developed websites and apps that provide product lists and pricing, reviews of dispensaries and products, and educational materials. Many of these companies get their start by bringing solutions from other industries and modifying those solutions to work in the cannabis sector.

Media Companies

Cannabis-oriented media companies existed for decades prior to legalization, including *High Times Magazine* which was founded in 1974. As legalization has spread, a variety of new media companies have entered the market, many through online channels.

Other Ancillary Businesses

Many other companies exist that specialize in cannabis cultivation equipment, extraction equipment, packaging and packaging equipment, glassware, tourism, and events.

Cannabis Purchase Channels

There are multiple channels or locations through which cannabis products can be purchased, and most are quite different from those of traditional prescription drugs or over-the-counter medicine in terms of who is eligible to purchase, what products are available for purchase, when and where purchases can take place, and how the purchase process happens. Each channel is subject to a variety of federal, state, and local rules and regulations that can vary significantly between jurisdictions, as described below.

Medical Dispensary Channel

Medical dispensaries are the most prevalent option for the purchase of legal cannabis since many more states and countries have legalized medical cannabis than adult-use cannabis.

Who Can Purchase

In states and countries that have legalized medical cannabis, only a specific set of qualified individuals have legal access to purchase through the medical dispensary channel. Typically, these individuals must be 18 years old or older with a valid medical card. Some U.S. states, such as Nevada, provide reciprocity to out-of-state cannabis patients with a valid medical card from their home state. A unique aspect of various state medical cannabis programs is that patients can designate another individual, known as a "caregiver," who can purchase cannabis on their behalf and transport it to them for consumption. The caregiver role originated as a legal way for one individual to grow medical cannabis on behalf of another individual who had qualifying medical conditions but was unable or uninterested in growing their own. Through court challenges and revised regulation, it has been extended to encompass the commercial purchase of medical cannabis.

In Illinois, for example, medical marijuana dispensaries can only sell to an individual who "presents an active registered qualifying patient, provisional patient, or designated caregiver card issued by the Department of Public Health ("DPH").[10] The requirements to obtain a patient or provisional patient card include being age 18 or older, proving in-state Illinois residency, approval by a physician with a bona fide relationship to the patient, the physician's conclusion that the customer had a qualifying medical condition, and payment of an annual registration fee.[11]

The caregiver designation has also been used to provide access to cannabis patients who are under 18 and have both parental and physician approval. For example, under Maryland's program those under the age of 18 are required to have at least one designated caregiver and a maximum of two and those individuals must be their parents or legal guardians.[12]

10 Under The Compassionate Use of Medical Cannabis Program Act of 2019, Opioid Alternative Pilot Program (OAPP) participants were added to the list of eligible purchasers. 410 Ill. Comp. Stat. 130/7.
11 68 Ill. Admin. Code § 1290.300(m)(4).
12 For a description of Maryland's caregiver program see <u>https://mmcc.maryland.gov/pages/caregivers.aspx</u>

What Can be Purchased

All products available for sale through licensed medical dispensaries are required to originate from licensed businesses within the same jurisdiction to ensure a level of consistency in tracking and oversight and avoid legal issues with interstate commerce or import/export restrictions. Many jurisdictions have banned certain types of cannabis products such as edibles in shapes or packaging that appear designed to appeal to children. In some jurisdictions where both medical and recreational cannabis have been legalized, such as Colorado, the range of approved cannabis products also differs between the medical and recreational markets, with some medical products allowed to have greater potency. In contrast to a traditional pharmacy transaction, where the type and quantity of product that can be purchased is usually specified the patient's prescription, a medical marijuana card is generally valid for an extended time period and does not provide any guidance as to the type of cannabis product that can or should be purchased. In some U.S. states, such as Colorado, the maximum quantity of medical cannabis that can be purchased can be increased based on physician recommendation.

When and Where Purchases Take Place

Most jurisdictions that have legalized medical cannabis define maximum daily operating hours that prevent medical dispensaries from being open 24/7 or late in the evening. For example, Illinois medical marijuana dispensaries cannot operate before 6 a.m. or after 8 p.m. local time. In terms of dispensary locations, jurisdictions have imposed restrictions in terms of minimum setbacks from schools and other landmarks such as day cares, parks, and even churches, and in some cases, setbacks from the nearest dispensary to prevent clustering. These restrictions are in addition to any standard zoning restrictions for commercial establishments that may apply. Further, most jurisdictions require that medical dispensaries not share the same exact commercial space as a recreational retail outlet (or other non-cannabis business), even if the two operations have common ownership. In some cases, medical and recreational outlets can still be located side by side with separate entrances within the same building. Dispensaries can vary significantly both in terms of size and style. Some offer a medical-style environment similar to a pharmacy, others seek to provide a high-end retail experience comparable to Starbucks or Apple, and some have an environment more consistent with the cannabis counterculture of the 1960s and 1970s.

How Purchases Take Place

The first step in the medical cannabis dispensary purchase process is for the customer to gain access to the facility by producing a valid medical cannabis card, and potentially a second piece of identification such as a driver's license, for inspection. Once verified, the individual is invited into the purchase area where products are typically displayed in an assortment of cabinets, display cases, or jars. Some jurisdictions may allow for handling of products prior to purchase, while others may not. Knowledgeable customers purchasing flowers may evaluate the smell as well as look for vibrant colors, visible trichomes, limited seeds and stems, and a certain feel or flower structure. Customers may consult dispensary staff, known as "budtenders," for advice on products and consumption methods in a manner somewhat similar to a patient seeking advice from a pharmacist. When it is time to complete a purchase, the quantity being purchased must conform to any program-wide or patient-specific quantity limits. The taxes assessed are a combination of both standard state and local taxes and potential additional taxes imposed specifically on medical cannabis. In California, unlike in most other jurisdictions, home delivery of medical cannabis has emerged as an alternative method of obtaining products in person at a licensed medical dispensary. Customers can place their orders with a specific dispensary remotely and then have the purchase delivered by in-house or third-party delivery services.

Adult-Use Channel

Adult-use or "recreational" cannabis stores share many similarities with medical dispensaries and, in some cases, are located side by side while sharing the same ownership. However, there are still notable differences in the purchase process at these locations as described below.

Who Can Purchase

In states and countries that have legalized adult-use cannabis, restrictions on purchases through the channel typically involve a minimum age of 18 (in the Canadian province of Alberta), 19 (for most other Canadian provinces) or 21 (all legal U.S. states and the Canadian province of Quebec). Some, but not all, jurisdictions also require proof of residency. In contrast to medical dispensaries, physician approval plays no role in determining purchase eligibility.

What Can be Purchased

As with medical dispensaries, all products available for sale through adult-use outlets are required to originate from licensed businesses within the same jurisdiction. Many jurisdictions have banned certain types of cannabis products that may appeal to children. Over time, some jurisdictions have defined required standardized amounts of THC for each serving portion and maximum quantities of THC in each purchased package. Colorado, for example, requires serving portions of 10mg and a maximum THC per purchased package of 100mg. In contrast, initial Canadian regulations for edible products have set the maximum THC content per purchased item at 10mg (Hristova, 2019). These standardization requirements are intended to help customers understand the expected potency of cannabis products across product types and brands and to limit excess consumption. However, additional product packaging may also be required. All jurisdictions also impose some transaction level or daily limit on purchase quantity, usually set to correspond to jurisdictional legal possession limits and reduce the likelihood that legal purchases will be diverted to other jurisdictions where cannabis is not yet legalized. In Colorado, adult-use purchases are limited to 1 ounce per day, whereas in Nevada and Illinois the limit is 2.5 ounces every 14 days. A surprising aspect of some state adult-use programs such as Colorado is that the sale of non-marijuana food products that do not contain THC has been prohibited in these outlets. This rule has had the effect of preventing not just the sale of other food products but also the sale of CBD-only products with minimal THC content.

When and Where Purchases Take Place

As with medical dispensaries, most jurisdictions that have legalized adult-use cannabis set maximum daily operating hours and impose restrictions on physical outlet locations. Local counties and municipalities may be even more restrictive. Depending on the jurisdiction, adult-use retail outlets may or may not be allowed to locate adjacent to a co-owned medical dispensary. As with medical cannabis dispensaries, the size of adult-use retail outlets can vary from a few hundred square feet to megastores such as those found in Las Vegas, Nevada with over 15,000 square feet of retail space.

How Purchases Take Place

The first step in the purchase process for an adult-use customer is to gain access to the facility by providing a government ID that establishes sufficient age, and potentially, residency. Once verified, the individual is invited into the purchase area and may ask a "budtender" for advice. As with medical purchases, the quantity being purchased must conform to any quantity limits. Specific adult-use cannabis taxes in addition to standard state and local taxes are common and often higher than for medical cannabis. As with home delivery of medical cannabis, California has also been an early leader in allowing home delivery of adult-use cannabis purchased from licensed retail outlets. California residents can have their purchases from licensed retail outlets delivered to their residence, and delivery services can operate in regions that don't allow dispensaries, except in locations that have banned deliveries altogether.

Traditional Pharmacy Channel

While dispensaries are the most prevalent channel for legal cannabis purchases, pharmacies have a limited role in the jurisdictions such as the United States, Uruguay, and Europe. In the United States, there are a limited number of Food & Drug Administration (FDA)-approved prescription cannabis products available for purchase through traditional U.S. pharmacies. In Uruguay, legal cannabis for both medical or recreational use is available exclusively through government pharmacies. In Germany, pharmacies have been distributing medical cannabis since 2017, filling 27,000 prescriptions that year and 95,000 in 2018 (Griffin, 2019).

Who Can Purchase

In the United States, as with any other prescription drug purchase at a pharmacy, the ability to purchase is determined by possession of a valid prescription from a physician rather than a medical cannabis card. In Uruguay, access is limited to those 18 or older. In Germany, purchasers require a doctor's prescription that is only issued after other medicines have been tried.

What Can be Purchased

In the United States, only four products derived from cannabis have been approved by the FDA: Epidiolex, Marinol, Syndros, and Cesamet. Epidiolex is a cannabis-derived drug product approved for treatment of two seizure conditions—Dravet syndrome and Lennox-Gastaut syndrome. Marinol (dronabinol), a synthetic cannabis-related drug product, first received FDA approval in 1985 for nausea and vomiting associated with chemotherapy. Two other synthetic cannabis-related drug products, Syndros (dronabinol) and Cesamet (nabilone), have also received FDA approval. Another product, Sativex (nabixmols), has been approved in the UK but has not yet been approved by FDA. In Uruguay, customers can purchase up to 10 grams, or 0.35 ounces, of cannabis per week. In Germany, both domestic and international producers can receive authorization to provide cannabis in dried form, as an extract, or as an oil in a product. The amount that can be purchased varies across the 16 German states, and the pharmacy must have some interaction with the product, whether grinding flower or formulating a custom tincture, rather than merely selling it as a finished product (Griffin, 2019).

When and Where Purchases Take Place

These products can be purchased during standard operating hours at any pharmacy that carries the products.

How Purchases Take Place

In all jurisdictions, the purchase process in pharmacies is quite similar to that of any other prescription drug. Pharmacists have access to national government guidelines on the prescription and consumption of approved products.

General Retail Outlets

While the Schedule 1 status of cannabis has prevented marijuana products from being sold outside of the three channels described above, changes in the 2014 and 2018 U.S. Farm Bill have led to industrial hemp-derived CBD products being sold in additional channels, including general retail outlets such as convenience stores, gas stations, and department stores that also sell a variety of non-cannabis products. Large-scale retailers including Ulta Cosmetics, Neiman Marcus, Sephora, Barney's, DSW, CVS, Walgreens, Kroger, American Eagle Outfitters, and Abercrombie & Fitch have already carried CBD products on a pilot or ongoing basis (Skelly, 2019). However, neither the U.S. federal government nor individual U.S. states have developed comprehensive regulation for the sale of industrial hemp products. As a result, the description below reflects current practices rather than a specific legal standard.

Who Can Purchase

Unlike the previous three channels above, no federal or state law sets a particular restriction on who is eligible to purchase these CBD products in terms of age, residency, or medical condition.

What Can be Purchased

The key distinction among CBD products sold in general retail is that they meet the standard established in the 2018 Farm Bill for industrial hemp of containing less than 0.3 percent THC by dry weight. This determination involves considerable uncertainty since there are a variety of ways to test THC content in plant matter and substances, and THC levels can vary across different parts of the same plant as well as between different plants of the same crop, shipment, or strain. No purchase quantity limits have been established, and no standards for other product characteristics such as CBD levels or the presence of pesticides or contaminants have been set.

When and Where Purchases Take Place

These products can be purchased during standard operating hours at any general retailer that has them in stock.

How Purchases Take Place

The purchase process is identical to that of other products in these stores. Store staff may or may not have any knowledge of the nature and application of the CBD products for sale, and the FDA and state regulators provide no guidance to these retailers regarding sale and consumption.

Mail Order Channel

The mail order channel for cannabis product purchases relies on the same standard postal or courier delivery services used to deliver a wide variety of other non-cannabis products. The legal availability of this channel is a factor of both the type of cannabis product being purchased and the jurisdiction in which the customer lives. In Canada, mail order was the primary legal purchase channel for medical cannabis during the period before adult use of cannabis was legalized in October 2018. Since that time, it continues to be an available channel for both medical and adult-use purchases. In the United States, the Schedule 1 status of marijuana dating back to the 1970s has been a primary obstacle to legal mail order purchases. However, as with the general retail channel above, industrial hemp-derived CBD products have begun to be sold through this channel due to changes in federal treatment of industrial hemp resulting from the 2014 and 2018 Farm Bills.

Who Can Purchase

In Canada, the mail order channel is available to individuals who qualify under either the medical or adult-use programs. In the United States, unlike the previous three channels above, no federal or state law sets a particular restriction on who is eligible to purchase these CBD products in terms of age, residency, or medical condition.

What Can be Purchased

In Canada, the same set of products are legally permitted to be sold via mail order and physical stores. Any variation in product availability is due to inventory and stock keeping differences rather than legal limitations. In the United States, the key distinction among CBD products sold by mail order is the same as for general retail: Products must meet the standard established in the 2018 Farm Bill for industrial hemp of containing less than 0.3 percent THC by dry weight. No purchase quantity limits exist and no standards for other product characteristics such as CBD levels or the presence of pesticides or contaminants are in place.

When and Where Purchases Take Place

In Canada, marijuana products are typically purchased through a provincial government website that offers products from a wide variety of products from multiple producers. In the United States, CBD products are typically ordered directly from the producer or a CBD retailer through their website or phone line.

How Purchases Take Place

Two key limitations for the mail order channel relate to product—inspection and timeliness. Customers do not have the option of physically examining products before purchase although they may have access to online reviews and other product information to inform their purchase decision. Remote access to trained staff is also a possibility. Mail order also requires waiting for product delivery rather than having immediate access after purchase.

Future Outlook

While significant progress has been made towards widespread cannabis legalization, the process is still in its early stages. As a result, predicting the future outlook for cannabis businesses is a challenging task. However, events to date provide some clues as to potential developments.

First, the legal environment for cannabis businesses is likely to continue expanding into new U.S. states and new countries. No jurisdictions which have legalized cannabis in the past 10–15 years have chosen to reverse course, and public support for legalization continues to grow in almost all locations. Local, state, and national governments have built elaborate regulatory systems to enable legalization, and cannabis businesses have become increasingly established and accepted in legal jurisdictions. At the U.S. state level, efforts to legalize cannabis through state legislatures continue to prove much more difficult than efforts focused on ballot initiatives, so states without a viable mechanism for ballot initiatives will likely be last to legalize non-medical use. At the U.S. federal level, expanded legal protections for state-legal cannabis businesses, such as greater legal banking access, are a likely precursor to full national legalization that will require significant political effort. Internationally, many countries have legalized medical use of cannabis, and many of those are candidates to join Uruguay and Canada in also legalizing adult use.

Second, as legal barriers to multi-state businesses and interstate commerce are reduced, expanded legalization should enable the emergence of national and international businesses and brands. International import and export of varius forms of cannabis is also likely to expand and to include the United States for the first time.

Third, given how little integration currently exists between legal cannabis and traditional medicine, increased integration seems likely. Canada provides a potential model for other jurisdictions, with a national cannabis regulatory system that grants a significant role to Health Canada, the national health regulator comparable to the U.S. FDA. However, even in Canada, further progress is needed before medical professionals and their patients approach the medical use of cannabis in a manner similar to other medical options. In the United States, an expanded role for the FDA could lead to additional cannabis-based FDA-approved drugs but also greater concern and scrutiny over the potential harms of cannabis and further restrictions on non-medical sales channels in particular. Throughout the world, cannabis businesses and their customers stand to benefit from the results of expanded medical research into the effects of cannabis consumption in its various forms.

Fourth, as laws regulating marijuana are loosened, it seems likely that industrial hemp-derived CBD will face increasing regulation. The current U.S. environment, in which neither state nor local governments provide significant oversight of CBD, has led to a spike in production and consumer access, but also appears sub-optimal in many ways. In the past, physical similarities between hemp and marijuana plants and a lack of understanding or interest in the compositional differences caused both plants to be regulated (or banned) in the same manner. Given the non-intoxicating nature of CBD products and the increasing prevalence and acceptance, a more moderate regulatory structure for CBD will likely emerge but with additional restrictions on allowable health and wellness claims.

Fifth, the level of diversity and inclusion in the cannabis business has much room for improvement. Increasing recognition of this reality and the implementation of intentional programs to address it in jurisdictions such as Massachusetts and Oakland, California offer a reason to expect further change in the future.

Together, these changes should serve to further expand the prevalence and impacts of cannabis businesses while resulting in a gradual reduction of stigma associated with cannabis (Lashley and Pollock, 2019). A few decades ago, the idea of legal cannabis businesses operating in plain sight and with the support of a large portion of their communities was hard to imagine in most parts of the world. Significant societal change has already occurred to make such a situation a reality, and many additional surprises and changes are to be expected. As society develops a clearer understanding of cannabis consumption and its potential benefits and risks, stakeholders will continue to hold differing views on their preferred future scenarios for cannabis legalization. However, it appears increasingly likely that legal cannabis businesses will remain a part of the business environment for many years to come.

References

Caulkins, J. P. (2018). Editorial: Advertising restrictions on cannabis products for nonmedical use: Necessary but not sufficient? *American Journal of Public Health*, *108*(1), 19–21.

Everson, E. M., Dilley, J. A., Maher, J. E., & Mack, C. E. (2019). Post-legalization opening of retail cannabis stores and adult cannabis use in Washington State, 2009–2016. *American Journal of Public Health*, *109*(9), 1294–1301.

Fiala, S. C., Dilley, J. A., Firth, C. L., & Maher, J. E. (2018). Exposure to marijuana marketing after legalization of retail sales: Oregonians' experiences, 2015–2016. *American Journal of Public Health*, *108*(1), 120–127.

Griffin, B. (2019, November 18). German medicinal cannabis: Pharmacies serve key roles for distribution. *Cannabyte*. Retrieved from https://newfrontierdata.com/cannabis-insights/german-medicinal-cannabis-pharmacies-serve-key-roles-for-distribution/

Hristova, B. (2019, October 29). Health experts praise 10 mg cannabis edibles, but will consumers bite? The Growth Op. Retrieved from https://www.thegrowthop.com/cannabis-news/day-49-health-experts-praise-10-mg-cannabis-edibles-but-will-consumers-bite

Landau, N. J., & Wright, J. W. (2019). Cannabis patents, trademarks, and other forms of intellectual property face difficulties. *Intellectual Property & Technology Law Journal*, *31*(7), 8–11.

Lashley, K., & Pollock, T. G. (2019). Waiting to inhale: Reducing stigma in the medical cannabis industry. *Administrative Science Quarterly*. doi:10.1177%2F0001839219851501.

Rahwanji, M. (2019). Hash'ing. *Out inequality in the legal recreational cannabis industry. Northwestern Journal of International Law and Business*, *39*(3), 333–357.

Schencker, L. (2019, November 29). More Illinois doctors using marijuana as medicine. "It's going to be part of any family primary care practice". Chicago Tribune. Retrieved from https://www.chicagotribune.com/business/ct-biz-marijuana-doctors-offices-legalization-20191127-ljocchb6c5djtl2nwixz4c3lkq-story.html

Schuster, W. M., & Wroldsen, J. (2018). Entrepreneurship and legal uncertainty: Unexpected federal trademark registrations for marijuana derivatives. *American Business Law Journal*, *55*(1), 117–166.

Seaborn, P., & Miller, W. (2014). Medical Marijuana Industry Group: Outdoor advertising in Denver. Case Research Journal, *34*(4), 119–127.

Skelly, C. (2019, March 18). *Retailers are going after CBD*. Retrieved from https://blog.brightfieldgroup.com/retailers-enter-cbd

Van Leynseele, A. (2019). Washington: Vertical integration: What it is and why it matters to Cannabis. Cannabis Law Journal. Retrieved from https://journal.cannabislaw.report/washington-vertical-integration-what-it-is-and-why-it-matters-to-cannabis/

Cannabis as Medicine: Research, Practice and Future Directions

Part Two

Chapter 5

The Endocannabinoid System (ECS)

Gary Starr and Stephen Dahmer

Introduction

Most medical practitioners, in the modern, Western world, were trained in the doctrines of the biomedical model of disease. The biomedical model of disease is based on an established language which regards the human body as a collection of parts (anatomy), systems (physiology), and functions performed by those parts and systems. While these all overlap and work together, it has proven useful to separate them in order to better understand how the body works and to validate the biomedical model with objective evidence (Giblett, 2008). This reductionist manner of contemplating the physical human condition is a foundation of modern Western medicine, is coherent with the paradigms of scientific theory (Winther, 2016), and has served us well in understanding the many complexities of the human body and human health.

The world's best-selling medical textbook, the Merck Manual, is divided like most medical textbooks, by chapter, into organ systems (Porter et al., 2006). Listed there, we find the numerous systems that make up our current understanding of human physiology: cardiovascular, gastrointestinal, endocrinological, musculoskeletal, etc. The manual offers useful summaries supporting our understanding of disease. For the most part, the categories within this body of knowledge closely match the many "specialties" within the field of medicine and encompass what is taught in modern medical schools. All readily observable body parts, organs, and functions fit nicely into this model, with each system doing its "own thing" to contribute the whole. Many diseases can be attributed, via evidence-based research, to a dysfunction of one or more of these systems.

The distinct correlation between organs and body systems is not so simple, however. The immune system illustrates an example wherein no readily visible single organ or anatomical part is responsible for the system's activity. It was first described around 60 years ago (Moulin, 1989) when technology facilitated its discovery. Scientists were able to observe cellular functions that were, in aggregate, performing a body function. Prior to the discovery of this system, we lacked a framework and language to discover and describe immune-specific diseases. By virtue of naming and studying this system, scientists could use available technology to make observations and update past models, incorporating new data. Similarly, the nascent field of human psychoneuroimmunology has emerged as an interdisciplinary effort to understand and explain the links between brain, behavior, and the immune system (Irwin, 2008). Around the same time as the discovery of the immune system, another system and its unique functions were being observed. Despite the discovery of key endogenous chemicals linked to it which impact diverse and multiple body tissues, standard medical texts do not list this important body system: the Endocannabinoid System (ECS).

The ECS is deeply involved in critical physiological functions at an *inter*cellular and *intra*cellular level. ECS physiology is comprised of various signaling pathways with numerous, linked feedback and regulation processes. It has been referred to as a homeostatic super modulatory system, and its salient homeostatic effects on the human body have been summed up in five words: "relax, eat, sleep, forget, and protect" (DiMarzo, 1998). At present, this system is still widely unknown and even misunderstood by the majority of healthcare practitioners. More than a half-century after its discovery, it is exciting to offer this chapter on what is currently understood about this key physiologic system.

What Is the ECS?

The ECS refers to a physiologic system present in all chordates. The term derives from ligands and corresponding receptors identified at a cellular and intercellular level, which have been referred to as *cannabinoids* and *cannabinoid receptors*. The cannabinoid receptor ligands produced in our own bodies are often referred to as *endo*cannabinoids. Other structurally similar exogenous molecular ligands, produced by plants which can interact with our cellular cannabinoid receptors, are referred to distinctly as *phyto*cannabinoids. Endocannabinoids, the enzymes that form and metabolize them, along with the associated cell membrane receptors they bind to (and a host of other molecules that interact directly and indirectly with the receptors), are collectively referred to as the endocannabinoid system (ECS).

Over the last 90 years, scientists have been observing and publishing new information about cannabinoids and the ECS (once it was recognized), yet there remain many unanswered questions about the "how" and even the "what" of this system and its related compounds. The definition of the ECS has expanded significantly as new discoveries have been made and as our understanding has grown (DiMarzo et al., 2015). Our current incomplete understanding of this system and its vast interactions with the other physiological systems in our body is rapidly evolving. Readers are referred to other well-documented and thorough reviews of the ECS (Pertwee, 2015;

Meccariello 2016) and encouraged to remain vigilant and to continue to seek new information as it becomes available.

ECS History

The ECS was not discovered in one fell swoop. Our knowledge about the ECS has been informed and influenced by 5,000 years of medical, religious, and commercial experience (and heated debate) about the plant *Cannabis sativa* L. (cannabis). It is widely recognized that the cannabis plant has been used medicinally for thousands of years and in multiple cultures worldwide. A more detailed history of cannabis in an ethnomedical context is provided in Chapter 1. Contrary to the message conveyed by accumulated negative stigma and the marginalization from respected discourse, cannabis has played a key role as a healing plant-medicine throughout human history. A recent piece in that history contrasts the current viewpoint from that of just 100 years ago. In the latter half of the 19th century, Sir William Osler, often regarded as the "father of modern medicine" and a founder of the John Hopkins School of Medicine, viewed cannabis treatments as the best remedy for migraine headaches in *The Principles and Practice of Medicine* (1892).

In subsequent decades, despite increasing political pressure to the contrary, the American Medical Association defended the medical use of cannabis in front of Congress (Schaffer Library of Drug Policy, n.d.). Medicinal cannabis products were produced by pharmaceutical firms such as Eli Lilly, Squibb, Parke-Davis (Pfizer), Merck, Abbott Laboratories and more prior to the 1940s and cannabis remained in the United States Pharmacopoeia (USP) until 1942 (*The Antique Cannabis Book*, 2018).

In the second half of the 19th century, physicians and scientists endeavored to know more about the medical properties of the cannabis plant which had been observed in clinical use in India. At the time, it was common to conclude that effects produced by cannabis were likely due to alkaloids in the plant. While this was, ultimately, not the case for cannabis, attempts to extract and isolate alkaloids were, nevertheless, undertaken. In 1896, cannabinol (CBN), not an alkaloid, but a degradation product of Δ-9-tetrahydrocannabinol (THC), was the first cannabinoid to be isolated from the cannabis plant (Wood et al., 1896; Mechoulam et al., 2000). The structure of CBN was noted in the 1930s. In 1940, organic chemist Roger Adams isolated a second cannabinoid, cannabidiol (CBD), from the plant, and two years later, THC was extracted from cannabis by H. J. Wollner and his team at the U.S. Bureau of Narcotics. An Israeli chemist, Raphael Mechoulam, discovered the chemical structures for CBD and THC in 1963 and 1964 respectively. During the following years, numerous additional phytocannabinoids were isolated from cannabis and identified.

From the 1940s onward, animal studies, largely done on rodents and rabbits, helped identify some of the physiological activities affected by individual phytocannabinoids. These early studies and many subsequent investigations in animals and humans helped further our understanding that THC appeared to be responsible for the altered sensorium noted in human subjects. Likely as a consequence of cultural influence, political incentive, and funding, researchers in the 1960s and 1970s were largely focused on understanding cannabis as a drug of abuse with associated potential harms.

Even today, a majority of published scientific literature and information in the popular press (in the U.S.) is often biased towards the negative aspects of cannabis use. The National Institute of Drug Abuse (NIDA), whose mission "is to lead the nation in bringing the power of science to bear on drug abuse and addiction" funds more than 90% of all research on many of the most commonly used recreational drugs (Rudroff et al., 2017). This research bias is arguably responsible for current widespread misunderstanding about the current state of research into the ECS. Once THC was implicated as the agent responsible for the "high" produced by cannabis, various theories were postulated to explain this effect. Naturally, researchers wondered whether THC might interact with existing human cellular receptors (opiate, for example) or if it simply interacted with cell membranes themselves to cause the observed effects.

In the late 1980s, our collective scientific understanding of cellular signaling via G-protein-coupled receptors (described later) advanced. At the same time, new experimental techniques employing radiolabeled ligands facilitated the identification of THC-associated receptor sites in cellular tissue. Once "CP 55,940," a more soluble, synthetic THC analog was produced with radiolabeling, it wasn't long before researchers identified specific cellular receptors to which THC binds (Herkenham et al., 1991). Between 1991 and 1993 these newly identified receptors were cloned and ultimately identified as G-protein-coupled receptors. These G-protein-coupled receptors were the binding sites researchers were looking for and were subsequently named cannabinoid receptors (CB1 and CB2). The heated debate was resolved and the existence of a completely new receptor as the target for THC in the human body was proven. This was the beginning of our understanding that these cellular level interactions constituted part of a whole-body system, essential for health and present in all of us.

Dr. Mechoulam and his contemporaries pursued answers to logical follow-up questions to their initial work. If our bodies contained a previously undiscovered ubiquitous cell membrane receptor that has such a great affinity for THC, a molecule from a plant, then surely this receptor must normally bind to something else in us humans—something generated within us. It was reasonable to suspect that this endogenous G-protein receptor wasn't lying around inside us, waiting for us to consume THC from cannabis in order to activate it. Why was this receptor there? What function required its presence? What human ligands normally bound to it?

Utilizing the advancing technology of the time, additional animal model studies in 1992 helped identify an endogenously produced material that proved to be a partial agonist of the CB1 receptor. Subsequent investigations and synthesis of this material identified it as arachidonoyl ethanolamide (AEA). The researchers named the molecule *anandamide* from 'ananda,' the Sanskrit word for 'bliss' or 'joy.' This was the first endogenous cannabinoid or *endo*cannabinoid to be discovered. In the 1990s, additional fatty acid derivatives were found in mammalian tissue which also behaved as endocannabinoids. The most well studied of these additional endocannabinoids is 2-arachidonoyl glycerol (2-AG).

In the following two decades, a deluge of new information reinforcing the complexity of the ECS and its interactions with other body systems has been revealed, but far more questions than answers remain. The ECS appeared evolutionarily over 500 million years ago. It is present in all vertebrates as well as some non-vertebrates, and it plays an essential role in almost all other physiological systems. It is estimated that the ECS contains more individual neurochemical receptors than any other neurochemical receptor type in the nervous system in addition to its wide presence in tissue outside the nervous system.

Cannabinoids

*Phyto*cannabinoids are cannabinoids produced by plants, chiefly cannabis. They are organic compounds encountered mostly in the flowering portions of cannabis but also, to a lesser and varying degree, in the leaves and non-flowering parts of the plant. At least 113 different cannabinoids have been isolated from the cannabis plant with THC being the primary psychoactive cannabinoid (Aizpurua-Olaizola et al., 2016). Other species known to produce smaller amounts of various cannabinoids include *Echinacea purpurea*, *Echinacea angustifolia*, *Acmella oleracea*, *Helichrysum umbraculigerum*, and *Radula marginata*. The cannabinoids found in these species are less studied than the more well-known molecules CBD and THC, occurring in higher quantities in cannabis (Bauer et al., 2008).

Though the word "cannabinoid" was first used in 1967 by Dr. Mechoulam's group as they studied the chemically active compounds in cannabis, it now also describes similar chemical compounds found elsewhere in nature. The most notable example is endocannabinoids, which are produced in our bodies. A discussion about the ECS is made simpler if we categorize these different cannabinoids based on where we find them in nature, rather than by their exact chemical structure.

Phytocannabinoids found in cannabis can be usefully categorized into various classes following the pathways of their natural synthesis. The main classes of phytocannabinoids derive from cannabigerol (CBG)-type compounds and differ mainly in the way CBG is cyclized by different plant enzymes. Many phytocannabinoids, including THC and CBD, are derived from their respective carboxylic acids via a process called decarboxylation. The carboxylic acid form of a particular cannabinoid is usually indicated by including an "A" (for acid) after the normal abbreviation. An example of this for CBD would be CBDA or cannabidiolic acid.

Decarboxylation of these carboxylic acids is catalyzed by heat (including during combustion of plant material), light, or alkaline conditions. Some phytocannabinoids have homologues with a smaller carbon side chain. These propyl (3-carbon) side chain versions usually have very different chemical and biological activity than the "normal" pentyl (5-carbon) side chain phytocannabinoids. Propyl cannabinoids have names with the suffix -varin added. An example for the THC homologue would be tetrahydrocannabivarin (THCV). In addition, the propyl homologues are biosynthesized from cannabigerovarinic acid (CBGVA) instead of cannabigerolic acid (CBGA). From there, the synthesis of other propyl homologue cannabinoids mirrors the same pathways used for the more common pentyl cannabinoids.

The primary classes of phytocannabinoids can be found in Table 5.1 along with key notes regarding each. There are many other related minor cannabinoids which are not detailed here. The biosynthesis pathway for phytocannabinoids is shown in Figure 5.1 (Hanus et al., 2005).

Terpenes and terpenoids are found with abundance in nature and are expressed with significant variety in cannabis. It has been observed that the clinical effectiveness of cannabis in various medical conditions is improved when the many terpenes, terpenoids, flavonoids, minor cannabinoids, and potential other compounds found in the plant are consumed along with the primary cannabinoids, THC and CBD. This is often referred to as the "entourage effect," and it refers to the suspected positive interaction of the combination of various chemicals with the ECS (Russo, 2011a). Terpenes and their terpenoid derivatives are chemically distinct from the phytocannabinoids but have a common starting point (Figure 5.1). There is some evidence to suggest that some terpenes and terpenoids also interact with elements of the ECS. A list of those with ECS interactivity can be found in Table 5.2. This list may grow substantially as additional research into the nature of the ECS progresses.

Endocannabinoids are chemical compounds produced in the human body which bind to or affect other ligands binding to our cannabinoid receptors. Though these produce similar biological effects to those observed when phytocannabinoids bind these same receptors, endocannabinoids are not structurally identical to the phytocannabinoids. In fact, their structure can appear quite different. The primary endocannabinoids, AEA and 2-AG are members of a family of signaling lipids called N-acylethanolamines. This family also includes palmitoylethanolamide (PEA) and oleoylethanolamide (OEA). These latter two possess anti-inflammatory and anorexigenic effects, but do not appear to interact directly with the known cannabinoid

Table 5.1 Primary classes of phytocannabinoids can be found in along with key notes regarding each

Phytocannabinoid Type	Molecular Model	Examples	Key notes
Cannabigerol-type CBG		CBGA CBG CBGV CBGVA	Non-psychoactive. Precursor molecule derived from the combination of geranyl pyrophosphate and olivetol.
Cannabichromene-type CBC		CBCA CBC CBCV CBCVA	Non-psychoactive. Acts on the ECS TRPV1 and TRPA1 receptors, interfering with their ability to break down endocannabinoids.
Cannabidiol-type CBD		CBDA CBD CBDV CBDVA	Non-psychoactive. Acts as an indirect antagonist of ECS cannabinoid agonists.
Tetrahydrocannabinol & Cannabinol-type THC, CBN	Δ⁹-THC CBN	THCA THC THCV THCVA CBN	Cannabinol (CBN) is the primary product of THC degradation. CBN is mildly psychoactive and partial agonist of CB1 and CB2 THC is the primary psychoactive phytocannabinoid and is a partial agonist of CB1 and CB2.

(Continued)

Table 5.1 Continued (Primary classes of phytocannabinoids can be found in along with key notes regarding each

Phytocannabinoid Type	Molecular Model	Examples	Key notes
Cannabielsoin-type CBE		CBE	Non-psychoactive. Degradation byproduct of CBD
Cannabicyclol-type CBL		CBL	Non-psychoactive. Degradation byproduct of CBC when exposed to light.
Cannabicitran-type CBT		CBT	A unique tetracyclic and di-ether molecule without alcohol groups. Isolated in 1971, but recently re-gained attention. Very little research done.

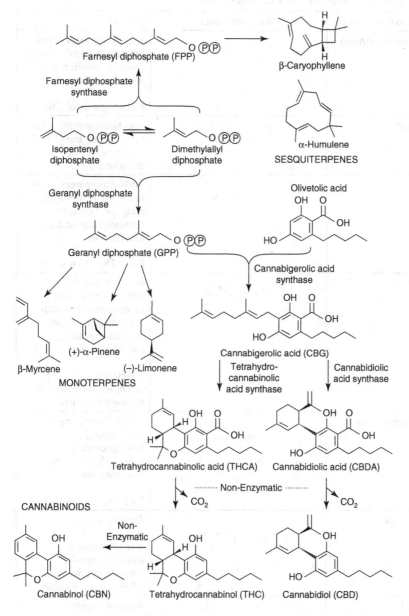

Figure 5.1 Biosynthesis pathway for key phytocannabinoids, terpenes and their terpenoid derivatives

Table 5.2 A list of terpenes with ECS interactivity

Terpenoid or Terpene	Molecular Model	Key notes
(+)-(R)-Limonene		Anti-inflammatory, anti-tumorigenic, anti- oxidant, immunostimulant, anti-microbial, anxiolytic. Partial agonist of CB2.
(±)-α-Pinene	(+)-α-pinene (−)-α-pinene	Anti-inflammatory, anti-tumorigenic, anxiolytic, neuroprotective, bronchodilator.
β-Myrcene		Anti-inflammatory, anti-tumorigenic, sedative, analgesic. Lowers resistance across blood-brain barrier. Binds TRPV1 receptor.
Linalool		Anti-tumorigenic activity, anti-oxidant, cardioprotective, anti-microbial, anxiolytic, anti- inflammatory, anti-nociceptive. Affects voltage gated and ligand mediated ion channels in neurons.
β-caryophyllene		Anti-inflammatory, anti-tumorigenic, neuroprotective hypocholesterolemic, anti- microbial. Partial agonist of CB2.
Nerolidol		Antioxidant, anti-microbial, anti- ulcerogenic, anti-tumorigenic, anti- nociceptive, anti-inflammatory, insecticidal.
Phytol		Anti-nociceptive, anti-inflammatory, anti- oxidant.

receptors, so they are not currently categorized as cannabinoids. PEA and OEA bind to a nuclear receptor and thereby instigate a variety of biological effects, some related to chronic inflammation and pain (O'Sullivan, 2016). N-acylethanolamines have also been found in plant seeds and some mollusks (Chapman et al., 1999; Sepe et al., 1998).

Similar to THC, AEA binds as a partial agonist to CB1 in the central nervous system and, to a lesser extent, CB2 in the peripheral tissue as well as transiently to receptor potential vanilloid 1 receptor (TRPV1) (Zygmunt, 1999). AEA is found in nearly all body tissues and has also been found in some plants, including chocolate (Martin et al., 1999; di Tomaso et al., 1996). The small amount of AEA in consumed chocolate has been shown to break down via the enzyme fatty acid amide hydrolase (FAAH) before it ever reaches the brain to exert any effect. (Di Marzo et al., 1996). The second endocannabinoid, 2-AG, binds as an agonist to both the CB1 and CB2 receptors with similar affinity (Grotenhermen, 2005). A third, ether-type endocannabinoid, 2-arachidonyl glyceryl ether (noladin ether), has been identified, but much remains unknown about this molecule's endogenous role (Hanus et al., 2001). It binds primarily to the CB1 and only weakly to the CB2 receptor.

Two other endocannabinoids have been discovered since the year 2000. N-Arachidonoyl dopamine (NADA) binds the CB1 and TRPV1 receptors. Virodhamine, or O-arachidonoyl-ethanolamine (OAE), was discovered in 2002. It is a full CB2 agonist and a partial CB1 agonist in vitro. Yet again, highlighting the complexity of the ECS, it behaves differently in vivo, as a CB1 antagonist. In 2012, Lysophosphatidylinositol (LPI) was identified as an endogenous ligand to the novel endocannabinoid receptor GPR55 (described later). Pending additional research, LPI may warrant designation as the sixth endocannabinoid (Porter et al., 2002; Piñeiro et al., 2012). The molecular structures of the endocannabinoids along with some key notes are shown in Table 5.3.

The synthesis and degradation of endocannabinoids as well as their various functional interactions in the ECS will be covered in greater detail in a later section. As we have discovered more about the role which endocannabinoids play in our bodies, various synthetic cannabinoids have been developed in an effort to mimic natural endocannabinoids. Synthetic cannabinoids are particularly useful in experiments designed to determine the relationship between the structure and activity of cannabinoid compounds. By making incremental modifications to synthetic designed cannabinoid molecules, the clinical or biological effects of different cannabinoid features can be measured (Lauritsen et al., 2016).

The motive for synthetic cannabinoid research is not limited to advantages in potency, specificity of effect, and patentable intellectual property. For more than 100 years, the legal quagmire surrounding the natural phytocannabinoids has forced innovation to facilitate compliance with various laws which prohibit the use of cannabis.

Table 5.3 The molecular structures of the endocannabinoids along with some key notes

Endocannabinoid	Molecular Model	Key notes
Anandamide, Arachidonoylethanolamine (AEA)		Partial agonist at CB1, very little activity at CB2. Full agonist of TRPV1 receptor. AEA negatively regulates 2- AG metabolism.
2-Arachidonoylglycerol (2-AG)		Full agonist at CB1 and CB2. 1000x > 2-AG than AEA in brain: postulated that this is the primary ECS ligand in the CNS.
2-Arachidonyl glyceryl ether (2-AGE, Noladin ether)		Binds CB1 primarily. Weak affinity for CB2.
N-Arachidonoyl dopamine (NADA)		Binds CB1 and TRPV1 receptors.
Virodhamine (O- arachidonoyl ethanolamine; O-AEA)		Binds CB2 as full agonist. Binds CB1 as partial agonist as well as antagonist in vivo.
Lysophosphatidylinositol (LPI, lysoPI)		Binds GPR55

A side effect of this pursuit has been covered extensively in the media as well as peer-reviewed research regarding the recreational abuse of synthetic cannabinoids (Funada et al., 2020; Roehler et al., 2020). Many synthetic cannabinoids present significant health dangers to users with more severe side effects than the natural cannabinoids, more significant withdrawal symptoms, and the risk of lethal overdose when consumed. To make matters more complicated, some synthetic cannabinoids are also the active pharmaceutical ingredients in some FDA-approved drugs (DEA 2014). Notable synthetic cannabinoids are listed in Table 5.4 below.

Table 5.4 Some notable synthetic cannabinoids

Synthetic cannabinoid	Molecular Model	Key notes
Dronabinol		Brand name Marinol, Syndros Synthetically produced Δ9-THC. FDA approved as an antiemetic and appetite stimulant
Nabilone		Brand name Cesamet,Canemes. Synthetic analogue ofdronabinol.
JWH-018		A synthetic cannabinoid; potent CB1 and CB2 receptor agonist. Used illegally and recreationally and referred to as "Spice".
JWH-073		Another potent agonist of CB1 and CB2. This compound and some of its derivatives have been abused recreationally.
CP 55,940		Developed by Pfizer to mimic THC. Used for researching the ECS. 45 times more potent than Δ9-THC

(Continued)

Table 5.4 (Continued) Some notable synthetic cannabinoids

Synthetic cannabinoid	Molecular Model	Key notes
HU-210		Developed by Dr. Mechoulam's team and used for ECS research. 100-800x more potent than Δ9-THC
HU-331		Synthetic derivative of CBD. Inhibits DNA topoisomerase II and shows promise as an antineoplastic drug.
SR 144528		Acts as a potent and selective CB2 receptor inverse agonist. Used for investigating CB2 function.
AM-2201		Recreational designer drug which is a full non-selective CB1, CB2 agonist. Several related cannabinoids have also been synthesized.

Cannabinoid Receptors

Our understanding of the ECS and its numerous interactions with other body systems is a model. Newtonian physics and quantum mechanics are also models that seek to explain the rules by which natural forces interact with matter. These are not perfect models that answer all questions about our observed world, but are useful for understanding the answer to isolated questions which trigger new and improved questions and, more importantly, can potentially help us in our daily lives. Similarly, our understanding of the ECS is incomplete and the model we review in this chapter will highlight the many unanswered questions that beckon scientists to study further.

The story of the discovery of the ECS itself is merely a refinement of our previous models of complex human physiology. This story began with the discovery of phytocannabinoids and evolved as we sought to better understand the clinical effects of cannabis which have been observed in humans for thousands of years. In the span of a couple decades, the ECS grew to encompass the cellular receptors which those phytocannabinoids bind to and the endocannabinoids which had been there all along, binding those same receptors present in each of us. Continued rapid expansion of our knowledge is further fueled by intense interest and expanding research regarding the possibility of numerous medical therapies targeting the ECS (Treister-Goltzman et al., 1999).

As noted in the previous section, the boundary delineating the ECS from other physiologic systems has grown blurry. Terpenoids, terpenes, flavonoids, and cannabinoid-like molecules are all being studied to better understand their place in this fluid puzzle. Some of these chemicals appear to directly bind cannabinoid receptors while others modulate the effect of known ECS ligands. Additionally, cannabinoids and some of these entourage of peripheral chemical actors interact with the biochemical mechanisms of other body systems—most notably neurotransmission, endocrine function, and the immune response. The first, and perhaps the most important, link between the various signaling ECS ligands and the effects we observe in our physiology are the cannabinoid receptors.

Cannabinoids are lipophilic. This physical property led scientists to initially suspect that cannabinoids acted by disrupting the lipid cell membrane. When Pfizer developed the synthetic cannabinoid in the 1970s, CP 55,940, it proved to be instrumental in the next chapter of ECS research. Radioactive tritium-labeled versions of this drug ($[^3H]$-CP55940) were used to identify where cannabinoids were attaching to cells. Unexpectedly, the destination turned out to be a previously unknown G-protein-coupled cell membrane receptor (GPCR).

G-proteins (guanine nucleotide-binding proteins) belong to a larger group of enzymes called GTP-ases and function as molecular switches inside eukaryotic cells. These bind and hydrolyze guanosine triphosphate (GTP) to guanosine diphosphate (GDP). Simplistically, when bound to GTP, the enzymes are "on," and, they are "off" when bound to GDP. G-proteins affect metabolic enzyme production, ion channel permeability, and other intracellular mechanics. The enzymes help regulate gene transcription, cellular motility, contractility, secretion, and even cellular proliferation which, in turn, affects diverse systemic functions such as embryonic development, memory, and homeostasis (Neves et al., 2002).

GPCRs are large proteins which are embedded in the lipid bilayer of cellular membranes. They extend all the way through the cell's outer surface and interface with the environment on both sides of the membrane. In general, there exists a large family of GPCRs that bind a wide range of ligands outside the cell. The transduction of the signal through the membrane by the GPCR is not completely understood. When bound to a ligand,

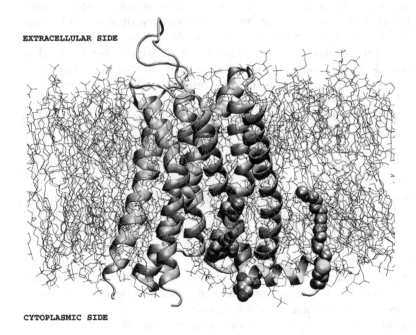

EXTRACELLULAR SIDE

CYTOPLASMIC SIDE

Figure 5.2 Graphical depiction of a generic transmembrane receptor

the conformational structure of the GPCR protein is changed and the internal portion of the GPCR then modulates coupled intracellular G-protein function. Consequently, internal signal transduction pathways and cellular activities are altered. In this way, GPCRs function a bit like remarkably complex snack machine buttons. Once the button is pushed, a variety of events happen on the other side of the door dependent on numerous other factors.

G-proteins are made up of alpha (α), beta (β) and gamma (γ) subunits and there are multiple G-protein subtypes, each with subtle functional differences. Figure 5.2 graphically depicts a generic transmembrane receptor and Figure 5.3 shows a simplified diagram detailing the cycle of GPCR activation and deactivation (Hurowitz et al., 2000).

The overall GPCR population likely exists in a constant flux between activated and deactivated states. Physiologically, when ligands bind to GPCRs, the overall equilibrium shifts. Ligands can be: 1) Agonists (full or partial), which shift the equilibrium towards the active state; 2) Inverse Agonists (full or partial), which shift the equilibrium towards inactive states; and 3) Neutral Antagonists, which bind the GPCR and keep other ligands from binding, but which do not affect the equilibrium of GPCR states.

The complexity of GPCR signaling is apparent when we consider the following: GPCRs can bind different ligands with different affinity and with

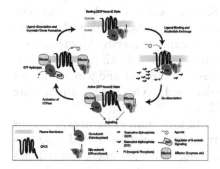

Figure 5.3 Cartoon depicting the Heterotrimeric G-protein activation-deactivation cycle in the context of GPCR signaling

different resulting conformational changes. Ligand binding can result in activation, deactivation, or neutral binding depending on the ligand and the specific coupled G-protein type. All these factors can be modulated by other cellular mechanisms, including the regulation of G-protein subtype concentrations, ligand production and degradation, and the acceleration or blockade of GTP recycling as GPCRs cycle between activation states (Wettschureck et al., 2005; Sprang et al., 2007; Rubenstein et al., 1998; Pertwee 2008; Elphick et al., 2001).

The ECS functions via multiple GPCRs which have been named cannabinoid receptors or CBRs. The cannabinoid receptor, CB1R (CB1), is encoded by the CNR1 gene and consists of 472 amino acids in humans. CB1 predominates in the central nervous system (CNS), but its presence in the brain is not uniform. The cerebral cortex, septum, amygdala, hypothalamus, and parts of the brainstem and the dorsal horn of the spinal cord have moderate concentrations, but some regions like the thalamus and the ventral horn of the spinal cord have very low expression of CB1. Receptor density and location are key variables that ultimately affect the safety profile of cannabinoids—especially as pertaining to non-lethality. Due to the paucity of CB1 receptors in the respiratory center of the brainstem, cannabis exposure is not associated with respiratory depression (Davis, 2014), the underlying etiology for the vast number of opioid-related deaths.

CB1 receptors are primarily located in the cell membrane of the presynaptic neuron at a nerve synapse. In the CNS, lower concentrations of CB1 expression have also been found in astrocytes, oligodendrocytes, and microglial cells. CB1 expression in the peripheral nervous system (PNS) and in some regional tissues is also well documented. In the PNS, CB1 expression occurs at sympathetic nerve terminals, in the trigeminal ganglion, dorsal root ganglion, and nerve endings of primary sensory neurons in the skin. In the gastrointestinal (GI) tract, CB1 is expressed in enteric nerves and in enteroendocrine cells, immune cells, and enterocytes.

CB1 expression is upregulated in the cardiovascular and hepatic system under pathologic conditions, and the expression of CB1 has also been reported in adipose cells, skeletal muscle, bone, dermal and ocular tissue, the reproductive tissues and several types of cancerous cells (Montecucco et al., 2012; Maccarrone et al., 2015). A CB1 variant, CB1Rb (with 33 amino acid deletion at the N-terminus), is expressed in the liver and pancreatic islet cells, and its function is not yet well understood (Ryberg et al., 2005; Shire et al.; 1995, Gonzalez-Mariscal et al., 2016).

CB2R (or CB2) is encoded by the CNR2 gene and, in humans, contains 360 amino acids. Two human CB2 subtypes have been discovered. CB2 was originally found to be present in splenic tissue, but subsequent research has demonstrated its moderate expression in many peripheral tissues (cardiovascular system, GI tract, liver, adipose tissue, bone, reproductive tissue, and the immune system). CB2 is expressed at very low levels in the cell membranes of CNS and PNS neurons, but its *intracellular* expression in certain areas of the brain may play an important role in neurologic activity.

The initial discovery of CB1 and CB2 helped focus the search for CBR expression within cell surface membranes. This is the most well understood manner in which CBRs participate in the ECS, but *intracellular* CBR expression is now understood to play an important role too. There are several distinct populations of intracellular CBRs. Intracellular subpopulations of CB1 are the best characterized to date. Some intracellular CB1 is present due to the continuous internalization of portions of the cellular plasma membrane with embedded CB1. A distinct pool of intracellular CB1 is present on intracellular endosome and lysosome organelles and does not appear to recycle with the cell membrane CB1 population. Finally, a subpopulation of CB1 receptors is expressed in some mitochondria (Zou et al., 2018).

Cannabinoids also can act as ligands for other protein receptors in addition to the novel CBRs. This blurs the line as to where the ECS ends and other body systems begin. Various cannabinoids directly bind the TRPV1 receptor as agonists. The TRPV1 receptor is a non-selective ion channel protein receptor which responds to certain physical and chemical stimuli. TRPV1 activation initiates a pain signal in response to heat, chemical exposure (such as capsaicin), acidic conditions, etc. Cannabinoid modulation of the TRPV1 receptor is one of various mechanisms by which the ECS regulates pain perception (Everaerts et al., 2011; Andradas, 2013).

Other GPCRs have been identified which bind cannabinoids, but consensus has not been reached on whether to classify these receptors as "endocannabinoid receptors" due partially to the complexity of interaction and, to some degree, because not enough data exists. GPR-55 was cloned in 1999 and is the most notable candidate. Phytocannabinoids and endocannabinoids bind this receptor, which appears to play a role in the body's response to cancer.

Finally, indirect evidence has shown that certain cannabinoids bind brain tissue at an unknown receptor in the absence of CB1. This evidence suggests an additional CBR is present in brain tissue which has not yet been identified, but which some researchers have dubbed "CB3."

ECS Interactions and Other Neurochemical Mediators

The interactions between cannabinoids, cannabinoid receptors, and other chemical mediators within the ECS are, as noted earlier, complex and an intense topic of investigation. The primary signaling pathway is unique in that the signal is propagated in reverse between neurons at the nerve synapse. Normally, CNS nerve signal transmission progresses from the presynaptic to postsynaptic neuron; calcium ion influx through voltage-gated calcium channels in the presynaptic nerve terminus initiates the release of stored neurotransmitters that diffuse across the nerve synapse to the postsynaptic nerve.

ECS signaling begins with endocannabinoid production at the *post*synaptic nerve, followed by endocannabinoid diffusion across the synapse, and finally activation of CBRs on the *pre*synaptic neuron. This retrograde, synaptic transmission has been described as the primary way in which pain signals are modulated by the ECS (Dunlap et al., 1995; Olivera et al., 1994).

In this model, AEA and 2-AG are produced and released by postsynaptic nerves at the nerve terminal with repeated nerve stimulation. The enzyme diacylglycerol lipase-α (DAGLα) synthesizes 2-AG from the precursor, diacylglycerol (DAG). Similarly, AEA is enzymatically synthesized from its precursor, N-acyl-phosphatidylethanolamine (NAPE), by NAPE-specific phospholipase D (NAPE-PLD). These resulting lipophilic endocannabinoids then travel in a retrograde fashion across the nerve synapse where they can bind to CB1 receptors located on the presynaptic nerve terminal. Fatty acid binding protein 5 (FABP5) is essential for retrograde endocannabinoid signaling and may serve as a synaptic carrier for the hydrophobic endocannabinoids diffusing across synapses (Haj-Dahmane et al., 2018).

A postsynaptic nerve can effectively downregulate the signal it is receiving from the presynaptic nerve through this retrograde transmission. This homeostatic feedback model has been postulated as a mechanism by which the postsynaptic nerve is able to "shut off the spigot" when too much stimulatory signal is received over time. This is easiest to understand in the context of excitatory nerve overstimulation over longer periods of time, but endocannabinoids have been shown to suppress synaptic transmission through multiple other mechanisms, independent of the type of synapse or the duration of the neurostimulation (Kano et al., 2009; Castillo et al., 2012).

ECS nerve signal inhibition proceeds in the following way: Presynaptic CB1 receptors are bound *primarily* by 2-AG. G-proteins coupled to CB1 are then activated. The intracellular response includes: (a) modulation of adenylate cyclase activity to inhibit cAMP accumulation, (b) voltage-gated calcium channel closure, (c) potassium channel activation and, ultimately,

(d) the reduction of neurotransmitter release into presynaptic excitatory and inhibitory synapses (Kendall & Yudowski, 2017).

Once endocannabinoids are released into the synaptic cleft, they continue to bind available CBRs until degraded. Cannabinoid metabolism can also be altered by endogenous or synthetic compounds that target the intracellular enzymes which are responsible for the degradation process. Residual 2-AG in the synaptic cleft is absorbed into presynaptic neurons, via an unclear mechanism, and then metabolized to arachidonic acid (AA) and glycerol by the enzyme monoacylglycerol lipase (MAGL). AEA is primarily metabolized in the postsynaptic nerve by fatty acid amide hydrolase (FAAH). FAAH converts AEA to AA and ethanolamine (EtNH2). Figure 5.4 illustrates this process (Deutsch, 2016; Zou et al., 2018).

Other endocannabinoid signaling pathways have recently been identified. The specific enzymes, chemical mediators and downstream intracellular results for alternate mechanisms depend on the specific brain (or tissue) region and physiological conditions which are present. 2-AG is able to activate CB1 receptors located in astrocytes and facilitate the release of glutamate, in contrast to the inhibitory feedback cycle described above. AEA activates *intracellular* CB1 as well as TRPV1 resulting in the activation or inhibition of various cellular processes (Kendall & Yudowski, 2017; Zou et al., 2018).

Endocannabinoid-modulated synaptic transmission via CB1 activation is a primary model of ECS activity in the CNS, but the role CB2 plays is less clear. Additionally, the signal transduction pathways induced by CB2 receptor activation have not been as well defined. AEA and 2-AG can bind both CB1 and CB2 and modulate intracellular signal transduction pathways, such as the inhibition of cAMP-production, activation of protein kinase R (PKR)-like endoplasmic reticulum kinase (PERK), G-protein-coupled ion channel regulation (noted previously), nitric oxide production, etc.

CBR activation can also mediate intracellular activity via β-arrestin, or phosphatidylinositol-3-kinases (PI3K) rather than coupled G-proteins. These pathways have been linked to cellular survival versus death and have been implicated in the regulation of embryonic development. Numerous other intracellular effects have also been linked to these intracellular signaling cascades (Felder et al., 1995; Howlett et al., 2002; Demuth & Molleman, 2006l Hurowitz et al., 2000).

While CB1 is one of the most numerous GPCRs found in the CNS, CB2 exhibits a limited pattern of CNS expression. CB2 expression in immune system tissue is much more common. (Klein, 2005; Mackie, 2006; Dhopeshwarkar & Mackie, 2014; Atwood & Mackie, 2010). CNS CB2 receptors are often encountered in association with inflammatory processes and primarily expressed in microglia (CNS macrophages) (Mackie, 2008; Palazuelos et al., 2009).

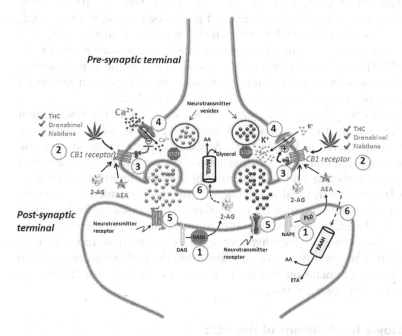

Figure 5.4 ECS retrograde signaling diagram. 1) neurotransmitter stimulation stimulates endocannabinoid synthesis in post synaptic cell, 2) endocannabinoids, phytocannabinoids and synthetic cannabinoids bind CBR on presynaptic cell, 3) GPCR activation results in multiple intracellular biochemical cascades including ion channel modulation, 4) altered ion concentrations shut down release of neurotransmitter, 5) neurotransmission to post synaptic cell is affected by neurotransmitter concentration in synaptic cleft, 6) 2-AG is degraded after absorption into presynaptic cell where MAGL converts it to AA and glycerol. AEA is primarily metabolized in the postsynaptic nerve by fatty acid amide hydrolase (FAAH). FAAH converts AEA to AA and ethanolamine (ETA) as illustrated in this figure. Source: © All Rights Reserved. Information for Health Care Professionals: Cannabis (marihuana, marijuana) and the cannabinoids). Health Canada. Adapted and reproduced with permission from the Minister of Health, 2020.

There are some notable differences that have been observed between CB1 and CB2 activation, however. CB2-associated G-proteins do not appear to couple to potassium channels. Additionally, the activation of CB2 receptors in the immune system can result in very different intracellular pathway activation than what is encountered in the CNS. The modulation of inflammation, both inhibitory and stimulatory has been observed when endocannabinoids activate CB2. This dichotomy may be due to different intracellular endocannabinoid metabolites formed in the process (Turcotte et al., 2016; Felder et al., 1995).

Modulation of CNS, PNS and immune system function are the most intensely researched and best understood physiologic domains of the ECS, but a final word on the overlap between the endocrine system and the ECS is warranted. Recent research has demonstrated that the activation of CB1, CB2, TRPV1 and possibly other ECS receptors within the hypothalamus, adrenal and pituitary glands, and other endocrine tissues is an important contributor to hormone regulation (DeLaurentiis et al., 2014).

An overarching theme predominates when we consider the vast amount of information on the role that ECS function plays in other physiologic systems. That theme is *homeostasis*. Much like the nervous system and immune system examples, the neuroendocrine system also demonstrates that the ECS often plays a homeostatic role. Endocannabinoids and can mitigate maladaptive hormonal axes function just as they modulate exaggerated nerve stimulation pathways and inflammatory cascades in the setting of disease. The ECS of the brain plays an important role in homeostasis by regulating hypothalamo-neurohypophyseal axis activity (DeLaurentiis et al., 12122010). Though it is an oversimplification, these observations have led to the oft-stated conclusion that the ECS is, to a large degree, a "buffer" or homeostasis physiological system.

Physiologic Implications of the ECS

At the onset of this chapter, the framework of physiologic body systems predicated on the biomedical model of disease was highlighted. As we attempt to link the various biochemical mechanisms of the ECS with observable physiologic outcomes, the biomedical model of disease has its shortcomings. It is important to remember that the reductionism inherent in explaining all things in the simplest subdivided fashion is *useful* for designing research and for seeking molecular targets for pharmaceutical development, but it can bias us, as observers, to overlook the complexity of the truth. A full understanding of the potential physiologic outcomes affected by the ECS requires understanding the many overlapping systems which the ECS modulates, as well as the less-well-defined impact of an individual person's genetics, diet, mood, past conscious experience, overall health, and more. Some of these variables may be objectively measurable, and some are clearly more subjective—but, perhaps, no less important—as they affect ECS function. While much more research into the holistic factors which affect ECS function is needed, an overview of the known physiologic implications of ECS modulation follows.

Therapeutic modulation of the ECS to treat disease can occur in a variety of dimensions, either by agonism or antagonism of cannabinoid receptors themselves, or by targeted interaction with the various endocannabinoid synthetic and degradative enzymes such as NAPE-PLD, FAAH, DAGLα and β, and MAGL (Kolb et al., 2019). Alteration of the endocannabinoid signaling system has been implicated in a vast array of human diseases (Di Marzo et al., 2004).

ECS modulation may play an important role in treating disease states where memory dysfunction is present. Memory processing and, specifically, the extinction of old memories can be facilitated through ECS action. The hippocampus is part of the brain's limbic system and plays important roles in the conversion of information from short-term memory to long-term memory. Hippocampal neuroprogenitor (NP) cell proliferation and differentiation are increased via CB1 activation (Jiang et al., 2005; Aguado et al., 2005; Christie & Cameron, 2006). The ECS's modulatory effect on memory process is being investigated as a potential avenue for treating diseases such as Post Traumatic Stress Disorder (PTSD) and Alzheimer's Dementia (AD) (Kendall & Yudowski, 2017).

Cannabinoid receptors are involved in the physiologic response to Traumatic Brain Injury (TBI) and 2-AG increases after TBI in animal models (Panikashvili et al., 2001; Mechoulam & Shohami, 2007). These findings have led to additional research on the neuroprotective implications of ECS-based therapies. While the safety and efficacy of such therapies will require more investigation, there is evidence to show that endocannabinoid activity may prevent nerve damage resulting from over excitation, can inhibit inflammatory cytokine production, and can augment stem cell migration and differentiation during nerve healing processes (Gruenbaum et al., 2016).

Disease states which affect neuromuscular interaction and muscle spasticity can also be affected by ECS neuromodulation. Multiple sclerosis (MS), Parkinson's Disease (PD), Huntington's Chorea, and Amyotrophic Lateral Sclerosis (ALS), to name a few, have all been associated with clinical improvements in some patients with ECS stimulation (primarily CB1 and CB2 activation) (Kendall & Yudowski, 2017; Di Iorio et al., 2013).

Academic focus on the potential for cannabinoid-based treatments for chronic pain states is well documented. ECS impact on the blockade or downregulation of various pain signals is an exciting physiologic target for patients with chronic pain. Multiple biochemical mechanisms are at play in pain modulation, including those described earlier. CBR and TRPV1 activation pathways have been shown to impact pain perception and pain signal transmission in both chronic neuropathic, cancer-associated, and inflammatory disease states (Saito et al., 2012; Fu & Taylor, 2015; Manzanares et al., 2006; Barrie & Manolios, 2017; Guindon & Hohmann 2011).

Promising physiologic results have also been demonstrated when targeting ECS pathways for mood disorders. Anxiety and depression states and their associated emotional responses can be buffered by the ECS (Huang et al., 2016; Ruehle et al., 2012). Current research continues to investigate effective treatment strategies which take advantage of this ECS physiologic effect.

In addition to the observed effects of the ECS on mood disorders, the ECS's impact on several other mental disease states has also been researched.

Schizophrenia, Autism, Turret's Syndrome, disorders of addiction, and other mental health disorders are among these. Evidence is still being gathered, and no consensus on the specific ECS mechanism or an ultimate risk/benefit analysis has been reached, but the ECS clearly has an impact when the mind suffers from these conditions. It is also important to note that ECS modulation has the potential to alter these conditions for better or worse depending on many variables which are still the topic of debate (Ibarra-Lecue et al., 2018; Sloane et al., 2019).

Popular culture references to the "anti-cancer" properties of phytocannabinoids are commonplace. Bridging the gap between the anecdotal reports from cannabis-using cancer patients and the empiric evidence required to definitively say an ECS modulating treatment "cures cancer" is an ongoing process, but evidence is accumulating. Cannabinoids and cannabis-like compounds demonstrate anti-proliferative properties and, for certain neoplasms such as brain (glioblastoma), breast, prostate and bone cancer, a therapeutic potential appears closer to reality (Guindon & Hohmann 2011; Hermanson & Marnett, 2011; Dumitru et al., 2018).

CBD has received significant attention for its anti-epileptic properties, and one of the few phytocannabinoid-based medications approved by the FDA counts CBD as its primary active pharmaceutical ingredient (API). The ECS effect on seizure manifestation is still not perfectly understood, but effective reductions in seizure frequency are achievable through ECS-mediated pathways (Cheung et al., 2019).

Cannabinoid administration has been shown to stimulate appetite and reduce nausea and has, therefore, been clinically indicated for the treatment of certain disease-related appetite disorders, cachexia, and nausea. This physiologic effect is largely attributable to CB1 activation. Endocannabinoids, phytocannabinoids, and synthetic cannabinoids have been studied as appetite stimulants and the first FDA-approved synthetic cannabinoids targeted appetite stimulation and antiemetic effect (Di Marzo & Matias, 2005; Koch, 2017; Smith et al., 2015).

Endocannabinoid signaling within the CNS can promote sleep effects through various neurologic and neuroendocrine pathways. Recent evidence demonstrates endocannabinoid-mediated CB1 activation is necessary for the stability of non-rapid eye movement (NREM) sleep cycles (Murillo-Rodríguez, 2008; Prospéro-García et al., 2016l Pava et al., 2016).

CB2-mediated anti-inflammatory effects within the ECS point to the immense therapeutic potential for ECS manipulation of various disease states where inflammation is a contributing factor. Many animal studies have successfully demonstrated a wide array of anti-inflammatory physiologic effects impacted by the ECS, but additional research is needed to know exactly when and how this can be most effectively used in human treatment protocols. Specific clinical examples of inflammatory diseases where ECS modulating treatments have shown promise for human application include

Inflammatory Bowel Disease (IBD), arthritis, atherosclerotic disease, and many neurologic disorders where neuroinflammation is present (Turcotte et al., 2016).

ECS effects on our gastrointestinal (GI) system and its interface with our neuroendocrine system are only recently being described. GI propulsion, secretion, and inflammation are modulated by ECS activity. The physiologic implications are numerous and include potential utility with irritable bowel syndrome (IBS) and other gut-motility disorders (Pertwee, 2001).

A clinical entity of CED—clinical endocannabinoid deficiency syndrome—has been postulated. The model of CED is best understood in the context of disease entities such as fibromyalgia, migraine headaches, and irritable bowel syndrome (IBS) but may also be applicable in many other manifestations of disease. CED syndrome postulates that since all humans have a basal presence of endocannabinoids and a baseline tone of ECS function, a deficiency in either can partially explain the presence of certain manifestations of disease. If CED proves to be a clinical syndrome or entity, the implication is that replacement of any deficiency may have clinical relevance (Russo, 2004, 2016).

This section has been focused on presenting an overview of some of the known physiologic impacts that are linked to ECS function. It is not the goal here to extrapolate on the many trials which have investigated the negative effects observed with cannabis and phytocannabinoid ingestion. A final note is needed, however, regarding the physiologic impact of exogenous cannabinoids on morbidity and mortality. Although treatment with cannabinoids has been associated with various side effects, most often after oral administration, the majority of these effects are mild and short-lasting (Vu˘ckovic´ et al., 2018). In animals, the LD50 of oral THC is 800–1900 mg/kgc in rats, and from 3000–9000 mg/kgc in dogs and monkeys. No acute fatal cases resulting from phytocannabinoid (THC or other) ingestion have been reported in humans, although some evidence suggests that THC may trigger myocardial infarction when predisposition exists (Tamba et al., 2020).

Future Research

As alluded to earlier, the field of cannabinoid medicine is growing rapidly, but many challenges remain on the road to better understanding and the development of safe, effective therapeutics. First and foremost is the debate surrounding "entourage" versus a single molecular therapeutic agent.

There exist vast interconnections, feedback and inhibition systems, and cross reactivity with other neurochemical systems within the biochemical pathways of the ECS. Considering this, the strategy of selective drug targeting with a single cannabinoid ligand in order to attain a specific, predictable, and beneficial clinical effect that is similar in all individuals is difficult to attain. Some available evidence suggests that an entourage of chemical mediators which each affect the ECS in different ways, but which mimic nature when administered together, have an improved clinical effect. This is the argument for developing therapeutic "whole plant" formulations of phytocannabinoids mixed with other non-cannabinoids found naturally in the cannabis plant. While the clinical outcomes associated with this approach are worthy of investigation, the specific biochemical pathways activated by an entourage of potential APIs in a botanical medication are not as easily defined.

The immediate challenge with investigations into the effect of exogenous modulators of the ECS is numerous. We must not only expand our current knowledge about ECS function, including exogenous agonists, antagonists, and inverse agonists, but must also characterize the many potential non-CB1 and non-CB2 sites of action for the exogenous chemicals in question. Large amounts of new information related to ECS function have been accumulated to date, but more questions than answers remain. Future investigations must piggyback on the results of previous work and expand our understanding of the roles endocannabinoids play in human physiology and pathology.

Additional studies must be developed to better determine which points of ECS activation or inhibition are most beneficial to overall health and at what point in life or during a disease process is the optimum timing of any potential therapeutic intervention. The question of which cannabinoid or other molecule (or entourage of molecules!) will best alter ECS function in an individual person or specific disease state remains an important unanswered question that is crucial for effective medical therapy.

Perhaps most importantly, research questions pertaining to ECS modulatory therapy will need to take the overall "risk versus benefit" into greater consideration as we seek to develop the most efficacious agents with the lowest adverse event rates. Since many of the positive and negative clinical effects reported to date are related to complex multiple-system interactions and amenable largely to personal, subjective analysis, new validated methods of comparing objective and subjective outcome data will be helpful.

Historical, political, and social constraints ultimately must be taken into consideration. Heightened concerns surrounding the intoxicating effects of the cannabis plant and CB1 agonism in general often raise significant concerns for patients and healthcare providers who do not consider such effects acceptable. Additional strategies to minimize this potential side effect despite ECS activation should be developed. Beneficial paths to ECS modulating pharmaceutical development will certainly include additional research into drug therapies with actions limited to peripheral tissues or which do not primarily act as CB1 agonists in the CNS.

Conclusion

The expansive mystery of the human body and all its interrelated systems is exposed by an examination of the ECS, which interfaces with the body's many facets as a regulator of homeostasis. The fact that, until now, the ECS has not been routinely acknowledged in modern medical curricula speaks to the continued need for improvements in the understanding of and education about the ECS.

Tremendous work accomplished by many scientists has paved a path to greater understanding, even in the face of societal opposition, and opened our eyes to new fields of medical research and new potential clinical applications. As is often the case when following the scientific method, answers have triggered more detailed questions related to the ECS and the exogenous plants and molecules that interact with it. We need to work diligently to fill in these important gaps in our understanding of this endogenous supermodulatory homeostatic system. The ECS is now, due to the accumulation of evidence, assuming its rightful place within the Western medical paradigm. Despite its daunting complexity, excitement brews regarding the tremendous future therapeutic potential of the ECS and the many agents that interact with it.

References

Aguado, T., Monory, K., Palazuelos, J., Stella, N., Cravatt, B., Lutz, B., ... Galve-Roperh, I. (2005). The endocannabinoid system drives neural progenitor proliferation. *FASEB Journal*, *19*(12), 1704–1706. https://doi.org/10.1096/fj.05-3995fje

Aizpurua-Olaizola, O., Soydaner, U., Öztürk, E., Schibano, D., Simsir, Y., Navarro, P., ... Usobiaga, A. (2016). Evolution of the cannabinoid and terpene content during the growth of *Cannabis sativa* Plants from different chemotypes. *Journal of Natural Products*, *79*(2), 324–331. https://doi.org/10.1021/acs.jnatprod.5b00949

Andradas, C., Caffarel, M. M., Pérez-Gómez, E., Guzmán, M., & Sánchez, C. (2013). The role of GPR55 in cancer. In M. E. Abood, R. G. Sorensen, & N. Stella (Eds.), *Endocannabinoids* (pp. 115–133). New York: Springer. https://doi.org/10.1007/978-1-4614-4669-9_5

The Antique Cannabis Book (rev. 2018). Appendix C, 2nd Ed. *Antiquecannabisbook.com*. Retrieved from 03/30/2020 from: http://antiquecannabisbook.com/Appendix/AppendixC.htm/

Atwood, B. K., & Mackie, K. (2010). CB2: A cannabinoid receptor with an identity crisis: CB2 expression in neurons. *British Journal of Pharmacology*, *160*(3), 467–479. https://doi.org/10.1111/j.1476-5381.2010.00729.x

Barrie, N., & Manolios, N. (2017). The endocannabinoid system in pain and inflammation: Its relevance to rheumatic disease. *European Journal of Rheumatology*, *4*(3), 210–218. https://doi.org/10.5152/eurjrheum.2017.17025

Bauer, R., Woelkart, K., & Salo-Ahen, O. (2008). CB receptor ligands from plants. *Current Topics in Medicinal Chemistry*, *8*(3), 173–186. https://doi.org/10.2174/156802608783498023

Brailoiu, G. C., Deliu, E., Marcu, J., Hoffman, N. E., Console-Bram, L., Zhao, P., ... Brailoiu, E. (2014). Differential activation of intracellular versus plasmalemmal CB$_2$ cannabinoid receptors. *Biochemistry*, *53*(30), 4990–4999. https://doi.org/10.1021/bi500632a

Castillo, P. E., Younts, T. J., Chávez, A. E., & Hashimotodani, Y. (2012). Endocannabinoid signaling and synaptic function. *Neuron*, *76*(1), 70–81. https://doi.org/10.1016/j.neuron.2012.09.020

Chapman, K. D., Venables, B., Markovic, R., Blair, R. W., & Bettinger, C. (1999). N -Acylethanolamines in seeds. Quantification of molecular species and their degradation upon imbibition. *Plant Physiology, 120*(4), 1157–1164. https://doi.org/10.1104/pp.120.4.1157

Cheung, K. A., Peiris, H., Wallace, G., Holland, O. J., & Mitchell, M. D. (2019). The interplay between the endocannabinoid system, epilepsy and cannabinoids. *International Journal of Molecular Sciences, 20*(23), 6079. doi: 10.3390/ijms20236079

Christie, B. R., & Cameron, H. A. (2006). Neurogenesis in the adult hippocampus. *Hippocampus, 16*(3), 199–207. https://doi.org/10.1002/hipo.20151

Davis, M. P. (2014). Cannabinoids in pain management: CB1, CB2 and non-classic receptor ligands. *Expert Opinion on Investigational Drugs, 23*(8), 1123–1140. https://doi.org/10.1517/13543784.2014.918603

De Laurentiis, A., Fernández Solari, J., Mohn, C., Zorrilla Zubilete, M., & Rettori, V. (2010). Endocannabinoid system participates in neuroendocrine control of homeostasis. *Neuroimmunomodulation, 17*(3), 153–156. https://doi.org/10.1159/000258711

Demuth, D. G., & Molleman, A. (2006). Cannabinoid signalling. *Life Sciences, 78*(6), 549–563. https://doi.org/10.1016/j.lfs.2005.05.055

Deutsch, D. G. (2016). A personal retrospective: Elevating anandamide (AEA) by targeting fatty acid amide hydrolase (FAAH) and the fatty acid binding proteins (FABPs). *Frontiers in Pharmacology, 7.* https://doi.org/10.3389/fphar.2016.00370

Dhopeshwarkar, A., & Mackie, K. (2014). CB $_2$ cannabinoid receptors as a therapeutic target—What does the future hold? *Molecular Pharmacology, 86*(4), 430–437. https://doi.org/10.1124/mol.114.094649

Di Iorio, G., Lupi, M., Sarchione, F., Matarazzo, I., Santacroce, R., Petruccelli, F., … Di Giannantonio, M. (2013). The endocannabinoid system: A putative role in neurodegenerative diseases. *International Journal of High Risk Behaviors and Addiction. 100*, 2(3)–106. https://doi.org/10.5812/ijhrba.9222

Di Marzo, V. (1998). "Endocannabinoids" and other fatty acid derivatives with cannabimimetic properties: Biochemistry and possible physiopathological relevance. *Biochimica et Biophysica Acta (BBA) - Lipids and Lipid Metabolism, 1392*(2–3), 153–175. https://doi.org/10.1016/S0005-2760(98)00042-3

Di Marzo, V., & De Petrocellis, L. (2012). Why do cannabinoid receptors have more than one endogenous ligand? *Philosophical Transactions of the Royal Society of London Series B, 367*(1607), 3216–3228. https://doi.org/10.1098/rstb.2011.0382

Di Marzo, V., & Matias, I. (2005). Endocannabinoid control of food intake and energy balance. *Nature Neuroscience, 8*(5), 585–589. https://doi.org/10.1038/nn1457

Di Marzo, V., & Piscitelli, F. (2015). The endocannabinoid system and its modulation by phytocannabinoids. *Neurotherapeutics, 12*(4), 692–698. https://doi.org/10.1007/s13311-015-0374-6

Di Marzo, V., Sepe, N., De Petrocellis, L., Berger, A., Crozier, G., Fride, E., & Mechoulam, R. (1998). Trick or treat from food endocannabinoids? *Nature, 396*(6712), 636–636. https://doi.org/10.1038/25267

di Tomaso, E., Beltramo, M., & Piomelli, D. (1996). Brain cannabinoids in chocolate. *Nature, 382*(6593), 677–678. https://doi.org/10.1038/382677a0

Dumitru, C. A., Sandalcioglu, I. E., & Karsak, M. (2018). Cannabinoids in glioblastoma therapy: New applications for old drugs. *Frontiers in Molecular Neuroscience, 11*, 159. https://doi.org/10.3389/fnmol.2018.00159

Dunlap, K., Luebke, J. I., & Turner, T. J. (1995). Exocytotic Ca2+ channels in mammalian central neurons. *Trends in Neurosciences, 18*(2), 89–98.

Elphick, M. R., & Egertová, M. (2001). The neurobiology and evolution of cannabinoid signalling. *Philosophical Transactions of the Royal Society of London Series B, 356*(1407), 381–408. https://doi.org/10.1098/rstb.2000.0787

Everaerts, W., Gees, M., Alpizar, Y. A., Farre, R., Leten, C., Apetrei, A., ... Talavera, K. (2011). The capsaicin receptor TRPV1 is a crucial mediator of the noxious effects of mustard oil. *Current Biology, 21*(4), 316–321. https://doi.org/10.1016/j.cub.2011.01.031

Felder, C. C., Joyce, K. E., Briley, E. M., Mansouri, J., Mackie, K., Blond, O., ... Mitchell, R. L. (1995). Comparison of the pharmacology and signal transduction of the human cannabinoid CB1 and CB2 receptors. *Molecular Pharmacology, 48*(3), 443–450.

Fellermeier, M., Eisenreich, W., Bacher, A., & Zenk, M. H. (2001). Biosynthesis of cannabinoids: Incorporation experiments with 13 C-labeled glucoses. *European Journal of Biochemistry, 268*(6), 1596–1604. https://doi.org/10.1046/j.1432-1327.2001.02030.x

Fu, W., & Taylor, B. K. (2015). Activation of cannabinoid CB2 receptors reduces hyperalgesia in an experimental autoimmune encephalomyelitis mouse model of multiple sclerosis. *Neuroscience Letters, 595*, 1–6. https://doi.org/10.1016/j.neulet.2015.04.002

Funada, M., & Tomiyama, K. (2020). Dependence and cytotoxicity of components of cannabis. *YAKUGAKU ZASSHI, 140*(2), 205–214. https://doi.org/10.1248/yakushi.19-00195-4

Giblett, R. J. (2008). Machine body of modern western medicine. *The body of nature and culture* (pp. 19–36). Palgrave Macmillan. Retrieved from http://link.springer.com/book/10.1057/9780230595170

González-Mariscal, I., Krzysik-Walker, S. M., Doyle, M. E., Liu, Q.-R., Cimbro, R., Santa-Cruz Calvo, S., ... Egan, J. M. (2016). Human CB1 receptor isoforms, present in hepatocytes and β-cells, are involved in regulating metabolism. *Scientific Reports, 6*(1), 33302. https://doi.org/10.1038/srep33302

Grotenhermen, F. (2005). Cannabinoids. *Current Drug Target -CNS and Neurological Disorders, 4*(5), 507–530. https://doi.org/10.2174/156800705774322111

Gruenbaum, S. E., Zlotnik, A., Gruenbaum, B. F., Hersey, D., & Bilotta, F. (2016). Pharmacologic neuroprotection for functional outcomes after traumatic brain injury: A systematic review of the clinical literature. *CNS Drugs, 30*(9), 791–806. https://doi.org/10.1007/s40263-016-0355-2

Guindon, J., & Hohmann, A. G. (2011). The endocannabinoid system and cancer: Therapeutic implication: Cannabinoids and cancer. *British Journal of Pharmacology, 163*(7), 1447–1463. https://doi.org/10.1111/j.1476-5381.2011.01327.x

Haj-Dahmane, S., Shen, R.-Y., Elmes, M. W., Studholme, K., Kanjiya, M. P., Bogdan, D., ... Kaczocha, M. (2018). Fatty-acid–binding protein 5 controls retrograde endocannabinoid signaling at central glutamate synapses. *Proceedings of the National Academy of Sciences, 115*(13), 3482–3487. https://doi.org/10.1073/pnas.1721339115

Hanus, L., Abu-Lafi, S., Fride, E., Breuer, A., Vogel, Z., Shalev, D. E., ... Mechoulam, R. (2001). 2-arachidonyl glyceryl ether, an endogenous agonist of the cannabinoid CB1 receptor. *Proceedings of the National Academy of Sciences of the United States of America*, 98(7), 3662–3665. https://doi.org/10.1073/pnas.061029898

Hanus, L., & Mechoulam, R. (2005). Cannabinoid chemistry: An overview. In R. Mechoulam (Ed.), *Cannabinoids as therapeutics* (pp. 23–46). Birkhäuser Basel. Retrieved from https://www.researchgate.net/figure/A-tentative-biogenesis-of-the -plant-cannabinoids_fig1_263899667

Herkenham, M., Lynn, A. B., Johnson, M. R., Melvin, L. S., de Costa, B. R., & Rice, K. C. (1991). Characterization and localization of cannabinoid receptors in rat brain: A quantitative in vitro autoradiographic study. *Journal of Neuroscience: The Official Journal of the Society for Neuroscience*, 11(2), 563–583.

Hermanson, D. J., & Marnett, L. J. (2011). Cannabinoids, endocannabinoids, and cancer. *Cancer and Metastasis Reviews*, 30(3–4), 599–612. https://doi.org/10.1007/s10555-011-9318-8

Howlett, A. C., Barth, F., Bonner, T. I., Cabral, G., Casellas, P., Devane, W. A., ... Pertwee, R. G. (2002). International union of pharmacology. XXVII. Classification of cannabinoid receptors. *Pharmacological Reviews*, 54(2), 161–202. https://doi.org/10.1124/pr.54.2.161

Huang, W.-J., Chen, W.-W., & Zhang, X. (2016). Endocannabinoid system: Role in depression, reward and pain control (Review). *Molecular Medicine Reports*, 14(4), 2899–2903. https://doi.org/10.3892/mmr.2016.5585

Hurowitz, E. H., Melnyk, J. M., Chen, Y. J., Kouros-Mehr, H., Simon, M. I., & Shizuya, H. (2000). Genomic characterization of the human heterotrimeric G protein alpha, beta, and gamma subunit genes. *DNA Research: An International Journal for Rapid Publication of Reports on Genes and Genomes*, 7(2), 111–120. https://doi.org/10.1093/dnares/7.2.111

Ibarra-Lecue, I., Pilar-Cuéllar, F., Muguruza, C., Florensa-Zanuy, E., Díaz, Á., Urigüen, L., ... Callado, L. F. (2018). The endocannabinoid system in mental disorders: Evidence from human brain studies. *Biochemical Pharmacology*, 157, 97–107. https://doi.org/10.1016/j.bcp.2018.07.009

Irwin, M. R. (2008). Human psychoneuroimmunology: 20 years of discovery. *Brain, Behavior, and Immunity*, 22(2), 129–139. https://doi.org/10.1016/j.bbi.2007.07.013

Jiang, W., Zhang, Y., Xiao, L., Van Cleemput, J., Ji, S.-P., Bai, G., & Zhang, X. (2005). Cannabinoids promote embryonic and adult hippocampus neurogenesis and produce anxiolytic- and antidepressant-like effects. *The Journal of Clinical Investigation*, 115(11), 3104–3116. https://doi.org/10.1172/JCI25509

Kano, M., Ohno-Shosaku, T., Hashimotodani, Y., Uchigashima, M., & Watanabe, M. (2009). Endocannabinoid-mediated control of synaptic transmission. *Physiological Reviews*, 89(1), 309–380. https://doi.org/10.1152/physrev.00019.2008

Kendall, D. A., & Yudowski, G. A. (2017). Cannabinoid receptors in the central nervous system: Their signaling and roles in disease. *Frontiers in Cellular Neuroscience*, 10. https://doi.org/10.3389/fncel.2016.00294

Klein, T. W. (2005). Cannabinoid-based drugs as anti-inflammatory therapeutics. *Nature Reviews. Immunology*, 5(5), 400–411. https://doi.org/10.1038/nri1602

Koch, M. (2017). Cannabinoid receptor signaling in central regulation of feeding behavior: A mini-review. *Frontiers in Neuroscience*, 11, 293. https://doi.org/10.3389/fnins.2017.00293

Kolb, B., Saber, H., Fadel, H., & Rajah, G. (2019). The endocannabinoid system and stroke: A focused review. *Brain Circulation*, 5(1), 1. https://doi.org/10.4103/bc.bc_29_18

Kwan Cheung, K. A., Peiris, H., Wallace, G., Holland, O. J., & Mitchell, M. D. (2019). The interplay between the endocannabinoid system, epilepsy and cannabinoids. *International Journal of Molecular Sciences*, 20(23), 6079. https://doi.org/10.3390/ijms20236079

Laurentiis, A., Araujo, H., & Rettori, V. (2014). Role of the endocannabinoid system in the neuroendocrine responses to inflammation. *Current Pharmaceutical Design*, 20(29), 4697–4706. https://doi.org/10.2174/1381612820666140130212957

Lauritsen, K. J., & Rosenberg, H. (2016). Comparison of outcome expectancies for synthetic cannabinoids and botanical marijuana. *The American Journal of Drug and Alcohol Abuse*, 42(4), 377–384. https://doi.org/10.3109/00952990.2015.1135158

Liu, Q.-R., Pan, C.-H., Hishimoto, A., Li, C.-Y., Xi, Z.-X., Llorente-Berzal, A., … Uhl, G. R. (2009). Species differences in cannabinoid receptor 2 (*CNR2* gene): Identification of novel human and rodent CB2 isoforms, differential tissue expression and regulation by cannabinoid receptor ligands. *Genes, Brain and Behavior*, 8(5), 519–530. https://doi.org/10.1111/j.1601-183X.2009.00498.x

Maccarrone, M., Bab, I., Bíró, T., Cabral, G. A., Dey, S. K., Di Marzo, V., … Zimmer, A. (2015). Endocannabinoid signaling at the periphery: 50 years after THC. *Trends in Pharmacological Sciences*, 36(5), 277–296. https://doi.org/10.1016/j.tips.2015.02.008

Mackie, K. (2006). Mechanisms of CB1 receptor signaling: Endocannabinoid modulation of synaptic strength. *International Journal of Obesity*, 30(Suppl.1), S19–S23. https://doi.org/10.1038/sj.ijo.0803273

Mackie, K. (2008). Cannabinoid receptors: Where they are and what they do. *Journal of Neuroendocrinology*, 20 (Suppl. 1), 10–14. https://doi.org/10.1111/j.1365-2826.2008.01671.x

Manzanares, J., Julian, M., & Carrascosa, A. (2006). Role of the cannabinoid system in pain control and therapeutic implications for the management of acute and chronic pain episodes. *Current Neuropharmacology*, 4(3), 239–257. https://doi.org/10.2174/157015906778019527

Martin, B. R., Mechoulam, R., & Razdan, R. K. (1999). Discovery and characterization of endogenous cannabinoids. *Life Sciences*, 65(6–7), 573–595. https://doi.org/10.1016/S0024-3205(99)00281-7

Marzo, V. D., Bifulco, M., & Petrocellis, L. D. (2004). The endocannabinoid system and its therapeutic exploitation. *Nature Reviews. Drug Discovery*, 3(9), 771–784. https://doi.org/10.1038/nrd1495

Meccariello, R., & Chianese, R. (Eds.) (2016). *Cannabinoids in health and disease.* InTech. https://doi.org/10.5772/61595

Mechoulam, R., & Hanuš, L. (2000). A historical overview of chemical research on cannabinoids. *Chemistry and Physics of Lipids*, 108(1–2), 1–13. https://doi.org/10.1016/S0009-3084(00)00184-5

Mechoulam, R., & Shohami, E. (2007). Endocannabinoids and traumatic brain injury. *Molecular Neurobiology*, 36(1), 68–74. https://doi.org/10.1007/s12035-007-8008-6

Merriam-Webster (2020). *Cannabinoid*. Retrieved from https://www.merriam-webst er.com/dictionary/cannabinoid

Montecucco, F., & Di Marzo, V. (2012). At the heart of the matter: The endocannabinoid system in cardiovascular function and dysfunction. *Trends in Pharmacological Sciences*, *33*(6), 331–340. https://doi.org/10.1016/j. tips.2012.03.002

Moulin, A. M. (1989). The immune system: A key concept for the history of immunology. *History and Philosophy of the Life Sciences*, *11*(2), 221–236.

Murillo-Rodríguez, E. (2008). The role of the CB1 receptor in the regulation of sleep. *Progress in Neuro-Psychopharmacology and Biological Psychiatry*, *32*(6), 1420–1427. https://doi.org/10.1016/j.pnpbp.2008.04.008

N-(1-amino-3-methyl-1-oxobutan-2-yl)-1-(cyclohexylmethyl)-1H-indazole-3-carb oxamide(AB-CHMINACA), N-(1-amino-3-methyl-1-oxobutan-2-yl)-1-pentyl-1H-indazole-3-carboxamide (AB-PINACA)and[1-(5-fluoropentyl)-1H-indazol-3-yl](naphthalen-1-yl)methanone(THJ-2201). CID=70969900. Pubchem.ncbi. nlm.nih.gov. Retrieved 03/30/2020 from: https://pubchem.ncbi.nlm.nih.gov/co mpound/70969900

National Center for Biotechnology Information. PubChem Database (2020).

Neves, S. R., Ram, P. T., & Iyengar, R. (2002). G protein pathways. *Science (New York, NY)*, *296*(5573), 1636–1639. https://doi.org/10.1126/science.1071550

Olivera, B. M., Miljanich, G. P., Ramachandran, J., & Adams, M. E. (1994). Calcium channel diversity and neurotransmitter release: The ω-conotoxins and ω-agatoxins. *Annual Review of Biochemistry*, *63*(1), 823–867. https://doi. org/10.1146/annurev.bi.63.070194.004135

O'Sullivan, S. E. (2016). An update on PPAR activation by cannabinoids: Cannabinoids and PPARs. *British Journal of Pharmacology*, *173*(12), 1899–1910. https://doi.org/10.1111/bph.13497

Palazuelos, J., Aguado, T., Pazos, M. R., Julien, B., Carrasco, C., Resel, E., … Galve-Roperh, I. (2009). Microglial CB2 cannabinoid receptors are neuroprotective in Huntington's disease excitotoxicity. *Brain*, *132*(11), 3152–3164. https://doi. org/10.1093/brain/awp239

Panikashvili, D., Simeonidou, C., Ben-Shabat, S., Hanuš, L., Breuer, A., Mechoulam, R., & Shohami, E. (2001). An endogenous cannabinoid (2-AG) is neuroprotective after brain injury. *Nature*, *413*(6855), 527–531. https://doi.org/10.1038/35097089

Pava, M. J., Makriyannis, A., & Lovinger, D. M. (2016). Endocannabinoid signaling regulates sleep stability. *PLOS ONE*, *11*(3), e0152473. https://doi.org/10.1371/ journal.pone.0152473

Pertwee, R. G. (2001). Cannabinoids and the gastrointestinal tract. *Gut*, *48*(6), 859–867. https://doi.org/10.1136/gut.48.6.859

Pertwee, R. G. (2008). The diverse CB1 and CB2 receptor pharmacology of three plant cannabinoids: Delta9-tetrahydrocannabinol, cannabidiol and delta9-tetrahydrocannabivarin. *British Journal of Pharmacology*, *153*(2), 199–215. https://doi.org/10.1038/sj.bjp.0707442

Pertwee, R. G. (Ed.) (2015). *Endocannabinoids* (vol. 231). Springer International Publishing. https://doi.org/10.1007/978-3-319-20825-1

Pertwee, R. G., & Ross, R. A. (2002). Cannabinoid receptors and their ligands. *Prostaglandins, Leukotrienes and Essential Fatty Acids (PLEFA)*, *66*(2–3), 101–121. https://doi.org/10.1054/plef.2001.0341

Piñeiro, R., & Falasca, M. (2012). Lysophosphatidylinositol signalling: New wine from an old bottle. *Biochimica Et Biophysica Acta*, 1821(4), 694–705. https:// doi.org/10.1016/j.bbalip.2012.01.009

Porter, A. C., Sauer, J.-M., Knierman, M. D., Becker, G. W., Berna, M. J., Bao, J., ... Felder, C. C. (2002). Characterization of a novel endocannabinoid, Virodhamine, with antagonist activity at the CB1 receptor. *Journal of Pharmacology and Experimental Therapeutics*, 301(3), 1020–1024. https://doi.org/10.1124/ jpet.301.3.1020

Porter, R. S., Kaplan, J. L., Lynn, R. B., Reddy, M. T., & Merck & Co. (2018). *The Merck manual of diagnosis and therapy* (20 ed.). Merck & Company, Incorporated.

Próspero-García, O., Amancio-Belmont, O., Becerril Meléndez, A. L., Ruiz-Contreras, A. E., & Méndez-Díaz, M. (2016). Endocannabinoids and sleep. *Neuroscience and Biobehavioral Reviews*, 71, 671–679. https://doi.org/10.1016/j. neubiorev.2016.10.005

Rodriguez De Fonseca, F., & Schneider, M. (2008). The endogenous cannabinoid system and drug addiction: 20 years after the discovery of the CB1 receptor: Guest editorial. *Addiction Biology*, 13(2), 143–146. https://doi. org/10.1111/j.1369-1600.2008.00116.x

Roehler, D. R., Hoots, B. E., & Vivolo-Kantor, A. M. (2020). Regional trends in suspected synthetic cannabinoid exposure from January 2016 to September 2019 in the United States. *Drug and Alcohol Dependence*, 207, 107810, https://doi. org/10.1016/j.drugalcdep.2019.107810

Rubenstein, L. A., & Lanzara, R. G. (1998). Activation of G protein-coupled receptors entails cysteine modulation of agonist binding. *Journal of Molecular Structure: THEOCHEM*, 430, 57–71. https://doi.org/10.1016/S0166-1280(98)90217-2

Rudroff, T., & Honce, J. M. (2017). Cannabis and multiple sclerosis—The way forward. *Frontiers in Neurology*, 8, 299. https://doi.org/10.3389/ fneur.2017.00299

Ruehle, S., Rey, A. A., Remmers, F., & Lutz, B. (2012). The endocannabinoid system in anxiety, fear memory and habituation. *Journal of Psychopharmacology*, 26(1), 23–39. https://doi.org/10.1177/0269881111408958

Russo, E. B. (2004). Clinical endocannabinoid deficiency (CECD): Can this concept explain therapeutic benefits of cannabis in migraine, fibromyalgia, irritable bowel syndrome and other treatment-resistant conditions? *Neuro Endocrinology Letters*, 25(1–2), 31–39.

Russo, E. B. (2008). Clinical endocannabinoid deficiency (CECD): Can this concept explain therapeutic benefits of cannabis in migraine, fibromyalgia, irritable bowel syndrome and other treatment-resistant conditions? *Neuro Endocrinology Letters*, 29(2), 192–200.

Russo, E. B. (2011a). Taming THC: Potential cannabis synergy and phytocannabinoid-terpenoid entourage effects: Phytocannabinoid-terpenoid entourage effects. *British Journal of Pharmacology*, 163(7), 1344–1364. https:// doi.org/10.1111/j.1476-5381.2011.01238.x

Russo, E. B. (2011b). Taming THC: Potential cannabis synergy and phytocannabinoid-terpenoid entourage effects: Phytocannabinoid-terpenoid entourage effects. *British Journal of Pharmacology*, 163(7), 1344–1364. https:// doi.org/10.1111/j.1476-5381.2011.01238.x

Russo, E. B. (2016). Clinical endocannabinoid deficiency reconsidered: Current research supports the theory in migraine, fibromyalgia, irritable bowel, and other treatment-resistant syndromes. *Cannabis and Cannabinoid Research*, 1(1), 154–165. https://doi.org/10.1089/can.2016.0009

Ryberg, E., Vu, H. K., Larsson, N., Groblewski, T., Hjorth, S., Elebring, T., … Greasley, P. J. (2005). Identification and characterisation of a novel splice variant of the human CB1 receptor. *FEBS Letters*, 579(1), 259–264. https://doi.org/10.1016/j.febslet.2004.11.085

Saito, M., V., Rezende, M., R., Teixeira, L., & A. (2012). Cannabinoid modulation of neuroinflammatory disorders. *Current Neuropharmacology*, 10(2), 159–166. https://doi.org/10.2174/157015912800604515

Schaffer Library of Drug Policy (n.d.). *Statement of Dr. William C. Woodward, legislative counsel, American medical association*. Retrieved from www.druglbrary.com, Retrieved 03/30/2020 from: http://www.druglibrary.org/schaffer/hemp/taxact/woodward.htm

Sepe, N., De Petrocellis, L., Montanaro, F., Cimino, G., & Di Marzo, V. (1998). *1389*. Bioactive long chain N-acylethanolamines in five species of edible bivalve molluscs. *Biochimica et Biophysica Acta (BBA) - Lipids and Lipid Metabolism*, 2(2), 101–111. https://doi.org/10.1016/S0005-2760(97)00132-X

Shire, D., Carillon, C., Kaghad, M., Calandra, B., Rinaldi-Carmona, M., Fur, G. L., … Ferrara, P. (1995). An amino-terminal variant of the central cannabinoid receptor resulting from alternative splicing. *Journal of Biological Chemistry*, 270(8), 3726–3731. https://doi.org/10.1074/jbc.270.8.3726

Sloan, M. E., Grant, C. W., Gowin, J. L., Ramchandani, V. A., & Le Foll, B. (2019). Endocannabinoid signaling in psychiatric disorders: A review of positron emission tomography studies. *Acta Pharmacologica Sinica*, 40(3), 342–350. https://doi.org/10.1038/s41401-018-0081-z

Smith, L. A., Azariah, F., Lavender, V. T., Stoner, N. S., & Bettiol, S. (2015). Cannabinoids for nausea and vomiting in adults with cancer receiving chemotherapy. *Cochrane Database of Systematic Reviews*. https://doi.org/10.1002/14651858.CD009464.pub2

Sprang, S. R., Chen, Z., & Du, X. (2007). Structural basis of effector regulation and signal termination in heterotrimeric Galpha proteins. *Advances in Protein Chemistry*, 74, 1–65. https://doi.org/10.1016/S0065-3233(07)74001-9

Tamba, B. I., Stanciu, G. D., Urîtu, C. M., Rezus, E., Stefanescu, R., Mihai, C. T., … Alexa-Stratulat, T. (2020). Challenges and opportunities in preclinical research of synthetic cannabinoids for pain therapy. *Medicina*, 56(1), 24. https://doi.org/10.3390/medicina56010024

Treister-Goltzman, Y., Freud, T., Press, Y., & Peleg, R. (2019). Trends in publications on medical cannabis from the year 2000. *Population Health Management*, 22(4), 362–368. https://doi.org/10.1089/pop.2018.0113

Turcotte, C., Blanchet, M.-R., Laviolette, M., & Flamand, N. (2016). The CB2 receptor and its role as a regulator of inflammation. *Cellular and Molecular Life Sciences*, 73(23), 4449–4470. https://doi.org/10.1007/s00018-016-2300-4

Vučković, S., Srebro, D., Vujović, K. S., Vučetić, Č., & Prostran, M. (2018). Cannabinoids and pain: New insights from old molecules. *Frontiers in Pharmacology*, 9, 1259. https://doi.org/10.3389/fphar.2018.01259

Wettschureck, N., & Offermanns, S. (2005). Mammalian G proteins and their cell type specific functions. *Physiological Reviews*, *85*(4), 1159–1204. https://doi. org/10.1152/physrev.00003.2005

Wilson, R. I., & Nicoll, R. A. (2002). Endocannabinoid signaling in the brain. *Science*, *296*(5568), 678–682. https://doi.org/10.1126/science.1063545

Winther, R. G. (2016). The structure of scientific theories. In E. N. Zalta (Ed.), The Stanford encyclopedia of philosophy (winter 2016 edition). Retrieved 03/30/2020 from: https://plato.stanford.edu/entries/structure-scientific-theories/

Wood, T. B., Spivey, W. T. N., & Easterfield, T. H. (1896). XL.—Charas. The resin of Indian hemp. *Journal of the Chemical Society, Transactions*, *69*(0), 539–546. https://doi.org/10.1039/CT8966900539

Zhang, H.-Y., Bi, G.-H., Li, X., Li, J., Qu, H., Zhang, S.-J., ... Liu, Q.-R. (2015). Species differences in cannabinoid receptor 2 and receptor responses to cocaine self-administration in mice and rats. *Neuropsychopharmacology*, *40*(4), 1037–1051. https://doi.org/10.1038/npp.2014.297

Zou, S., & Kumar, U. (2018). Cannabinoid receptors and the endocannabinoid system: Signaling and function in the central nervous system. *International Journal of Molecular Sciences*, *19*(3), 833. https://doi.org/10.3390/ijms19030833

Zygmunt, P. M., Petersson, J., Andersson, D. A., Chuang, H., Sørgård, M., Di Marzo, V., ... Högestätt, E. D. (1999). Vanilloid receptors on sensory nerves mediate the vasodilator action of anandamide. *Nature*, *400*(6743), 452–457. https://doi. org/10.1038/22761

Chapter 6

Medical Cannabis for Children and Adolescents

Bonni S. Goldstein

Although considered controversial, the use of phytocannabinoid medicine in the pediatric population has become popular during the past decade. Due to the continued Schedule I categorization of phytocannabinoids in the Controlled Substances Act, clinical trials on the therapeutic benefits of phytocannabinoid medicines are still highly restricted. Historically, state laws, namely in California and Colorado, allowed parents to seek medical cannabis treatment for children with certain qualifying conditions. Internet forums, social media, and documentaries about the "miraculous" improvement of seriously ill children resulted in desperate parents treating their children, often without medical supervision. This societal interest has led to changes in state policy, with the passage of legislation allowing for the use of cannabis in children with certain severe illnesses. Moreover, it has led to many clinical trials for pediatric epilepsy and autism. Although expanded research is needed, the preliminary findings are quite promising.

The Endocannabinoid System

Research shows that the endocannabinoid system (ECS) plays a fundamental role from early stages of gestation and throughout the life of a developing organism. The presence of cannabinoid CB1 receptors as early as the pre-implantation period in the embryonal mouse and at gestation day 11 has been documented (Paria & Dey, 2000; Buckley et al., 1997). Subsequent research reveals "atypical distribution patterns" of CB1 receptors between gestational day 21 and postnatal day 5 in areas of the brain where none are found in adulthood, suggesting a role for the ECS during early brain development (Fernández-Ruiz et al., 2000); Biegon & Kerman, 2001). In human embryos, CB1 receptors were detected at week 14 of gestation (Biegon & Kerman, 2001). High concentrations of functionally active CB1 receptors were found on several white matter neuronal tracts of the fetus, which disappeared by infancy (Mato et al., 2003). That study reported a progressive increase in the concentrations of CB1 receptors in the frontal cortex, hippocampus, basal ganglia, and cerebellum during development from fetus to adulthood.

Anandamide (arachidonyl ethanol amide) and 2-AG (2-arachidonoyl glycerol), the two most studied endocannabinoids, are found in the fetus, with significantly higher concentrations of the latter during the fetal period Fernández-Ruiz et al., 2000). Interestingly, anandamide increases throughout development until adult levels are reached, but fetal 2-AG levels are comparable to those in young and adult brains (Berrendero et al., 1999). Endocannabinoids are also found in animal and human breast milk, with research demonstrating that activation of CB1 receptors by these endocannabinoids triggers milk sucking critical for survival of the newborn (Fride et al., 2001; Fride et al., 2003).

The presence of the endocannabinoids and their receptors from early developmental stages is thought to play a key role in the following functions:

- Embryonal development
- Nervous system development
- Neuroprotection
- Food intake and survival in the newborn period
- Development of prefrontal cortex (Fride, 2004).

Mice research shows that the gradual increase of anandamide and CB1 receptors from infancy to adulthood is accompanied by a parallel maturing response to the intoxicating effects of delta-9-tetrahydrocannabinol (Δ^9-THC) (Fride & Mechoulam, 1996). This finding correlates to findings from experiences using Δ^8-THC (an isomer of Δ^9-THC that has intoxicating effects albeit less than Δ^9-THC) in children undergoing cancer chemotherapy and Δ^9-THC in children with severe neurological disease (Abrahamov et al.,1995; Lorenz, 2004)). The pediatric patients in these reports found significant improvement in symptoms with minimal or no side effects, implying that cannabinoid therapy is well-tolerated in children with few to no intoxicating effects, likely due to an immature but functional ECS.

Evidence of endocannabinoid system deficiency or dysfunction as a root cause of illness was first hypothesized by Russo in 2004 (Russo, 2008). Since that time, research has confirmed that underlying endocannabinoid system deficiencies play a role in many conditions such as epilepsy, autism, anxiety, depression, neurodegenerative disorders, and schizophrenia, as well as the three conditions noted in Russo's paper—migraine, fibromyalgia, and irritable bowel syndrome (Romigi et al., 2010; Chakrabarti et al., 2015; Viveros et al., 2005; Vinod & Hungund, 2006; Micale et al., 2007; Fernandez-Esejo et al., 2009; Smith & Wagner, 2014). There are many anecdotal reports of patients with these conditions improving with the use of cannabis, which may be replacing lower than normal levels of endocannabinoids, thus restoring balance to the ECS. This chapter will discuss the latest evidence on the ECS in pediatric conditions and the use of cannabinoids as medicine for this vulnerable population.

Epilepsy

Epilepsy is the most frequent neurologic condition in childhood, affecting 0.5%-1% of children (Aaberg et al., 2017). Despite the availability of almost 30 different anti-seizure medications, approximately 30% of epilepsy patients continue to have seizures, called intractable or treatment-resistant epilepsy. Uncontrolled seizures and side effects of seizure medications are associated with severe morbidity and increased mortality. The safety and side effect profile of antiepileptic medications has improved over the past few decades; however, side effects, especially those related to the central nervous system, are commonly experienced and can negatively affect quality of life (Perucca & Gilliam, 2012).

Anecdotal reports of the antiepileptic effects of cannabis go back to the 11th century. In 1843, Dr. William O'Shaughnessy reported on the benefits of "hemp" in a 40-day-old infant with convulsive epilepsy (1843). More recently, a CNN documentary in 2013 about medical cannabis highlighted the successful antiepileptic effects of cannabidiol-rich cannabis by a young girl with Dravet syndrome, a devastating genetic pediatric epilepsy. Since that time, interest in the antiepileptic effects of the phytocannabinoids, especially cannabidiol (CBD), has exploded, resulting in thousands of parents exploring cannabinoid treatment for their children, as well as FDA approval of the first plant-derived cannabinoid-based pharmaceutical in 2018.

Evidence of ECS Impairment in Epilepsy

The ECS plays a significant role in the regulation of seizures because of its well-known function of balancing excessive neuronal excitability. Wallace et al. found that both Δ^9-THC and the synthetic CB1 receptor agonist WIN55,212 completely abolished spontaneous epileptic seizures (2003). CB1 antagonists caused the development of status epilepticus, which could be reversed with high doses of CB1 agonists (Deshpande et al., 2007). The hippocampus in brain tissue surgically removed from patients with epilepsy showed 60% down-regulation of CB1 receptor mRNA and 60% reduction of the diacylglycerol lipase-α, which is responsible for synthesis of the endocannabinoid 2-AG when compared to control tissue from non-epileptic brain (Ludányi et al., 2008). Additionally, the same study reported a reduction in CB1 receptors on glutaminergic axon terminals; these findings taken together demonstrate that the neuroprotection conferred by the ECS is impaired in the hippocampus in the epileptic brain, and that the down-regulation of crucial components of this system contributes to increased neuroexcitability. Romigi et al. (2010) revealed a significant reduction of anandamide in the cerebral spinal fluid of patients with new onset untreated temporal lobe epilepsy compared to healthy controls, further supporting the theory of impairment of the ECS as a factor in epilepsy.

Preclinical Evidence

Both cannabidiol (CBD) and delta-9-tetrahydrocannabinol (Δ^9-THC) have antiepileptic effects in preclinical models of epilepsy (Hill et al., 2013). An excellent review, seen in Figure 6.1, of the preclinical studies investigating modulators of the ECS, cannabinoid receptor agonists and antagonists (both synthetic and plant-derived) reveals CBD and the phytocannabinoid, cannabidivarin (CBDV), had "consistently beneficial therapeutic effects in preclinical models of seizures, epilepsy, epileptogenesis, and neuroprotection" (Rosenberg et al., 2017).

Therapeutic effects of cannabinoids in animal models of seizures, epilepsy, epileptogenesis, and epilepsy-related neuroprotection. *Epilepsy & Behavior, 70(B)*, 319–327 with permission.

Human Studies

Only a few clinical trials assessing the antiepileptic effects of CBD have been published. Although limited by small sample size and lack of methodological details, these reports affirm the clinical potential of CBD as a safe and well-tolerated antiepileptic agent. Table 6.1 summarizes these studies, as well as other retrospective studies.

Epidiolex for Pediatric Epilepsy

In June 2018, the FDA-approved Epidiolex (GW Pharmaceuticals), a plant-derived pharmaceutical-grade CBD product, for two types of severe pediatric epilepsies, Dravet syndrome and Lennox-Gastaut syndrome. The DEA placed Epidiolex in Schedule V of the Controlled Substances Act, the least restrictive category, although all other CBD products remain in the Schedule I category. Epidiolex contains 99% cannabidiol mixed in dehydrated alcohol, sesame seed oil, strawberry flavor, and sucralose. Recommended dosing for Epidiolex starts with 5 mg/kg/day for the first week, followed by an increase to the therapeutic range of 10–20 mg/kg/day, depending on the response.

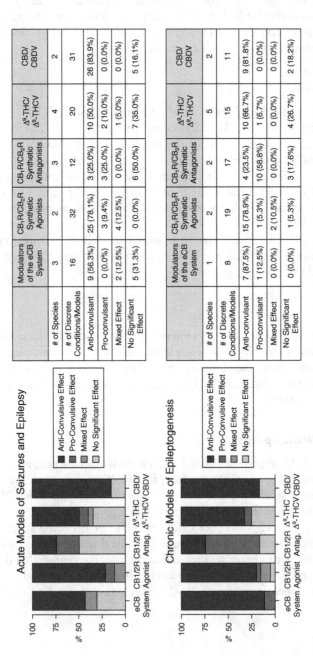

Acute Models of Seizures and Epilepsy

	Modulators of the eCB System	CB₁R/CB₂R Synthetic Agonists	CB₁R/CB₂R Synthetic Antagonists	Δ⁹-THC/Δ⁹-THCV	CBD/CBDV
# of Species	3	2	3	4	2
# of Discrete Conditions/Models	16	32	12	20	31
Anti-convulsant	9 (56.3%)	25 (78.1%)	3 (25.0%)	10 (50.0%)	26 (83.9%)
Pro-convulsant	0 (0.0%)	3 (9.4%)	3 (25.0%)	2 (10.0%)	0 (0.0%)
Mixed Effect	2 (12.5%)	4 (12.5%)	0 (0.0%)	1 (5.0%)	0 (0.0%)
No Significant Effect	5 (31.3%)	0 (0.0%)	6 (50.0%)	7 (35.0%)	5 (16.1%)

Chronic Models of Epileptogenesis

	Modulators of the eCB System	CB₁R/CB₂R Synthetic Agonists	CB₁R/CB₂R Synthetic Antagonists	Δ⁹-THC/Δ⁹-THCV	CBD/CBDV
# of Species	1	2	2	5	2
# of Discrete Conditions/Models	8	19	17	15	11
Anti-convulsant	7 (87.5%)	15 (78.9%)	4 (23.5%)	10 (66.7%)	9 (81.8%)
Pro-convulsant	1 (12.5%)	1 (5.3%)	10 (58.8%)	1 (6.7%)	0 (0.0%)
Mixed Effect	0 (0.0%)	2 (10.5%)	0 (0.0%)	0 (0.0%)	0 (0.0%)
No Significant Effect	0 (0.0%)	1 (5.3%)	3 (17.6%)	4 (26.7%)	2 (18.2%)

Legend: Anti-Convulsive Effect, Pro-Convulsive Effect, Mixed Effect, No Significant Effect

Figure 6.1 Therapeutic effects of cannabinoids in animal models of seizures, epilepsy, epileptogenesis, and epilepsy-related neuroprotection. Preclinical animal models of seizures, epilepsy, and epileptogenesis. Compiled data from synthetic and phytocannabinoids in 181 total animal models of A. Acute models of seizures and epilepsy. B. Chronic models of epileptogenesis. Preclinical interventions were subdivided into (1) Modulators of the Endocannabinoid System ("eCB System"), (2) CB1/CB2R Agonists, (3) CB1/CB2R Antagonists, (3) D9THC/THCV, and (4) CBD/CBDV. From Rosenberg et al. (2017).

Table 6.1 Summary of Studies: Anti Epileptic Effects of CBD

Source	Sample	Study Design	CBD Dose	Outcome
Mechoulam & Carlini, 1978	9 patients with treatment-resistant epilepsy, temporal focus	Double-blind Placebo-controlled	200 mg/day for 3 months Adjunct to other AEDs	3 of 4 improved with CBD (2 with seizure freedom); no improvement with placebo; no toxic side effects reported
Cunha et al., 1980	15 patients with treatment-resistant epilepsy	Double-blind Placebo-controlled Peer-reviewed	200–300 mg/day for 8–18 weeks Adjunct to other AEDs	7 of 8 improved with CBD; 1 of 7 improved with placebo; no toxic side effects reported
Ames et al., 1986	12 patients with epilepsy	Placebo-controlled	300 mg/day for 4 weeks	No improvements reported; only side effect reported was mild sedation in CBD group
Porter & Jacobson, 2013	19 pediatric patients with treatment-resistant epilepsy	Retrospective survey	CBD dosing ranged from <0.5 mg/kg/day–28.6 mg/day; all were using artisanal CBD-rich extract	16 of 19 (84%) reported reduction in seizures; 2 had seizure freedom; side effects reported were drowsiness (37%) and fatigue (16%)
Gedde & Maa, 2013	11 pediatric patients with treatment-resistant epilepsy	Retrospective survey	4–12 mg/kg/day; all were using artisanal CBD-rich extract	100% reported reduction of seizures; at 3 months, 5 of 11 were seizure free; side effects reported were sedation and unsteadiness
Hussain et al., 2015	117 pediatric patients with treatment-resistant epilepsy	Retrospective survey	Median dose 4.3 mg/kg/day	Overall 85% reported reduction of seizures; 14% reported seizure freedom; side effects reported included somnolence, increased appetite and increase seizure; benefits included more alertness, better mood, and better sleep *(Continued)*

Table 6.1 (Continued)

Source	Sample	Study Design	CBD Dose	Outcome
Tzadok et al., 2016	74 pediatric patients with treatment-resistant epilepsy	Retrospective survey	1–20 mg/kg/day for 3–12 months	Overall 89% reported reduction of seizures with one patient reporting seizure free; side effects included
Sulak et al., 2017	272 patients (mostly pediatric) with treatment-resistant epilepsy in three U.S. states	Retrospective survey	Varied dosing; some patients were also taking THC and/ or THCA extracts	Overall 86% reported reduction of seizures with 10% reporting seizure free; side effects included sedation, decreased appetite, sleep disturbance; benefits included better sleep, mood and alertness
Porcari et al., 2018	108 pediatric patients	Retrospective survey	0.18–50 mg/kg/day of artisanal CBD oil	Addition of CBD to regimen resulted in 39% having >50% reduction of seizures; 10% reporting seizure free; most common side effect sedation; benefits included increased alertness and verbal interactions

Clinical trials on Epidiolex revealed the following results:

- Dravet syndrome: Percentage of patients who had at least 50% reduction in convulsive seizure frequency was 43% with CBD compared to 27% with placebo (p=0.08) (Devinsky et al., 2017).
- Lennox-Gastaut syndrome: Median percentage reduction in monthly drop seizure frequency from baseline was 43.9% with CBD and 21.8% with placebo (p=0.0135) (Thiele et al., 2018).
- Drug-drug interactions: 39 adults and 42 children given Epidiolex dosing between 5–50 mg/kg/day had increased levels of topiramate, rufinamide, N-desmethlyclobazam and decreased clobazam; however, all changes were within accepted therapeutic range except for clobazam and N-desmethlyclobazam. A small number of patients on valproic acid had elevated liver transaminases (Gaston et al., 2017).

Side effects of Epidiolex include diarrhea, worsening seizures, sedation, decreased appetite, and elevated liver transaminases (in those on concurrent valproic acid). It is important to note that there is no evidence of elevated liver transaminases in children taking artisanal whole-plant CBD-rich cannabis oil. This discrepancy is likely due to the higher dosing of Epidiolex when compared to artisanal CBD oils. There are ongoing trials for tuberous sclerosis, Aicardi syndrome, Doose syndrome, and other severe pediatric epilepsies.

Autism Spectrum Disorder

According to the World Health Organization, 1 in 160 children have an autism spectrum disorder (ASD); in the United States, the prevalence is 1 in 59 (Baio et al., 2018). ASD is a heterogeneous neurodevelopmental disorder characterized by three core types of symptoms: various degrees of impaired communication, impaired reciprocal social interaction, and restrictive-repetitive behaviors and interests. Neuro-inflammation and neuro-immune abnormalities have been established as critical factors in the development and maintenance of ASD (Siniscalco et al., 2018). ASD is also associated with increased risk of seizures, gastrointestinal disorders, sleep disturbances, anxiety, depression, and attention issues. The underlying pathogenesis remains undefined, making curative treatments quite difficult. Diagnosis is made clinically, often between the ages of 2–4 years. Studies show that early intervention with different types of therapy, such as applied behavioral analysis (ABA), speech, and occupational therapy, can improve outcomes for these children. Two FDA-approved pharmaceuticals that treat irritability associated with autism are available; however, these do not address the core symptoms and often have significant adverse side effects. Initial investigations into the use of medicinal cannabis for autism have revealed benefits for core symptoms as well as an acceptable safety profile.

Evidence of ECS Impairment in ASD

The endocannabinoid system, specifically CB1 receptors, is expressed in the same areas of the brain implicated in abnormalities of ASD, namely the cerebellum, basal ganglia, and hippocampus Bauman & Kemper, 2005). As previously mentioned, CB1 receptors are involved in early brain development, driving axon guidance and establishing synaptogenesis. An impairment in this process has been hypothesized to be an underlying cause of ASD (McFadden & Minshew, 2013).

In the last decade, investigations into the relationship of the ECS and the symptoms of ASD in humans have revealed interesting findings. In a case report, a 6-year-old child with ASD was given dronabinol, a synthetic THC medication; compared to baseline, he showed significant improvement in hyperactivity, irritability, stereotypy, and speech (p=0.043) on a total daily dose of 3.62 mg dronabinol (synthetic THC) with no adverse effects (Kurz & Blaas, 2010). Subsequent research documents abnormalities in the ECS of children with ASD. Siniscalco et al. (2013) demonstrated dysregulation of CB2 receptors in peripheral blood mononuclear cells, suggesting a correlation between ECS-mediated immune dysfunction and ASD pathophysiology. In 2018, plasma anandamide levels were found to be lower in 59 children with ASD (p=0.034), and significantly differentiated ASD cases from controls such that those with lower anandamide levels were more likely to have ASD (Karhson et al., 2018). In a larger sample in 2019, similar findings of lower serum levels of circulating endocannabinoids were reported in children with ASD (Aran et al., 2019). Both reports suggest the possibility of plasma anandamide levels as a biomarker for early diagnosis of ASD, which currently is a diagnosis made clinically after symptoms arise. Early diagnosis would allow for early treatment, thereby improving outcomes for these children. It is important to note that the ECS represents a physiologic connection between the central nervous system and the immune system, both of which show abnormalities in autism (Carrier et al., 2005).

Recent research investigating the link between acetaminophen and ASD has implicated underlying involvement of the ECS. Acetaminophen produces analgesia through an indirect interaction with cannabinoid receptors, potentially disrupting normal ECS processes occurring during brain development, resulting in ASD (Schultz, 2010). Interestingly, the rates of ASD increased in the United States after the CDC warned against aspirin use in children in 1980. Rates of ASD decreased in 1982 and 1986 when acetaminophen use decreased after poisonings resulted from malicious tampering of the drug (Becker & Schultz, 2010). Despite evidence to the contrary, parents often view vaccines as the cause of ASD; however, the precipitating event may actually be the use of acetaminophen to treat vaccine-induced side effects in young children.

Preclinical Evidence

There are numerous clues from animal models suggesting ECS involvement in the pathogenesis of autism. Földy et al. (2013) found an autism-associated mutation in a set of genes involved in neurodevelopmental processes were associated with deficits in social behavior and disrupted ECS signaling. In a valproic acid rat model of autism, multiple alterations in the components of the ECS resulted in autistic-type behavioral abnormalities (Kerr et al., 2013). Two mouse models of ASD (BTBR and fmr1$^{-/-}$) showed the activity of anandamide was increased by blockage of FAAH (fatty acid amide hydrolase), the enzyme that degrades anandamide. This resulted in a complete reversal of social impairment in both mouse models (Wei et al., 2016). Another report demonstrated that *in vitro* monocyte-derived macrophagic cells, obtained from individuals with ASD, showed ECS dysfunction, possibly explaining the immune system abnormalities seen in those with ASD (Siniscalco et al., 2014).

Human Studies

Unfortunately, there are very few clinical trials using cannabinoid treatment for autism. However, there are two published reports from Israel showing significant benefits with overall minimal side effects. Sixty children with ASD and severe aggression were recruited to receive CBD-rich artisanal cannabis oil with a ratio of 20:1 (Aran et al., 2019). Dosing began at 1 mg/kg/day and was titrated up to 10 mg/kg/day. For those that did not respond well to this ratio (29 patients), THC was added to lower the ratio to CBD:THC of 6:1 with maximum dosing of 5 mg/kg/day. In this latter group, 13 patients showed "much better" responses, 7 patients "slightly better," no change in 6 patients, and worse behaviors in 3 patients. Using the Caregiver Global Impression of Change (CGIC) scale, behavioral outbreaks were "improved or very much improved" in 61% of patients, anxiety was improved or very much proved in 39%, and communication issues were improved or very much improved in 47%. Disruptive behaviors were improved by 29%. At the end of the study, 73% of patients continued with cannabinoid treatment. Irritability, difficulties giving the oil, low efficacy, or unwanted side effects were the reasons given for discontinuation. The range of dosing for CBD was 0.1–6.4 mg/kg/day and THC 0.2–0.5 mg/kg/day.

In another report, 188 patients with ASD were treated with 20:1 CBD:THC oil three times a day. Some patients (24.4%) took extra THC oil for insomnia. The most prevalent symptoms reported by parents were restlessness, rage attacks, and agitation. Dosing ranges were on average 79.5 ± 61.5 mg CBD and 4.0 ± 3.0 mg THC, three times a day. After one month, 179 patients were still using the treatment with 48.7% reporting significant improvement, 31.1% reporting moderate improvement, and 14.3% no benefit; only 5.9% experienced side effects. Follow-up at six months revealed 8.3% stopped treatment, 4.9% switched products, and 86.6% continued treatment. In the latter group, 30.1% reported significant improvement, 53.7% reported moderate improvement, 6.4% slight improvement, and 8.6% no change. Good quality of life was reported by 31.3% before treatment, and at six months good quality of life was reported by 66.8% ($p<0.001$). Other factors that showed statistically significant improvements were positive mood, ability to dress and shower independently, good sleep, and good concentration. Restlessness and rage attacks were improved in more than 90% of patients who reported these prior to treatment. Side effects were reported by 25.2% of patients: restlessness (6.6%), sleepiness (3.2%), psychoactive effect (3.2%), increased appetite (3.2%), digestion problems (3.2%), dry mouth (2.2%), and lack of appetite (2.2%). Overall

80% of parents reported significant or moderate improvement (Schleider et al., 2019).

Cancer

Cancer is diagnosed yearly in approximately 175,000 children aged 14 and under worldwide. It is the leading cause of death by disease in U.S. children who are past infancy. The most common cancers in children are leukemia (29% of pediatric cancers), brain and spinal cord tumors (26% of pediatric cancers), with neuroblastoma, lymphoma, bone cancers, and other solid tumors making up the rest. Approximately 12% of children diagnosed with cancer do not survive, and 60% of those who do survive suffer devastating late effects such as secondary cancers, infertility, and other debilitating medical issues. The incidence of childhood cancer has been steadily increasing over the last few decades, from 13 children per 100,000 in 1975 to over 17 children per 100,000 since 2007 (curesearch.org).

Preclinical Evidence

In addition to reducing side effects related to cancer, phytocannabinoids have anti-cancer properties.

Symptom Relief—Nausea and Vomiting

Considerable preclinical evidence exists that the endocannabinoid system plays a role in regulating nausea, vomiting, and pain, which are common side effects of cancer and cancer treatment. Cannabinoid agonists have been shown to reduce vomiting in numerous animal models including cats, ferrets, pigeons, and shrews, while CB1 receptor antagonists promote vomiting (McCarty & Borison, 1981; Simoneau et al., 2001; Feigenbaum et al., 1989; Darmani & Johnson, 2004). Both THC and CBD suppress conditioned gaping reactions (nausea) in rats (Limebeer & Parker, 1999; Parker & Mechoulam, 2003; Rock et al., 2010). The mechanisms by which cannabinoids reduce or eliminate nausea and vomiting include reduction of serotonin release from enterochromaffin cells in the small intestine, direct agonism of the CB1 receptor, FAAH inhibition, and vanilloid TRPV1 receptor agonism (Sharkey et al., 2014; Darmani, 2001; Ray et al., 2009; Van Sickle et al., 2005; Sharkey et al., 2007).

Symptom Relief—Cancer Pain

Cannabinoids were demonstrated to increase the threshold at which pain was perceived in mice with carcinoma (Guerrero et al., 2008). Additionally, multiple studies show synthetic cannabinoid agonists attenuated tumor-induced pain in mice through peripheral cannabinoid receptor action (Potenzieri et al., 2008; Hamamoto et al., 2007).

Anti-cancer Effects

The first mention of the anti-proliferative properties of phytocannabinoids was in 1975, when it was demonstrated that Δ^9-THC inhibited the growth of lung adenocarcinoma cells both *in vitro* and in mice (Munson et al., 1975). Preclinical trials since have shown cannabinoid efficacy against various cancer cell types such as breast, skin, colon, gliomas, lymphoma, leukemia, pancreas, and prostate (Blasco et al., 2018; Simmerman et al., 2019; Raup-Konsavage et al., 2018; López-Valero et al., 2018; Pham et al., 2016; Lombard et al., 2005; Carracedo et al., 2006; Roberto & Venkateswaran, 2017). The main mechanisms are through induction of apoptosis, inhibition of tumor growth, inhibition of metastasis, and inhibition of angiogenesis (Velasco et al., 2016a; Ramer & Hinz, 2015). These effects occur via signaling pathways such as mitogen-activated protein kinase (MAPK), ERK, Akt, phosphoinositide 3-kinase (PI3K), p8–trib-3and hypoxia inducible factor 1 (HIF1), and others (Velasco et al., 2016b; Javid et al., 2016). Preclinical studies related to the anti-cancer efficacy of cannabinoids number in the thousands, thus a complete review is beyond the scope of this chapter. However, since over 50% of pediatric cancers are leukemia and brain cancers, evidence of efficacy of phytocannabinoids against these and other malignancies justifies further investigation and human trials.

Human Studies

There are more than 50 published reports of the efficacy of synthetic and phytocannabinoids for nausea and vomiting from cancer chemotherapy and radiation therapy. There are also at least 15 published reports of the use of cannabinoids for cancer-related pain. The National Academies of Sciences, Engineering, and Medicine (NASEM), in an exhaustive review of the literature and assessment of the quality of the research, found "conclusive or substantial evidence of effect" for the use of cannabinoids for chemotherapy-induced nausea and vomiting and for chronic pain (NASEM, 2017; Abrams, 2018). Two studies investigated the use of cannabinoids for pediatric patients for symptomatic relief of nausea and vomiting, one with a synthetic cannabinoid and the other with Δ^8-THC, both of which showed efficacy (Abrahamov et al., 1995; Chan et al., 1987).

There are only two published human clinical trials investigating efficacy of phytocannabinoids as chemotherapy, both for patients with glioblastoma multiforme (GBM). Researchers in Spain directly administered THC into GBM cancer cells in terminal patients and found inhibition of tumor cell proliferation without any adverse side effects (Guzman et al., 2006). A two-part safety and exploratory efficacy double-blind, placebo-controlled trial combining CBD and THC with the chemotherapy Temozolomide in patients with recurrent GBM found one year survival of 83% with combination treatment versus 44% for placebo, with side effects of vomiting and dizziness reported in the treatment group (Short & Little, 2017).

Unfortunately, there are no human clinical trials of the chemotherapeutic or anti-proliferative effects of phytocannabinoids in pediatric cancer. The author of this chapter has treated many children with terminal cancers—including relapsed leukemia, metastatic Wilms tumor, metastatic osteosarcoma, rhabdomyosarcoma, and anaplastic ependymoma—who achieved remission with high doses of combination oral cannabinoids. Some patients had cannabinoids added to conventional chemotherapy, and others started cannabinoid treatment after chemotherapy was withdrawn due to lack of efficacy. In general, these pediatric patients tolerated the cannabinoids well with minimal side effects. All had extended survival beyond the oncologists' prognosis, and a few are approaching the 5-year survival anniversary with no evidence of disease despite a prior terminal diagnosis. These anecdotal cases of successful treatment of advanced cancers in children should serve to underscore the desperate need for human clinical trials.

Neuroprotection

The neuroprotective potential of compounds that interact with the ECS is the focus of extensive research around the globe. Cannabinoids have been shown to diminish the effects of cytotoxic insults including inflammation, oxidative stress and excitotoxicity, and promoting cell survival (Hassell et al., 2015). Pediatric patients with hypoxic-ischemic encephalopathy (HIE), traumatic brain injury, and neurodegenerative disorders have very few treatment options for neuroprotection and neuroinflammation. Cannabinoids, in their ability to interact with multiple targets not only within the ECS but also outside this system at other neuromodulatory sites, offer promise to mitigate neuronal damage with little toxicity of their own.

Preclinical Evidence

Much research has demonstrated that Δ^9-THC and endocannabinoids have neuroprotective effects (Pryce et al., 2003; Croxford et al., 2008; Hernández-Torres et al., 2014; .Bernal-Chico et al., 2015). The anti-inflammatory effects of cannabinoids are equally well documented (Klein, 2005; Nagarkatti et al., 2009; Rettori et al., 2012). The following is a summary of the research and multiple mechanisms by which cannabinoids provide neuroprotection and reduction of neuroinflammation for HIE and TBI:

Hypoxic-Ischemic Encephalopathy

- A synthetic CB1/CB2 receptor agonist (WIN55212-2) reduced cell death, decreased glutamate and cytokine release, and decreased inducible nitric oxide synthase expression in newborn rat forebrain slices subject to oxygen and glucose deprivation (Fernandez et al., 2006).
- Post-insult administration of a synthetic CB1/CB2 receptor agonist (WIN55212-2) in fetal lambs resulted in improved cerebral blood flow and reduced neuronal cell death (Alonso-Alconada et al., 2012).
- CBD administered 15–30 minutes after hypoxia-ischemia insult in newborn pigs lessened the death of neurons and astrocytes. EEG showed preserved brain activity as well as seizures were prevented. Neurobehavioral performance was improved at 72 hours post insult (Alvarez et al., 2008; Lafuente et al., 2011; Pazos et al., 2013).
- CBD administered 15 minutes after hypoxia-ischemia insult in newborn rats reduced brain damage and resulted in long-lasting improvement of neurobehavioral function (Pazos et al., 2012).
- CB2 and adenosine receptors mediated the neuroprotective effects of CBD in mice with HIE (Castillo et al., 2010).

Traumatic Brain Injury

- Activation of CB1 and CB2 receptors minimized damage to the blood brain barrier, decreased inflammation, and reduced neurodegeneration (Mauler et al., 2003; Amenta et al., 2012; Panikashvili et al., 2005).
- Blockade of NMDA receptors with a synthetic cannabinoid given after closed head injury resulted in less brain edema and improved cognitive function (Shohami et al., 1995).
- Activation of TRPV1 receptors by an endocannabinoid-like compound resulted in less edema, reduced lesion volume, and prevention of hypothermia (Cohen-Yeshurun et al., 2011).
- Activation of CB1 receptor, CB2 receptor and TRPV1 receptor by an endocannabinoid-like compound improved neurobehavioral function continuously for six weeks post-TBI (Cohen-Yeshurun et al., 2013).

Human Studies

Unfortunately, there are no published clinical trials assessing the neuroprotective properties of cannabinoids in the pediatric population. There is limited evidence of neuroprotection from cannabinoids in adults.

In a 2002 phase II randomized, placebo-controlled clinical trial, a synthetic cannabinoid HU-211 was given to 67 patients sustaining severe head injuries. Patients receiving the drug had better intracranial pressure/cerebral perfusion pressure control with no deleterious effect on blood pressure.

The authors also observed "a trend toward faster and better neurologic outcome" (Knoller et al., 2002). In a multi-center phase III randomized, placebo-controlled clinical trial, 846 patients from 15 countries were randomized to receive a single intravenous dose of HU-211 or placebo within six hours of severe traumatic brain injury. No differences were found between the treatment group and the placebo group (Maas et al., 2006). A retrospective study of adults with TBI presenting to a trauma center found that, after adjusting for differences between the study cohorts, a positive toxicology screen for THC was associated with a decreased mortality (p=0.049), suggesting a neuroprotective effect (Nguyen et al., 2014).

Clinical trials of cannabinoids in adults with neurodegenerative disorders, such as Parkinson's disease, have focused on symptom relief, not on the underlying neuronal pathophysiology. The FDA has granted orphan drug and fast track designation to a British pharmaceutical company for an intravenous form of CBD for the treatment of HIE in newborns. A completed phase I trial in healthy adult volunteers has been reported at the time of this writing.

Other Conditions Affecting Pediatric Patients

ADHD

Attention deficit hyperactivity disorder is characterized by persistent and disabling symptoms of inattention, hyperactivity, and impulsivity, and is often co-morbid with emotional dysregulation, cognitive impairments, and other psychiatric diagnoses. Three subtypes have been categorized: predominant inattention, predominant hyperactive-impulsive, and combined. These three subtypes have been associated with different neurotransmitter issues, namely dopamine, norepinephrine, and serotonin. Mechanisms by which cannabinoids may offer therapeutic benefits are enhanced dopaminergic transmission, similar to the mechanism by which stimulant medications decrease ADHD symptoms (Bossong et al., 2015).

There are many accounts of self-medication with cannabinoids by those with ADHD who report feeling calmer, less restless, and having better focus and sleep (Milz & Grotenhermen, 2015). Unfortunately, there are no clinical trials on the use of cannabinoid treatment in children. However, a recent randomized, placebo-controlled trial in 30 adults with ADHD using a 1:1 CBD:THC sublingual spray (Sativex, GW Pharmaceuticals) found no significant improvement in cognitive performance but did demonstrate some improvement in hyperactivity/impulsivity (p = 0.03) and a trend towards improvement for inattention (p = 0.10) and emotional lability (p = 0.11). No cognitive impairment was found (Cooper et al., 2017). Clinically the author has found success in treating children who struggle with ADHD symptoms using both CBD, THC, and THCA in various ratios and doses based on individual response.

Tourette Syndrome

Gilles de la Tourette syndrome (GTS) is a neuropsychiatric movement disorder that is characterized by motor and vocal tics. Often there are co-morbid conditions including ADHD, obsessive-compulsive disorder, anxiety, depression, impulsivity, and self-injurious behaviors. Most experts agree that current treatment modalities are unsatisfactory in efficacy and side effects. The underlying cause of GTS is still in question; however, imbalances in the dopaminergic system within key areas of the cortico-striato-thalamo-cortical circuitry are suspected.

There are numerous published case reports of patients using THC for GTS. In 1988, three male patients aged 15 years, 17 years, and 39 years who did not respond to conventional treatment found reduction of tics, less premonitory urges, less self-injurious behavior, and better attention with inhaled cannabis (Sandyk & Awerbuch, 1988). Additional case reports demonstrate similar outcomes, although only one adolescent is included in these case reports (Hemming & Yellowlees, 1993; Müller-Vahl et al., 1999; Müller-Vahl et al., 2002; Brunnauer et al., 2011; Hasan et al., 2010). A prospective survey by Müller-Vahl et al., found 82% of GTS sufferers using cannabis reported an improvement in symptoms (1997). A more recent retrospective survey of 19 GTS patients using cannabis found 95% reported an average of 60% improvement in tics without serious adverse side effects (Abi-Jaoude et al., 2017).

One case report of a 7 year old with disabling tics and ADHD who did not respond to any behavioral or pharmaceutical intervention found significant improvement with high dose THC in combination with risperidone and guanfacine with no adverse side effects (Szejko et al., 2018). Vaporized cannabis combined with oral THC was found to be effective in a 12-year-old boy with GTS who had severe insomnia from the tics. This patient had almost complete resolution of tics, as well as improved sleep with no reported adverse effects (Szejko et al., 2019).

Two randomized double-blind placebo-controlled studies in adults reported efficacy of THC for GTS far superior to placebo with no detrimental effects on cognitive function, memory, verbal learning, and other measurements of neuropsychological performance. Adverse effects were mild and resolved without intervention (Müller-Vahl et al., 2002; Müller-Vahl et al., 2003). The European and Canadian Societies for the study of Tourette syndrome recommend a trial of cannabinoid-based medication for GTS patients who have not improved with first-line treatments.

Spasticity

Spasticity is defined as "velocity-dependent increase in tonic stretch reflexes (muscle tone) with exaggeration tendon jerks, resulting from hyperexcitability of the stretch reflex" (Young, 1994). Approximately two-thirds of all children with cerebral palsy suffer with spasticity. This debilitating symptom also may occur in children with brain injuries, spinal cord injuries, or certain genetic syndromes.

Numerous studies support the use of cannabinoids for spasticity. Sativex (GW Pharmaceuticals), an oromucosal spray containing THC and CBD in a 1:1 ratio, has been available for many years and is effective for the treatment of spasticity in adults with multiple sclerosis (Giacoppo et al., 2017). In an open, uncontrolled retrospective study, 16 children and young adults with severe treatment-resistant spasticity were treated with dronabinol. Twelve patients reported abolishment or marked improvement of symptoms with no serious adverse effects (Kuhlen et al., 2016).

One other case report in the literature documented significant improvement with dronabinol treatment in spasticity in a child suffering from a rare terminal genetic condition, neuronal ceroid lipofuscinosis (also known as Batten disease) (Lorenz, 2002).

Risks of Cannabis Use in the Pediatric Patient

It is crucial to point out that recreational use of THC-rich cannabis by teenagers cannot be compared to medicinal use of cannabis for individuals struggling with chronic and debilitating medical conditions, especially when these conditions may have underlying ECS dysfunction as part of its etiology.

During adolescence, the central nervous system has an increased vulnerability to changes and exposures in its environment. Endocannabinoids are crucial in influencing neurotransmitters during this time, promoting proper circuitry, new cell growth, and maturation to the adult brain. Disruption in the ECS during this vulnerable time, for instance with heavy use of THC, may result in dysregulation of the normal maturation processes, which is why teenagers without chronic and serious illnesses should avoid recreational cannabis use.

Two studies of human adolescents aged 12–18 years who were heavy users of THC-rich cannabis reported increased risk of anxiety disorders, impulsivity issues, memory, decision-making and attention problems, and lowered verbal and overall IQ. First-time cannabis use after the age of 18 years was not associated with lowered IQ or neurocognitive performance (Renard et al., 2014; Meier et al., 2012). Additionally, there has been concern of schizophrenia in adolescents that use THC. Although the literature is conflicting, it appears teenagers who have increased risk factors, such as schizophrenia or severe mental illness in a first-degree family member and who use THC heavily from a young age, have an increased risk of developing schizophrenia (Arseneault et al., 2002; Stefanis et al., 2004; Sugranyes et al., 2009).

Interestingly, recent data from twin studies reported "youth who used cannabis at age 18 had lower IQ in childhood, prior to cannabis initiation, and had lower IQ at age 18, but there was little evidence that cannabis use was associated with IQ decline from age 12–18" and "although cannabis use was associated with lower IQ and poorer executive functions at age 18, these associations were generally not apparent within pairs of twins from the same family, suggesting that family background factors explain why adolescents who use cannabis perform worse on IQ and executive function tests." The researchers concluded that their findings suggest that the long-accepted premise that cannabis causes lower IQ and impairs executive function is now in question, even when amount of THC use reaches levels of dependence Meier et al., 2018).

Case Report

One of the author's patients, a 7-year-old male who presented with a history of seizures since infancy was also diagnosed with autism at the age of 3. He was trialed on 10 antiepileptic medications, some singly and some in combination, without improvement. He struggled with sleep, learning, memory, and behavioral issues, as well as various side effects from the two AEDs he was taking at the time of presentation. He began using CBD-rich cannabis with a CBD:THC ratio of 27:1, beginning at 1 mg/kg/day, with instructions to titrate up by 1 mg/kg/day every two weeks.

He began having less frequent seizures approximately two months into treatment, and by four months, seizures completely stopped. He continued to have symptoms of autism, mostly behavioral, as well as difficulty sleeping. Low-dose THC was introduced at this time, and he began sleeping well and having less tantrums, with no evidence of intoxication. The antiepileptic medications were weaned one at a time over a few months, and by the time they were discontinued, he was more alert and interactive with less unwanted behaviors. His parents reported that he seemed happier and was finally making progress at school, with teacher and behavioral therapists reporting better focus and learning. He was able to completely discontinue antiepileptic medications after eight months of CBD and THC treatment and has remained seizure free for the past five years with no reported side effects from medicinal cannabis treatment. His current dosing is 5.5 mg/kg/day of CBD-rich cannabis oil and 10 mg THC at night for sleep.

It is important to point out that this patient is within approximately 10% of children with intractable seizure disorders who have achieved seizure freedom with CBD-rich oil. Although this group is small, historically these patients faced a lifetime of disability with significant morbidity. Treatment with cannabis appears to be changing this almost certain poor prognosis for the better. Many patients who do not become fully seizure free are also showing significant improvement, with less frequency, less severity, and shorter duration of seizures, as well as quicker recovery after seizures with medicinal cannabis, potentially impacting future prognoses. Parents and physicians are also seeing similar improvements in the quality of life of children struggling with the other conditions discussed in this chapter.

As the cannabis industry and changes in policy march forward, so does the demand for meaningful clinical research. For healthcare professionals to properly advise parents and patients, robust investigation must be allowed. With proper knowledge, policies, and regulation, cannabis can be an effective and safe therapeutic tool in the practitioner's toolbox.

References

Aaberg, K. M., Gunnes, N., Bakken, I. J., Søraas, C. L., Berntsen, A., Magnus, P., ... Surén, P. (2017). Incidence and prevalence of childhood epilepsy: A nationwide cohort study. *Pediatrics, 139*(5), e20163908.

Abi-Jaoude, E., Chen, L., Cheung, P., Bhikram, T., & Sandor, P. (2017). Preliminary evidence on cannabis effectiveness and tolerability for adults with Tourette syndrome. *The Journal of Neuropsychiatry and Clinical Neurosciences, 29*(4), 391–400.

Abrahamov, A., Abrahamov, A., & Mechoulam, R. (1995). An efficient new cannabinoid antiemetic in pediatric oncology. *Life Sciences, 56*(23–24), 2097–2102.

Abrams, D. I. (2018). The therapeutic effects of cannabis and cannabinoids: An update from the national academies of sciences, engineering and medicine report. *European Journal of Internal Medicine, 49*, 7–11.

Alonso-Alconada, D., Alvarez, A., Alvarez, F. J., Martinez-Orgado, J. A., & Hilario, E. (2012). The cannabinoid WIN 55212-2 mitigates apoptosis and mitochondrial dysfunction after hypoxia ischemia. *Neurochemical Research, 37*(1), 161–170.

Alvarez, F. J., Lafuente, H., Rey-Santano, M. C., Mielgo, V. E., Gastiasoro, E., Rueda, M., ... Martinez-Orgado, J. (2008). Neuroprotective effects of the nonpsychoactive cannabinoid cannabidiol in hypoxic-ischemic newborn piglets. *Pediatric Research, 64*(6), 653–658.

Amenta, P. S., Jallo, J. I., Tuma, R. F., & Elliott, M. B. (2012). A cannabinoid type 2 receptor agonist attenuates blood–brain barrier damage and neurodegeneration in a murine model of traumatic brain injury. *Journal of Neuroscience Research, 90*(12), 2293–2305.

Ames, F. R., & Cridland, S. (1986). Anticonvulsant effect of cannabidiol. *South African Medical Journal, 69*(1), 14.

Aran, A., Cassuto, H., Lubotzky, A., Wattad, N., & Hazan, E. (2019). Brief report: Cannabidiol-rich cannabis in children with autism spectrum disorder and severe behavioral problems—A retrospective feasibility study. *Journal of Autism and Developmental Disorders, 49*(3), 1284–1288.

Aran, A., Eylon, M., Harel, M., Polianski, L., Nemirovski, A., Tepper, S., ... Tam, J. (2019). Lower circulating endocannabinoid levels in children with autism spectrum disorder. *Molecular Autism, 10*(1), 2.

Arseneault, L., Cannon, M., Poulton, R., Murray, R., Caspi, A., & Moffitt, T. E. (2002). Cannabis use in adolescence and risk for adult psychosis: Longitudinal prospective study. *Blood, 325*(7374), 1212–1213.

Baio, J., Wiggins, L., Christensen, D. L., Maenner, M. J., Daniels, J., Warren, Z., ... Durkin, M. S. (2018). Prevalence of autism spectrum disorder among children aged 8 years—Autism and developmental disabilities monitoring network, 11 sites, United States, 2014. *MMWR Surveillance Summaries*, 67(6), 1.

Bauman, M. L., & Kemper, T. L. (2005). Neuroanatomic observations of the brain in autism: A review and future directions. *International Journal of Developmental Neuroscience*, 23(2–3), 183–187.

Becker, K. G., & Schultz, S. T. (2010). Similarities in features of autism and asthma and a possible link to acetaminophen use. *Medical Hypotheses*, 74(1), 7–11.

Bernal_ Chico, A., Canedo, M., Manterola, A., Victoria Sánchez-Gómez, M., Pérez-Samartín, A., Rodríguez-Puertas, R., ... Mato, S. (2015). Blockade of monoacylglycerol lipase inhibits oligodendrocyte excitotoxicity and prevents demyelination in vivo. *Glia*, 63(1), 163–176.

Berrendero, F., Sepe, N., Ramos, J. A., Di Marzo, V., & Fernández-Ruiz, J. J. (1999). Analysis of cannabinoid receptor binding and mRNA expression and endogenous cannabinoid contents in the developing rat brain during late gestation and early postnatal period. *Synapse*, 33(3), 181–191.

Biegon, A., & Kerman, I. A. (2001). Autoradiographic study of pre-and postnatal distribution of cannabinoid receptors in human brain. *Neuroimage*, 14(6), 1463–1468.

Blasco-Benito, S., Seijo-Vila, M., Caro-Villalobos, M., Tundidor, I., Andradas, C., García-Taboada, E., ... Gordon, M. (2018). Appraising the "entourage effect": Antitumor action of a pure cannabinoid versus a botanical drug preparation in preclinical models of breast cancer. *Biochemical Pharmacology*, 157, 285–293.

Bossong, M. G., Mehta, M. A., van Berckel, B. N., Howes, O. D., Kahn, R. S., & Stokes, P. R. (2015). Further human evidence for striatal dopamine release induced by administration ofΔ 9-tetrahydrocannabinol (THC): Selectivity to limbic striatum. *Psychopharmacology*, 232(15), 2723–2729.

Brunnauer, A., Segmiller, F. M., Volkamer, T., Laux, G., Müller, N., & Dehning, S. (2011). Cannabinoids improve driving ability in a Tourette's patient. *Psychiatry Research*, 190(2–3), 382–382.

Buckley, N. E., Hansson, S., Harta, G., & Mezey, E. (1997). Expression of the CB1 and CB2 receptor messenger RNAs during embryonic development in the rat. *Neuroscience*, 82(4), 1131–1149.

Carracedo, A., Gironella, M., Lorente, M., Garcia, S., Guzmán, M., Velasco, G., & Iovanna, J. L. (2006). Cannabinoids induce apoptosis of pancreatic tumor cells via endoplasmic reticulum stress–related genes. *Cancer Research*, 66(13), 6748–6755.

Carrier, E. J., Patel, S., & Hillard, C. J. (2005). Endocannabinoids in neuroimmunology and stress. *Current Drug Targets-CNS and Neurological Disorders*, 4(6), 657–665.

Castillo, A., Tolón, M. R., Fernández-Ruiz, J., Romero, J., & Martinez-Orgado, J. (2010). The neuroprotective effect of cannabidiol in an in vitro model of newborn hypoxic–ischemic brain damage in mice is mediated by CB2 and adenosine receptors. *Neurobiology of Disease*, 37(2), 434–440.

Chakrabarti, B., Persico, A., Battista, N., & Maccarrone, M. (2015). Endocannabinoid signaling in autism. *Neurotherapeutics*, 12(4), 837–847.

Chan, H. S., Correia, J. A., & MacLeod, S. M. (1987). Nabilone versus prochlorperazine for control of cancer chemotherapy-induced emesis in children: A double-blind, crossover trial. *Pediatrics, 79*(6), 946–952.

Cohen-Yeshurun, A., Trembovler, V., Alexandrovich, A., Ryberg, E., Greasley, P. J., Mechoulam, R., … Leker, R. R. (2011). N-arachidonoyl-L-serine is neuroprotective after traumatic brain injury by reducing apoptosis. *Journal of Cerebral Blood Flow and Metabolism, 31*(8), 1768–1777.

Cohen-Yeshurun, A., Willner, D., Trembovler, V., Alexandrovich, A., Mechoulam, R., Shohami, E., & Leker, R. R. (2013). N-arachidonoyl-L-serine (AraS) possesses proneurogenic properties in vitro and in vivo after traumatic brain injury. *Journal of Cerebral Blood Flow and Metabolism, 33*(8), 1242–1250.

Cooper, R. E., Williams, E., Seegobin, S., Tye, C., Kuntsi, J., & Asherson, P. (2017). Cannabinoids in attention-deficit/hyperactivity disorder: A randomised-controlled trial. *European Neuropsychopharmacology, 27*(8), 795–808.

Croxford, J. L., Pryce, G., Jackson, S. J., Ledent, C., Giovannoni, G., Pertwee, R. G., … Baker, D. (2008). Cannabinoid-mediated neuroprotection, not immunosuppression, may be more relevant to multiple sclerosis. *Journal of Neuroimmunology, 193*(1–2), 120–129.

Cunha, J. M., Carlini, E. A., Pereira, A. E., Ramos, O. L., Pimentel, C., Gagliardi, R., … Mechoulam, R. (1980). Chronic administration of cannabidiol to healthy volunteers and epileptic patients. *Pharmacology, 21*(3), 175–185.

Darmani, N. A. (2001). Δ 9- tetrahydrocannabinol and synthetic cannabinoids prevent emesis produced by the cannabinoid CB1 receptor antagonist/inverse agonist SR 141716A. *Neuropsychopharmacology, 24*(2), 198–203.

Darmani, N. A., & Johnson, J. C. (2004). Central and peripheral mechanisms contribute to the antiemetic actions of delta-9-tetrahydrocannabinol against 5-hydroxytryptophan-induced emesis. *European Journal of Pharmacology, 488*(1–3), 201–212.

Deshpande, L. S., Sombati, S., Blair, R. E., Carter, D. S., Martin, B. R., & DeLorenzo, R. J. (2007). Cannabinoid CB1 receptor antagonists cause status epilepticus-like activity in the hippocampal neuronal culture model of acquired epilepsy. *Neuroscience Letters, 411*(1), 11–16.

Devinsky, O., Cross, J. H., Laux, L., Marsh, E., Miller, I., Nabbout, R., … Wright, S. (2017). Trial of cannabidiol for drug-resistant seizures in the Dravet syndrome. *New England Journal of Medicine, 376*(21), 2011–2020.

Feigenbaum, J. J., Richmond, S. A., Weissman, Y., & Mechoulam, R. (1989). Inhibition of cisplatin-induced emesis in the pigeon by a non-psychotropic synthetic cannabinoid. *European Journal of Pharmacology, 169*(1), 159–165.

Fernandez-Espejo, E., Viveros, M. P., Núñez, L., Ellenbroek, B. A., & De Fonseca, F. R. (2009). Role of cannabis and endocannabinoids in the genesis of schizophrenia. *Psychopharmacology, 206*(4), 531–549.

Fernández-López, D., Martínez-Orgado, J., Nuñez, E., Romero, J., Lorenzo, P., Moro, M. Á., & Lizasoain, I. (2006). Characterization of the neuroprotective effect of the cannabinoid agonist WIN-55212 in an in vitro model of hypoxic-ischemic brain damage in newborn rats. *Pediatric Research, 60*(2), 169–173.

Fernández-Ruiz, J., Berrendero, F., Hernández, M. L., & Ramos, J. A. (2000). The endogenous cannabinoid system and brain development. *Trends in Neurosciences, 23*(1), 14–20.

Földy, C., Malenka, R. C., & Südhof, T. C. (2013). Autism-associated neuroligin-3 mutations commonly disrupt tonic endocannabinoid signaling. *Neuron, 78*(3), 498–509.

Fride, E. (2004). The endocannabinoid-CB receptor system: Importance for development and in pediatric disease. *Neuroendocrinology Letters, 25*(1/2), 24–30.

Fride, E., Foox, A., Rosenberg, E., Faigenboim, M., Cohen, V., Barda, L., … Mechoulam, R. (2003). Milk intake and survival in newborn cannabinoid CB1 receptor knockout mice: Evidence for a "CB3" receptor. *European Journal of Pharmacology, 461*(1), 27–34.

Fride, E., Ginzburg, Y., Breuer, A., Bisogno, T., Di Marzo, V., & Mechoulam, R. (2001). Critical role of the endogenous cannabinoid system in mouse pup suckling and growth. *European Journal of Pharmacology, 419*(2–3), 207–214.

Fride, E., & Mechoulam, R. (1996). Ontogenetic development of the response to anandamide and Δ9-tetrahydrocannabinol in mice. *Developmental Brain Research, 95*(1), 131–134.

Gaston, T. E., Bebin, E. M., Cutter, G. R., Liu, Y., Szaflarski, J. P., & UAB CBD Program (2017). Interactions between cannabidiol and commonly used antiepileptic drugs. *Epilepsia, 58*(9), 1586–1592.

Gedde, M., & Maa, E. (2013, December). Whole cannabis extract of high concentration cannabidiol may calm seizures in highly refractory pediatric epilepsies. In Washington, DC: American Epilepsy Society Annual Meeting.

Giacoppo, S., Bramanti, P., & Mazzon, E. (2017). Sativex in the management of multiple sclerosis-related spasticity: An overview of the last decade of clinical evaluation. *Multiple Sclerosis and Related Disorders, 17*, 22–31.

Guerrero, A. V., Quang, P., Dekker, N., Jordan, R. C., & Schmidt, B. L. (2008). Peripheral cannabinoids attenuate carcinoma-induced nociception in mice. *Neuroscience Letters, 433*(2), 77–81.

Guzman, M., Duarte, M. J., Blazquez, C., Ravina, J., Rosa, M. C., Galve-Roperh, I. … González-Feria, L. (2006). A pilot clinical study of Δ 9-tetrahydrocannabinol in patients with recurrent glioblastoma multiforme. *British Journal of Cancer, 95*(2), 197–203.

Hamamoto, D. T., Giridharagopalan, S., & Simone, D. A. (2007). Acute and chronic administration of the cannabinoid receptor agonist CP 55,940 attenuates tumor-evoked hyperalgesia. *European Journal of Pharmacology, 558*(1–3), 73–87.

Hasan, A., Rothenberger, A., Münchau, A., Wobrock, T., Falkai, P., & Roessner, V. (2010). Oral Δ9-tetrahydrocannabinol improved refractory Gilles de la Tourette syndrome in an adolescent by increasing intracortical inhibition: A case report. *Journal of Clinical Psychopharmacology, 30*(2), 190–192.

Hassell, K. J., Ezzati, M., Alonso-Alconada, D., Hausenloy, D. J., & Robertson, N. J. (2015). New horizons for newborn brain protection: Enhancing endogenous neuroprotection. *Archives of Disease in Childhood-Fetal and Neonatal Edition, 100*(6), F541–F552.

Hemming, M., & Yellowlees, P. M. (1993). Effective treatment of Tourette's syndrome with marijuana. *Journal of Psychopharmacology, 7*(4), 389–391.

Hernández-Torres, G., Cipriano, M., Hedén, E., Björklund, E., Canales, Á., Zian, D. … Ortega-Gutiérrez, S. (2014). A reversible and selective inhibitor of monoacylglycerol lipase ameliorates multiple sclerosis. *Angewandte Chemie International Edition, 53*(50), 13765–13770.

Hill, A. J., Hill, T., & Whalley, B. (2013). The development of cannabinoid based therapies for epilepsy. In *Endocannabinoids: Molecular, pharmacological, behavioral, and clinical features* (pp. 164–204). Oak Park, IL: Bentham Science Publishers.

Hussain, S. A., Zhou, R., Jacobson, C., Weng, J., Cheng, E., Lay, J., ... Sankar, R. (2015). Perceived efficacy of cannabidiol-enriched cannabis extracts for treatment of pediatric epilepsy: A potential role for infantile spasms and Lennox–Gastaut syndrome. *Epilepsy and Behavior, 47*, 138–141.

Javid, F. A., Phillips, R. M., Afshinjavid, S., Verde, R., & Ligresti, A. (2016). Cannabinoid pharmacology in cancer research: A new hope for cancer patients? *European Journal of Pharmacology, 775*, 1–14.

Karhson, D. S., Krasinska, K. M., Dallaire, J. A., Libove, R. A., Phillips, J. M., Chien, A. S., ... Parker, K. J. (2018). Plasma anandamide concentrations are lower in children with autism spectrum disorder. *Molecular Autism, 9*(1), 18.

Kerr, D. M., Downey, L., Conboy, M., Finn, D. P., & Roche, M. (2013). Alterations in the endocannabinoid system in the rat valproic acid model of autism. *Behavioural Brain Research, 249*, 124–132.

Klein, T. W. (2005). Cannabinoid-based drugs as anti-inflammatory therapeutics. *Nature Reviews. Immunology, 5*(5), 400–411.

Knoller, N., Levi, L., Shoshan, I., Reichenthal, E., Razon, N., Rappaport, Z. H., & Biegon, A. (2002). Dexanabinol (HU-211) in the treatment of severe closed head injury: A randomized, placebo-controlled, phase II clinical trial. *Critical Care Medicine, 30*(3), 548–554.

Kuhlen, M., Hoell, J. I., Gagnon, G., Balzer, S., Oommen, P. T., Borkhardt, A., & Janßen, G. (2016). Effective treatment of spasticity using dronabinol in pediatric palliative care. *European Journal of Paediatric Neurology, 20*(6), 898–903.

Kurz, R., & Blaas, K. (2010). Use of dronabinol (delta-9-THC) in autism: A prospective single-case-study with an early infantile autistic child. *Cannabinoids, 5*(4), 4–6.

Lafuente, H., Alvarez, F. J., Pazos, M. R., Alvarez, A., Rey-Santano, M. C., Mielgo, V., ... Martinez-Orgado, J. (2011). Cannabidiol reduces brain damage and improves functional recovery after acute hypoxia-ischemia in newborn pigs. *Pediatric Research, 70*(3), 272–277.

Limebeer, C. L., & Parker, L. A. (1999).9-tetrahydrocannabinol interferes with the establishment and the expression of conditioned rejection reactions produced by cyclophosphamide: A rat model of nausea. *Delta. NeuroReport, 10*(18), 3769–3772.

Lombard, C., Nagarkatti, M., & Nagarkatti, P. S. (2005). Targeting cannabinoid receptors to treat leukemia: Role of cross-talk between extrinsic and intrinsic pathways in Δ9-tetrahydrocannabinol (THC)-induced apoptosis of Jurkat cells. *Leukemia Research, 29*(8), 915–922.

López-Valero, I., Torres, S., Salazar-Roa, M., García-Taboada, E., Hernández-Tiedra, S., Guzmán, M., ... Lorente, M. (2018). Optimization of a preclinical therapy of cannabinoids in combination with temozolomide against glioma. *Biochemical Pharmacology, 157*, 275–284.

Lorenz, R. (2002). A casuistic rationale for the treatment of spastic and myocloni in a childhood neurodegenerative disease: Neuronal ceroid lipofuscinosis of the type Jansky-Bielschowsky. *Neuro Endocrinology Letters*, 23(5–6), 387–390.

Lorenz, R. (2004). On the application of cannabis in paediatrics and epileptology. *Neuroendocrinology Letters*, 25(1/2), 40–44.

Ludányi, A., Erőss, L., Czirják, S., Vajda, J., Halász, P., Watanabe, M., ... Katona, I. (2008). Downregulation of the CB1 cannabinoid receptor and related molecular elements of the endocannabinoid system in epileptic human hippocampus. *Journal of Neuroscience*, 28(12), 2976–2990.

Maas, A. I., Murray, G., Henney III, H., Kassem, N., Legrand, V., Mangelus, M., ... Knoller, N. (2006). Efficacy and safety of dexanabinol in severe traumatic brain injury: Results of a phase III randomised, placebo-controlled, clinical trial. *The Lancet Neurology*, 5(1), 38–45.

Mato, S., Del Olmo, E., & Pazos, A. (2003). Ontogenetic development of cannabinoid receptor expression and signal transduction functionality in the human brain. *European Journal of Neuroscience*, 17(9), 1747–1754.

Mauler, F., Hinz, V., Augstein, K. H., Fasbender, M., & Horváth, E. (2003). Neuroprotective and brain edema-reducing efficacy of the novel cannabinoid receptor agonist BAY 38-7271. *Brain Research*, 989(1), 99–111.

McCarty, L. E., & Borison, H. L. (1981). Antiemetic activity of N-Methyllevonantradol and nabilone in cisplatin-treated cats. *The Journal of Clinical Pharmacology*, 21 (Suppl.1), 30S–37S, 94(5), 882–887.

McFadden, K., & Minshew, N. (2013). Evidence for dysregulation of axonal growth and guidance in the etiology of ASD. *Frontiers in Human Neuroscience*, 7, 671.

Mechoulam, R., & Carlini, E. A. (1978). Toward drugs derived from cannabis. *Naturwissenschaften*, 65(4), 174–179.

Meier, M. H., Caspi, A., Ambler, A., Harrington, H., Houts, R., Keefe, R. S., ... Moffitt, T. E. (2012). Persistent cannabis users show neuropsychological decline from childhood to midlife. *Proceedings of the National Academy of Sciences*, 109(40), E2657–E2664.

Meier, M. H., Caspi, A., Danese, A., Fisher, H. L., Houts, R., Arseneault, L., & Moffitt, T. E. (2018). Associations between adolescent cannabis use and neuropsychological decline: A longitudinal co-twin control study. *Addiction*, 113(2), 257–265.

Micale, V., Mazzola, C., & Drago, F. (2007). Endocannabinoids and neurodegenerative diseases. *Pharmacological Research*, 56(5), 382–392.

Milz, E., & Grotenhermen, F. (2015, September). Successful therapy of treatment resistant adult ADHD with cannabis: Experience from a medical practice with 30 patients. In *Abstract book of the Cannabinoid conference* (pp. 17–19).

Müller-Vahl, K. R., Kolbe, H., & Dengler, R. (1997). Gilles de la Tourette-Syndrom Einfluß von Nikotin, Alkohol und Marihuana auf die klinische Symptomatik. *Nervenarzt*, 68(12), 985–989.

Müller-Vahl, K. R., Schneider, U., & Emrich, H. M. (2002). Combined treatment of Tourette syndrome with Δ9-THC and dopamine receptor antagonists. *Journal of Cannabis Therapeutics*, 2(3–4), 145–154.

Müller-Vahl, K. R., Schneider, U., Koblenz, A., Jöbges, M., Kolbe, H., Daldrup, T., & Emrich, H. M. (2002). Treatment of Tourette's syndrome with Δ9-tetrahydrocannabinol (THC): A randomized crossover trial. *Pharmacopsychiatry*, 35(02), 57–61.

Müller-Vahl, K. R., Schneider, U., Kolbe, U., H., & Emrich, H. M. (1999). Treatment of Tourette's syndrome with delta-9-tetrahydrocannabinol. *American Journal of Psychiatry, 156*(3), 495–495.

Müller-Vahl, K. R., Schneider, U., Prevedel, H., et al. (2003). δ9-tetrahydrocannabinol (THC) is effective in the treatment of tics in Tourette syndrome: A 6-week randomized trial. *The Journal of Clinical Psychiatry, 64*(4), 459–465.

Munson, A. E., Harris, L. S., Friedman, M. A., Dewey, W. L., & Carchman, R. A. (1975).Antineoplastic activity of cannabinoids. *Journal of the National Cancer Institute, 55*(3), 597–602.

Nagarkatti, P., Pandey, R., Rieder, S. A., Hegde, V. L., & Nagarkatti, M. (2009). Cannabinoids as novel anti-inflammatory drugs. *Future Medicinal Chemistry, 1*(7), 1333–1349.

National Academies of Sciences, Engineering, and Medicine (2017). *The health effects of cannabis and cannabinoids: The current state of evidence and recommendations for research*. Washington, DC: National Academies Press.

Nguyen, B. M., Kim, D., Bricker, S., Bongard, F., Neville, A., Putnam, B., … Plurad, D. (2014). Effect of marijuana use on outcomes in traumatic brain injury. *American Surgeon, 80*(10), 979–983.

O'Shaughnessy, W. B. (1843). On the preparations of the Indian hemp, or Gunjah: Cannabis indica their effects on the animal system in health, and their utility in the treatment of tetanus and other convulsive diseases. *Provincial Medical Journal and Retrospect of the Medical Sciences, 5*(123), 363.

Panikashvili, D., Mechoulam, R., Beni, S. M., Alexandrovich, A., & Shohami, E. (2005). CB1 cannabinoid receptors are involved in neuroprotection via NF-κB inhibition. *Journal of Cerebral Blood Flow and Metabolism, 25*(4), 477–484.

Paria, B. c., & Dey, S. K. (2000). Ligand-receptor signaling with endocannabinoids in preimplantation embryo development and implantation. *Chemistry and Physics of Lipids, 108*(1–2), 211–220.

Parker, L. A., & Mechoulam, R. (2003). Cannabinoid agonists and antagonists modulate lithium-induced conditioned gaping in rats. *Integrative Physiological and Behavioral Science, 38*(2), 133–145.

Pazos, M. R., Cinquina, V., Gómez, A., Layunta, R., Santos, M., Fernández-Ruiz, J., & Martínez-Orgado, J. (2012). Cannabidiol administration after hypoxia–ischemia to newborn rats reduces long-term brain injury and restores neurobehavioral function. *Neuropharmacology, 63*(5), 776–783.

Pazos, M. R., Mohammed, N., Lafuente, H., Santos, M., Martínez-Pinilla, E., Moreno, E., … Hillard, C. J. (2013). Mechanisms of cannabidiol neuroprotection in hypoxic–ischemic newborn pigs: Role of 5HT1A and CB2 receptors. *Neuropharmacology, 71*, 282–291.

Perucca, P., & Gilliam, F. G. (2012). Adverse effects of antiepileptic drugs. *The Lancet Neurology, 11*(9), 792–802.

Pham, L., Chen, J., Tamayo, A., Bryant, J., Yang, D., & Ford Jr., R. J. (2016). Cannabinoid receptor signaling as a target for personalized therapy in aggressive B cell lymphomas. *Blood*. Retrieved from https://ashpublications.org/blood/articl e/128/22/4181/114331/Cannabinoid-Receptor-Signaling- As-a-Target-for

Porcari, G. S., Fu, C., Doll, E. D., Carter, E. G., & Carson, R. P. (2018). Efficacy of artisanal preparations of cannabidiol for the treatment of epilepsy: Practical experiences in a tertiary medical center. *Epilepsy and Behavior, 80*, 240–246.

Porter, B. E., & Jacobson, C. (2013). Report of a parent survey of cannabidiol-enriched cannabis use in pediatric treatment-resistant epilepsy. *Epilepsy and Behavior, 29*(3), 574–577.

Potenzieri, C., Harding-Rose, C., & Simone, D. A. (2008). The cannabinoid receptor agonist, WIN 55, 212–2, attenuates tumor-evoked hyperalgesia through peripheral mechanisms. *Brain Research, 1215*, 69–75.

Pryce, G., Ahmed, Z., Hankey, D. J., Jackson, S. J., Croxford, J. L., Pocock, J. M., … Cuzner, M. L. (2003). Cannabinoids inhibit neurodegeneration in models of multiple sclerosis. *Brain, 126*(10), 2191–2202.

Ramer, R., & Hinz, B. (2015). New insights into antimetastatic and antiangiogenic effects of cannabinoids. In *International review of cell and molecular biology*. Cambridge: Academic Press, *314*.

Raup-Konsavage, W. M., Johnson, M., Legare, C. A., Yochum, G. S., Morgan, D. J., & Vrana, K. E. (2018). Synthetic cannabinoid activity against colorectal cancer cells. *Cannabis and Cannabinoid Research, 3*(1), 272–281.

Ray, A. P., Griggs, L., & Darmani, N. A. (2009). Δ9-tetrahydrocannabinol suppresses vomiting behavior and Fos expression in both acute and delayed phases of cisplatin-induced emesis in the least shrew. *Behavioural Brain Research, 196*(1), 30–36.

Renard, J., Krebs, M. O., Le Pen, G., & Jay, T. M. (2014). Long-term consequences of adolescent cannabinoid exposure in adult psychopathology. *Frontiers in Neuroscience, 8*, 361.

Rettori, E., De Laurentiis, A., Zubilete, M. Z., Rettori, V., & Elverdin, J. C. (2012). Anti-inflammatory effect of the endocannabinoid anandamide in experimental periodontitis and stress in the rat. *Neuroimmunomodulation, 19*(5), 293–303.

Roberto, D., Klotz, L. H., & Venkateswaran, V. (2017). Cannabinoids as an anticancer agent for prostate cancer. *Journal of Urology and Research, 4*(3), 1090–1097.

Rock, E. M., Limebeer, C. L., Fletcher, P. J., Mechoulam, R., & Parker, L. A. (2010). *Cannabidiol (the non-psychoactive component of cannabis) may act as a 5-HT1A auto-receptor agonist to reduce toxin-induced nausea and vomiting.* Poster presented at the Society for Neuroscience meeting, San Diego, CA.

Romigi, A., Bari, M., Placidi, F., Marciani, M. G., Malaponti, M., Torelli, F., … Chiaramonte, C. (2010). Cerebrospinal fluid levels of the endocannabinoid anandamide are reduced in patients with untreated newly diagnosed temporal lobe epilepsy. *Epilepsia, 51*(5), 768–772.

Rosenberg, E. C., Patra, P. H., & Whalley, B. J. (2017). Therapeutic effects of cannabinoids in animal models of seizures, epilepsy, epileptogenesis, and epilepsy-related neuroprotection. *Epilepsy and Behavior, 70*(B), 319–327.

Russo, E. B. (2008). Clinical endocannabinoid deficiency (CECD): Can this concept explain therapeutic benefits of cannabis in migraine, fibromyalgia, irritable bowel syndrome and other treatment-resistant conditions? *Neuro Endocrinology Letters, 29*(2), 192–200.

Sandyk, R., & Awerbuch, G. (1988). Marijuana and Tourette's syndrome. *Journal of Clinical Psychopharmacology, 8*, 844.

Schleider, L. B. L., Mechoulam, R., Saban, N., Meiri, G., & Novack, V. (2019). Real life experience of medical cannabis treatment in autism: Analysis of safety and efficacy. *Scientific Reports, 9*(1), 1–7.

Schultz, S. T. (2010). Can autism be triggered by acetaminophen activation of the endocannabinoid system? *Acta neurobiologiae experimentalis, 70*(2), 227–231.

Sharkey, K. A., Cristino, L., Oland, L. D., Van Sickle, M. D., Starowicz, K., Pittman, Q. J., ... Di Marzo, V. (2007). Arvanil, anandamide and N-arachidonoyl-dopamine (NADA) inhibit emesis through cannabinoid CB1 and vanilloid TRPV1 receptors in the ferret. *European Journal of Neuroscience, 25*(9), 2773–2782.

Sharkey, K. A., Darmani, N. A., & Parker, L. A. (2014). Regulation of nausea and vomiting by cannabinoids and the endocannabinoid system. *European Journal of Pharmacology, 722*, 134–146.

Shohami, E., Novikov, M., & Bass, R. (1995). Long-term effect of HU-211, a novel non-competitive NMDA antagonist, on motor and memory functions after closed head injury in the rat. *Brain Research, 674*(1), 55–62.

Short, S. C., & Little, C. (2017). ACTR-56. A 2-part safety and exploratory efficacy randomised double-blind, placebo-controlled study OF A 1:1 ratio of cannabidiol and Delta-9-tetrahydrocannabinol (CBD: THC) plus dose-intense temozolomide in patients with recurrent glioblastoma multiforme (GBM). *Neuro-Oncology, 19* (Suppl. 6), vi13–vi13.

Simmerman, E., Qin, X., Jack, C. Y., & Baban, B. (2019). Cannabinoids as a potential new and novel treatment for melanoma: A pilot study in a murine model. *Journal of Surgical Research, 235*, 210–215.

Simoneau, I. I., Hamza, M. S., Mata, H. P., Siegel, E. M., Vanderah, T. W., Porreca, F., ... Malan, T. P. (2001). The cannabinoid agonist WIN55, 212–2 suppresses opioid-induced emesis in ferrets.

Siniscalco, D., Bradstreet, J. J., Cirillo, A., & Antonucci, N. (2014). The in vitro GcMAF effects on endocannabinoid system transcriptionomics, receptor formation, and cell activity of autism-derived macrophages. *Journal of Neuroinflammation, 11*(1), 78.

Siniscalco, D., Sapone, A., Giordano, C., Cirillo, A., de Magistris, L., Rossi, F., ... Antonucci, N. (2013). Cannabinoid receptor type 2, but not type 1, is up-regulated in peripheral blood mononuclear cells of children affected by autistic disorders. *Journal of Autism and Developmental Disorders, 43*(11), 2686–2695.

Siniscalco, D., Schultz, S., Brigida, A. L., & Antonucci, N. (2018). Inflammation and neuro-immune dysregulations in autism spectrum disorders. *Pharmaceuticals, 11*(2), 56.

Smith, S. C., & Wagner, M. S. (2014). Clinical endocannabinoid deficiency (CECD) revisited: Can this concept explain the therapeutic benefits of cannabis in migraine, fibromyalgia, irritable bowel syndrome and other treatment-resistant conditions? *Neuro Endocrinology Letters, 35*(3), 198–201.

Stefanis, N. C., Delespaul, P., Henquet, C., Bakoula, C., Stefanis, C. N., & Van Os, J. (2004). Early adolescent cannabis exposure and positive and negative dimensions of psychosis. *Addiction, 99*(10), 1333–1341.

Sugranyes, G., Flamarique, I., Parellada, E., Baeza, I., Goti, J., Fernandez-Egea, E., & Bernardo, M. (2009). Cannabis use and age of diagnosis of schizophrenia. *European Psychiatry, 24*(5), 282–286.

Sulak, D., Saneto, R., & Goldstein, B. (2017). The current status of artisanal cannabis for the treatment of epilepsy in the United States. *Epilepsy and Behavior, 70*(B), 328–333.

Szejko, N., Jakubovski, E., Fremer, C., Kunert, K., & Müller-Vahl, K. (2018). Delta-9-tetrahydrocannabinol for the treatment of a child with Tourette syndrome: Case report. EJMCR, 2, 39–41.

Szejko, N., Jakubovski, E., Fremer, C., & Müller-Vahl, K. R. (2019). Vaporized cannabis is effective and well-tolerated in an adolescent with Tourette syndrome. *Medical Cannabis and Cannabinoids*, 2(1), 60–64.

Thiele, E. A., Marsh, E. D., French, J. A., Mazurkiewicz-Beldzinska, M., Benbadis, S. R., Joshi, C., …Gunning, B. (2018). Cannabidiol in patients with seizures associated with Lennox-Gastaut syndrome (GWPCARE4): A randomised, double-blind, placebo-controlled phase 3 trial. *Lancet*, 391(10125), 1085–1096.

Tzadok, M., Uliel-Siboni, S., Linder, I., Kramer, U., Epstein, O., Menascu, S., … Dor, M. (2016). CBD-enriched medical cannabis for intractable pediatric epilepsy: The current Israeli experience. *Seizure*, 35, 41–44.

Van Sickle, M. D., Duncan, M., Kingsley, P. J., Mouihate, A., Urbani, P., Mackie, K., … Marnett, L. J. (2005). Identification and functional characterization of brainstem cannabinoid CB2 receptors. *Science*, 310(5746), 329–332.

Velasco, G., Hernández-Tiedra, S., Dávila, D., & Lorente, M. (2016a). The use of cannabinoids as anticancer agents. *Progress in Neuro-Psychopharmacology and Biological Psychiatry*, 64, 259–266.

Velasco, G., Sánchez, C., & Guzmán, M. (2016b). Anticancer mechanisms of cannabinoids. *Current Oncology*, 23(Suppl. 2), S23.

Vinod, K. Y., & Hungund, B. L. (2006). Role of the endocannabinoid system in depression and suicide. *Trends in Pharmacological Sciences*, 27(10), 539–545.

Viveros, M. P., Marco, E. M., & File, S. E. (2005). Endocannabinoid system and stress and anxiety responses. *Pharmacology, Biochemistry and Behavior*, 81(2), 331–342.

Wallace, M. J., Blair, R. E., Falenski, K. W., Martin, B. R., & DeLorenzo, R. J. (2003). The endogenous cannabinoid system regulates seizure frequency and duration in a model of temporal lobe epilepsy. *Journal of Pharmacology and Experimental Therapeutics*, 307(1), 129–137.

Wei, D., Dinh, D., Lee, D., Li, D., Anguren, A., Moreno-Sanz, G., … Piomelli, D. (2016). Enhancement of anandamide-mediated endocannabinoid signaling corrects autism-related social impairment. *Cannabis and Cannabinoid Research*, 1(1), 81–89.

Young, R. R. (1994). Spasticity: A review. *Neurology*, 44(11 Suppl. 9), S12–S20.

Chapter 7

Current and Future Uses of Medical Cannabis for Adults

Sherry Yafai

This chapter will provide the reader with a general overview of the medical use and indications for cannabis use for adults. This information is generally lacking in our current education for healthcare and human services professions, but it is necessary in order to properly educate patients and improve patient care and outcomes. This includes the use of both FDA and DEA approved medications, as well as artisanal cannabis formulations available in local dispensaries throughout the United States.

Content in this chapter is designed to teach the reader about indications for use and dosages available, where applicable, based on currently available research. After reading this chapter a clinician should be able to cite current available medical literature to help patients choose cannabis products with better treatment outcomes, in a shorter duration of time and minimize potential side effects. The end of the chapter looks at future directions for cannabis as a treatment strategy for the current opiate crisis.

The current approach for patients with significant medical illnesses is asking budtenders for recommendations about products to use, its dosage, and frequency. This all occurs without discussion about patients' other medications and/or medical histories. Unlike physicians, pharmacists, or nurses, budtenders have no educational prerequisites and can dispense any variety of cannabis medications including any dose, any quantity, and route of dosing within that state's laws. This is concerning, especially when older patients with multiple medical problems and multiple medications have begun to add in cannabis products to help their medical ailments without consideration for their other medications, in particular sedative-type medications. The reader should remember that diagnosis and dosage matters; giving a medication without addressing the diagnosis can be problematic. For example, Botox given for cosmetic purposes is dosed and administered differently than for the diagnosis and treatment of muscle spasms in patients with Multiple Sclerosis. Dosage also matters and is commonly focused on in Toxicology courses: Anything can be a toxin depending on dose and circumstance. Even water, when taken in large enough quantities can be deadly, causing swelling of the brain. Simply because we have not calculated the toxic dose or combination, does not mean that THC, CBD, or other cannabinoids do not have a lethal dose.

Common Medical Uses of Cannabis: Cancer

Currently there are several common medical indications that are widely accepted for cannabis usage including use as a cancer adjunct and for treatment of pain. Specifically, chronic pain, cancer-related pain, neuropathic pain, and musculoskeletal pain have been evaluated in numerous studies since the 1980s. Initially, studies involved with the pharmaceutical medication Dronabinol (trade name, Marinol), a synthetic pill form of THC, involved HIV/AIDS and cancer patients for the treatment of pain and appetite stimulation (Currier & Fliesler, 1995). These studies were incorporated into the initial Medical Marijuana Compassionate Care Act of 1996 in California. Despite decades of FDA and DEA legally regulated availability of Dronabinol, it has been used infrequently in the hospital or outpatient setting. Dronabinol is available in an oil capsule form in 2.5, 5, or 10 mg of synthetic THC with recommended dosing every 4–6 hours as needed for its given indication. Pain due to cancer that has been poorly controlled with opiates was evaluated in 2012 using Nabiximols (brand name, Sativex), a 1:1 CBD:THC oromucosal spray with 2.5 mg CBD: 2.7 mg THC per dose, with 26% improvement of pain compared with baseline (Portenoy, et al.).

Using cannabinoids, specifically low dose smoked THC, for treatment of nausea and vomiting related to chemotherapy, has been a standard indication for treatment in California since 1996. Interestingly, immune therapy is becoming used in cancer treatments more frequently, and the combination with cannabinoids is even more poorly understood. There have been reports citing the potential for cannabinoids to decrease the effectiveness of immune treatment but without an effect on overall remission (Taha et al., 2019). Breast cancer and glioblastoma are two of the most frequently reported types of cancer that have beneficial results in animal models, as documented in scientific journals by a range of cannabinoids and dosages.

Dr. Cristina Sanchez in Spain has been active in evaluating the use of cannabinoids in the treatment of breast cancer. In a review, she notes "these compounds exert anti-proliferative, pro-apoptotic, anti-migratory and anti-invasive actions in a wide spectrum of cancer cells in culture. Moreover, tumor growth, angiogenesis and metastasis are hampered by cannabinoids in xenograft-based and genetically engineered mouse models of cancer" (Caffarel et al., 2012). Unfortunately, currently there is no dose/frequency application to humans as these studies were performed on animal models using both THC and CBD.

Glioblastoma Multiforme is a type of very aggressive brain cancer that has received a considerable amount of attention for possible treatment related usage, as described by multiple articles (Galanti et al., 2008; McAllister et al.,

2005; Hashemi, Hashemi & Zali, 2016). GW pharmaceutical has also shown increase in life expectancy when using Temozolomide plus 1:1THC:CBD combination oil tinctures (www.gwpharm.com/about/news/gw-pharmaceut icals-achieves-positive-results-phase-2-proof-concept-study-glioma).

Of note, opiates are a mainstay of treatment for cancer pain. As a result of pain management focused on opiates, there is in an increasing likelihood of opiate addiction after cancer survival, with increasing rates of survivorship due to improved treatments available (Lawrence, 2017; Ward et al., 2019). This opens another avenue in which cannabinoids may be beneficial: The question of whether dependence on opiods for pain management can be decreased while using cannabinoids in parallel for chemotherapy adjunctive treatment of nausea, vomiting and anorexia.

Neuropathic Pain

University of California at San Diego (UCSD) created the Center for Medicinal Cannabis Research (CMCR) in 1999 after California's Medical Marijuana laws were implemented with a grant given to advance research in the field of cannabis. During the past 20 years, researchers at UCSD have found smoked THC products ranging from 1–4% THC have been effective for the treatment of neuropathic pain (Wilsey et al., 2013; Lee et al., 2018). Based on studies done at UCSD's CMCR and the efforts of Society of Cannabis Clinicians (SCC), a change in the California Medical Board's guidelines for medical cannabis recommendations was instituted in 2017. This change placed cannabis on an equal footing to pharmaceutical medications in the treatment guidelines for neuropathic pain (www.mbc.ca.gov/ Publications/guidelines_cannabis_recommendation.pdf).

Arthritic Pain

Pain due to arthritis potentially can be treated by two different modalities with cannabinoids. The first is through topical pathways, as first identified in 2016 by Hammell et al., (European Journal of Pain). That study showed the use of topical CBD on arthritic rats can reduce inflammation and pain-related behaviors as measured by significantly decreased joint swelling, limb posture scores as a rating of spontaneous pain, immune cell infiltration, and size of the synovial membrane in a dose-dependent manner. The second pathway is potentially through a systemic approach, such as inhaled, sublingual, or ingested cannabinoid. Currently there are no available rigorous control studies, only studies reviewing perspectives on potential treatment and possibilities which are varied and inconsistent (Lowin et al., 2019). In 2019, UCLA was awarded a grant under Dr. Veena Ranganath to study the use of oral CBD for the treatment of rheumatoid arthritis with results pending at the time of this publication.

Of note, narcotics are commonly used for treatment of arthritic pain, another avenue where cannabinoids may decrease the need for narcotic use (Hereford et al., 2018; Goodwin, Kraemer, & Bajwa, 2005).

Insomnia

The use of cannabis products for insomnia has been a long-discussed treatment pathway with many claims by the cannabis/hemp industry on treatment of insomnia both in terms of CBD and THC. CBD has been shown to be a wake-inducing compound that activates neurons, according to studies (Murillo-Rodríguez et al., 2008; Murillo-Rodríguez et al., 2014). A different study in 2012 showed CBD decreased anxiety-induced sleep disturbances but did not improve deep sleep overall (Hsiao et al., 2012). This has been frequently mis-advertised by CBD manufacturers, which consistently claim CBD as a treatment for insomnia. Often CBD-only products contain other ingredients such as melatonin, magnesium, and calming terpenes added in to help with sleep. However, sedation may be dose related and perhaps achieved with higher dosages of CBD. This dose-related effect is most notable in products such as Epidiolex, a pharmaceutical plant-based CBD, which has as a listed side effect "difficulty sleeping (insomnia, disordered sleep, and poor quality sleep)" (www.rxlist.com/epidiolex-side-effects-drug-ce nter.htm). Another study in 2019 showed that CBD disrupts the circadian rhythm in microglial cells, while THC does not (Lafaye et al., 2019).

This leads to consideration of THC for sleep. First identified in 1972, THC tends to have sedating effects with increases in deep sleep (NREM) (Pivik et al.,1972). A study evaluating Dronabinol, a THC isolate, identified sleep as a key side effect (Nicholson et al., 2004). A review of human studies through 2014 showed that THC does not seem to affect sleep in healthy patients but does seem helpful for those with a medical condition that has impacted their sleep. For example, patients with pain and spasticity show improvement in sleep with THC (Gates et al., 2014). These studies are consistent with clinical experience as well, with patients trying CBD as a sleep aid and getting occasional small benefits from large doses of CBD. Routinely changing patients to THC-based medications provides improved sleep consistently. This often requires starting at a low dose of THC (0.5–1 mg orally) and gradually increasing by small increments to desired effect, being mindful of other sedatives a patient is taking and consideration of decreasing other sedatives concurrently.

Another possible treatment for sleep is the usage of THC and CBD combination medications. A recent extension study of Sativex (1:1 CBD: THC) showed 20–50% of subjects were able to attain good sleep quality (Russo et al., 2007). This option is also useful for patients who have a history of negative side effects from THC alone. Unlike pharmaceutical medications, known as hypnosedatives, which cause most patients to have a complete "black out" sleep, THC and THC/CBD combination medications tend towards a more natural feeling of tiredness, desire to sleep, and allows for conscious wake-ups in the middle of the night with an easier time falling back to sleep.

Depending on the mode of administration, cannabis medications can be used to help with two aspects of sleep: falling asleep and staying asleep. Patients with difficulty falling asleep may be better assisted with a rapid onset medication, i.e. quick on and quick off, which can be achieved with an inhaled product. Patients with difficulty staying asleep may be better suited with a delayed onset medication, which in turn, lasts longer (roughly 6–8 hours), the length of time recommended for sleep. This can be achieved with an ingested product, with longer duration of action. For those who have difficulty with both aspects of sleep disorders, consider using a combination of medications or dose the ingested product 1–2 hours before bedtime to coincide with bedtime.

Parkinson's Disease

The use of cannabis for patients with Parkinson's is indicated for Parkinson's associated *symptoms*. For example, Parkinson's patients have increased rates of depression, pain, muscle stiffness and insomnia. In 2017, a study of 47 patients looked at the use of smokable THC (0.9 g average daily dose) with an improvement in falls, depression, pain, tremor, muscle stiffness, and sleep (Balash et al., 2017). Another study in 2014 evaluated 22 patients who smoked THC and showed improvement in tremor, rigidity, pain, sleep, and bradykinesia (Lotan et al., 2014). In both studies using inhaled THC only, there was an improvement in sleep.

Multiple Sclerosis

Multiple Sclerosis has also been studied with more interest overseas where medications such as Sativex, a 1:1 CBD:THC sublingual spray, is approved for the treatment of spasticity and has shown improvement in patient's quality of life (Giacoppo et al., 2017). One study in 2000, showed a decrease in muscle stiffness and pain in a double-blind placebo study of 279 using 5 mg–25 mg of THC daily (Zajicek et al., 2012).

Schizophrenia, CBD Only

Psychosis and induction of schizophrenia has long been considered a side effect of THC cannabis products. This has been studied again recently, with increasing or large doses of THC in smoke vape forms, known as "wax dabs" having increased potential to cause acute psychosis. (Pierre, 2017). On the other hand, CBD has recently been considered a potential treatment option for patients with schizophrenia. In 2012, CBD was noted to increase the amount of the body's circulating anandamide (natural endocannabinoid) which may contribute to antipsychotic effects (Leweke et al., 2012). It was not until 2017 when a randomized placebo control study tested the use of 1000 mg/day of CBD in schizophrenia patients resulting in a decrease in positive psychotic symptoms (McGuire et al., 2017).

Narcotic Alternative

Using cannabis-based products for decreasing or potentially removing opiates for pain management has been a much-discussed potential, especially in the backdrop of the current deadly opiate crisis in the United States that has been well documented by the Center for Disease Control (CDC) and well publicized due to the overwhelming number of deaths per day. The "solution" to this epidemic has not been found and, due to the nature of this epidemic, there has been a rise in the number of deaths every year (image below from the CDC website 11/9/2019: https://www.cdc.gov/drugoverdose/epidemic/index.html)

With increased mortality across the United States, many scientists and physicians have begun looking for alternatives for pain treatment. Due to

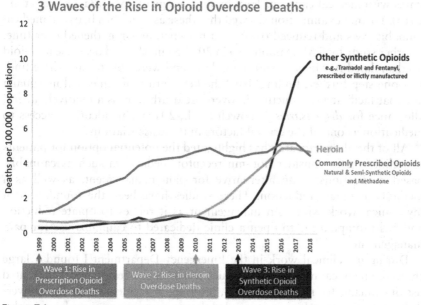

Figure 7.1

the current federal regulations, studies have looked at external markers of cannabis use as a self-mediated replacement for opiates. One study in 2016 evaluated medical cannabis use via a survey of patients (Boehnke, Litinas, & Clauw, 2016). In this study, 244 patients reported a 64% decrease in opioid use with overall improvements in quality of life (QOL) and a better side effect profile, an under-discussed aspect of patient care. Most notably, constipation is a key side effect of opiate use that causes abdominal pain, distention, and discomfort. Constipation due to opiates leads patients to seek medical care and additional medications in the form of laxatives, stool softeners, and suppositories. Severe constipation is a key missing side effect in the use of cannabinoid treatment.

In 2018, JAMA published a study showing a decrease in the number of prescription opiates filled in states with medical cannabis laws for the Medicare Part D population (Bradford et al., 2018). In the study, the authors showed a 2.11 million daily doses per year decrease (from average 23.08 million daily doses per year) when a state instituted any medical cannabis law. This was taken one step further to find that prescriptions for opiates then decreased by 3.742 million daily doses per year when medical cannabis dispensaries were opened in the state.

One would expect that if studies are showing reports of improvement in QOL and reported decreased opiate use followed by a decrease in number of prescription opiates filled, there should logically be a decrease in narcotic overdoses in those states with medical cannabis. In 2014, Bachhuber et al. showed a decrease in opioid mortality rates between 1999–2010 in states with medical cannabis laws by an average of 25% (Bachhuber et al., 2014). Further examination showed that these associations between medical cannabis laws and reduced opiate deaths generally strengthened over time. Another study by RAND published in 2015 again showed decrease in opioid deaths related to Medical Marijuana laws and were able to take these findings one step further, finding that "the key feature of a medical marijuana law that facilitates a reduction in overdose death rates is a relatively liberal allowance for *dispensaries*." (Powell et al., 2015) This identifies access to medication as one of the crucial factors in these associations.

All of the above research has highlighted the potential option for patients and clinicians to consider non-mu receptor medication such as cannabis-based medications as an alternative for pain management, as well as a method for opiate reduction. These studies have been the foundation of my clinical work with pain management as it relates to opiate reduction and has prompted me to open a clinic dedicated to cannabis use for pain management.

During my clinical work in the Emergency Department I found a large shortcoming in cannabis medical education and, as a result, poorly executed use of cannabis for medical patients, resulting in accidental non-lethal overdoses. Oncologists who recommended that patients use or consider cannabis would tell patients to "Google it." "Google-ing" a medication for treatment purposes is not the standard practice in any medical setting, and it should not be the standard for cannabis medicine. It was the culmination of these experiences and research—at a time when California's new Adult Use of Marijuana Act, allowing individuals over 21 to legally purchase cannabis for recreational purposes—that gave birth to my office, The ReLeaf Institute (TRI) in 2017.

TRI's mission to educate individuals on how to use cannabis products to accomplish their personal goals for medical treatment resulted in decreasing dosages and frequency of pharmaceutical medications prescribed. Within a few months of working at TRI, patients with pain who sought assistance became a substantial portion of my evaluations. The use of medical cannabis produced better, more consistent outcomes for these patients. Patients referred to the office with chronic pain and opiate, benzodiazepine, or hypnosedatives dependence have an option to decrease and/or remove medications which were not treating their pain, anxiety, or sleep well, rather than creating increased need for increased dose/frequency of pills. This increase in pain, referred to as Opioid Induced Hyperalgesia (Lee et al. 2011), can be the culprit of persistent and worsening pain despite opiate use for pain. Patients who seek medical attention to use cannabis frequently do not want to "get high" nor become physically dependent on another substance and are often out of options.

Currently, individuals are expected to decrease their narcotic use by 10% per week according to the CDC (Dowell et al. 2016) without any bridge therapy and are often not able to reduce by much. With the work done at TRI, I have found patients are able to reduce narcotics purposefully, by starting them on cannabis oils and edibles. In a dozen patients with history of chronic prescription opiate use from ages 30–70, weaning protocols were started with the addition of cannabis oils and edibles (all non-inhaled pathways), and all patients were able to stop all narcotics, except one who reduced prescription opiates by 50%. Patients were able to avoid nausea, vomiting, and diarrhea—all symptoms of active withdrawal from opiates. Patients were also able to reduce and/or remove opiates within a 3–4-month time frame (typically), decreasing by ~25% at each interval. Opiates that have been decreased to date are Percocet, Morphine, Oxycodone/Oxycontin, Norco, Fentanyl Patches, and Tramadol. Patients received daily phone calls with the physician, when appropriate, to ensure there were no negative side effects either from narcotic withdrawal or cannabis medication. Withdrawal symptoms were not all masked by treatment with cannabis-based medications. Symptoms that do remain are anxiety, mild pain, joint aches, and changes in bowel movements. Most often the changes in bowel movements are improvements, with decreases in need for stool softeners and laxatives while having increases in daily formed stools. Depending on the individual, cannabis was either continued or discontinued in part due to pain levels, sleep disorders and patient preference. For example, one patient required discontinuation of all cannabis products in order to return to his home, a state where cannabis was illegal. The patient later required modification of pain and was restarted on a Hemp CBD only liquid with reduction in pain. These results and conclusions parallel another recent study in 2019 by Takakuwa et al. in which cannabis-based medications were used instead of prescription opiates or as an adjunct to opiates to diminish pain for patients with chronic pain and chronic opiate use (www.liebertpub.com/doi/full/10.1089/can.2019.0039).

As identified in the Takakuwa et al. study above, another avenue for those with prescription opiate dependence could be the use of cannabis medications as an adjunct to prescription opiates for persistent pain management (Cooper et al., 2018). Consider many patients who are on X mg of Morphine or Oxycodone with 7/10 pain with increased pain despite their current opiate regimen. Currently our treatment strategies are to increase the dosage or frequency or add in another opiate to treat the patient's pain, for example, adding in Percocet three times a day in addition to Oxycodone twice daily. Another option to consider would be to add on cannabis medications, based on research studies by Abrams et al. (2011); Grenald et al. (2017); and Cooper et al. (2018) (www.nature.com/articles/s41386-018-0011-2/), which show synergistic effects of THC and opiates. The study by Abrams et al. showed that in twenty-one patients the use of inhaled THC used three times a day along with prescription opiates gave an average of 27% decrease in pain. In all three studies, THC use plus opiates decreased pain sensation.

Future Directions

While this chapter has provided insight on available research on cannabinoids such as THC and CBD, more rigorous double-blind placebo studies are needed to further enhance our clinical knowledge of patient treatment for a variety of diagnoses. Medical indications continue to increase with time, with the Farm Bill of 2019 opening many avenues for research on Hemp CBD. This Bill has decreased the roadblocks to cannabis and has allowed for an increase in research on CBD. In 2019, three million dollars in grant funding was awarded from the UCSD CMCR department to five groups with focuses on CBD isolates (https://ucsdnews.ucsd.edu/pressrelease/uc-san-diegos-center-for-medicinal-cannabis-research-awards-grants-for-five-novel-studies). As research results are presented, it is important to remember that CBD and THC, as well as the multitude of other cannabinoids and terpenes, may provide beneficial effects when given together. This concept, referred to commonly as "the entourage effect," has still not been clearly elucidated. Consider this in practice: Adding in small amounts of THC or other cannabinoids may effectively lead a patient to using smaller dosages of CBD to obtain the same end effect and vice versa. Adding in terpenes that are stripped from these research products or isolates may again provide an advantage to natural plant products as compared to research products. Ultimately, effective dose and ratio are yet to be determined.

Overall, there is a trend towards cannabis being treated more frequently like other medications with medical indications, benefits, and acceptable known side effects. To overstate either the benefits, indications, or negative side effects would only be advantageous to the companies creating, selling, or manufacturing products, which has always been the challenge between the prescriber and the dispenser. Potential use of cannabis prior to the initiation, removal, or minimization of opiate usage is a future potential that has already been shown to have positive outcomes. There will continue to be the need for large, randomized, double-blind studies to evaluate these medications in the format of a scientific model to eliminate positive and negative bias that tends to be prevalent in this field.

References

Abrams, D. I., Couey, P., Shade, S. B., Kelly, M. E., & Benowitz, N. L. (2011). Cannabinoid-opioid interaction in chronic pain. *Clinical Pharmacology and Therapeutics*, *90*(6), 844–851. Retrieved 11 11, 2019, from https://ncbi.nlm.nih.gov/pubmed/22048225

Bachhuber, M. A., Bachhuber, M. A., Saloner, B., Saloner, B., Cunningham, C. O., Barry, C. L., & Barry, C. L. (2014). Medical cannabis laws and opioid analgesic overdose mortality in the United States, 1999–2010. *JAMA Internal Medicine*, *174*(10), 1668–1673. Retrieved 9 20, 2019, from https://jamanetwork.com/journals/jamainternalmedicine/fullarticle/1898878

Balash, Y., Schleider, L. B.-L., Korczyn, A. D., Shabtai, H., Knaani, J., Rosenberg, A., ... Gurevich, T. (2017). Medical Cannabis in Parkinson disease: Real-life patients' experience. *Clinical Neuropharmacology*, *40*(6), 268–272. Retrieved 8 26, 2019, from https://insights.ovid.com/clinical-neuropharmacology/clneu/2017/11/000/medical-cannabis-parkinson-disease-real-life/8/00002826

Boehnke, K. F., Litinas, E., & Clauw, D. J. (2016). Medical cannabis use is associated with decreased opiate medication use in a retrospective cross-sectional survey of patients with chronic pain. *The Journal of Pain*, *17*(6), 739–744. Retrieved 9 20, 2019, from https://sciencedirect.com/science/article/abs/pii/s1526590016005678

Bradford, A. C., Bradford, W. D., Abraham, A. J., & Adams, G. B. (2018). Association between US state medical cannabis laws and opioid prescribing in the medicare part D population. *JAMA Internal Medicine*, *178*(5), 667–672. Retrieved 9 20, 2019, from https://jamanetwork.com/journals/jamainternalmedicine/fullarticle/2676999

Caffarel, M. M., Andradas, C., Pérez-Gómez, E., Guzmán, M., & Sánchez, C. (2012). Cannabinoids: A new hope for breast cancer therapy? *Cancer Treatment Reviews*, *38*(7), 911–918. Retrieved 8 26, 2019, from https://ncbi.nlm.nih.gov/pubmed/22776349

Cooper, Z. D., Bedi, G., Ramesh, D., Balter, R., Comer, S. D., & Haney, M. (2018). Impact of co-administration of oxycodone and smoked cannabis on analgesia and abuse liability. *Neuropsychopharmacology*, *43*(10), 1. Retrieved 12 2, 2019, from https://nature.com/articles/s41386-018-0011-2

Currier, J. S., & Fliesler, N. (1995). Dronabinol for anorexia in AIDS. *NEJM Journal Watch*, *1995*. Retrieved 9 3, 2019, from https://jwatch.org/ac199505010000010/1995/05/01/dronabinol-anorexia-aids

Dowell, D., Haegerich, T. M., & Chou, R. (2016). CDC guideline for prescribing opioids for chronic pain - United States, 2016. *MMWR Recommendations and Reports*, *65*(1), 1–49. Retrieved from https://www.cdc.gov/mmwr/volumes/65/rr/rr6501e1.htm. doi:10.15585/mmwr.rr6501e1

Galanti, G., Galanti, G., Fisher, T., Kventsel, I., Shoham, J., Gallily, R., ... Toren, A. (2008). Δ9-tetrahydrocannabinol inhibits cell cycle progression by downregulation of E2F1 in human glioblastoma multiforme cells. *Acta Oncologica*, *47*(6), 1062–1070. Retrieved 11 9, 2019, from https://ncbi.nlm.nih.gov/pubmed/17934890

Gates, P., Albertella, L., & Copeland, J. (2014). The effects of cannabinoid administration on sleep: A systematic review of human studies. *Sleep Medicine Reviews*, *18*(6), 477–487. Retrieved 9 15, 2019, from https://ncbi.nlm.nih.gov/pubmed/24726015

Giacoppo, S., Bramanti, P., & Mazzon, E. (2017). Sativex in the management of multiple sclerosis-related spasticity: An overview of the last decade of clinical evaluation. *Multiple Sclerosis and Related Disorders*, *17*, 22–31. Retrieved 11 11, 2019, from https://sciencedirect.com/science/article/pii/s2211034817301487

Goodwin, J. L., Kraemer, J. J., & Bajwa, Z. H. (2005). The use of opioids in the treatment of osteoarthritis: When, why, and how? *Current Pain and Headache Reports*, *9*(6), 390–398. Retrieved 12 2, 2019, from https://ncbi.nlm.nih.gov/pubmed/16282039

Grenald, S. A., Young, M. A., Wang, Y., Ossipov, M. H., Ibrahim, M. M., Largent-Milnes, T. M., & Vanderah, T. W. (2017). Synergistic attenuation of chronic pain using mu opioid and cannabinoid receptor 2 agonists. *Neuropharmacology*, *116*, 59–70. Retrieved 11 11, 2019, from https://ncbi.nlm.nih.gov/pubmed/28007501

Hammell, D., Zhang, L., Ma, F., Abshire, S., McIlwrath, S., Stinchcomb, A., & Westlund, K. (2016). Transdermal cannabidiol reduces inflammation and pain-related behaviours in a rat model of arthritis. *European Journal of Pain*, *20*(6), 936–948. doi:10.1002/ejp.818

Hashemi, F., Hashemi, M., & Zali, A. (2016). Cannabinoids as a promising therapeutic approach for the treatment of glioblastoma multiforme: A literature review. *International Clinical Neuroscience Journal*, *3*(3), 138–143. Retrieved 11 9, 2019, from http://journals.sbmu.ac.ir/neuroscience/article/view/13655

Hereford, T. E., Cryar, K. A., Edwards, P. K., Siegel, E. R., Barnes, C. L., & Mears, S. C. (2018). Patients with hip or knee arthritis underreport narcotic usage. *Journal of Arthroplasty*, *33*(10), 3113–3117. Retrieved 12 2, 2019, from https://sciencedirect.com/science/article/pii/s0883540318305163

Hsiao, Y.-T., Yi, P.-L., Yi, P.-L., Li, C.-L., Chang, F.-C., & Chang, F.-C. (2012). Effect of cannabidiol on sleep disruption induced by the repeated combination tests consisting of open field and elevated plus-maze in rats. *Neuropharmacology*, *62*(1), 373–384. Retrieved 9 3, 2019, from https://ncbi.nlm.nih.gov/pubmed/21867717

https://doi.org/10.1634/theoncologist.2018-0383. Epub 2019 Jan 22.

https://doi.org/10.1634/theoncologist.2018-0383. Epub 2019 Jan 22.

Lafaye, G., Desterke, C., Marulaz, L., & Benyamina, A. (2019). Cannabidiol affects circadian clock core complex and its regulation in microglia cells. *Addiction Biology*, 24(5), 921–934. Retrieved 11 9, 2019, from https://onlinelibrary.wil ey.com/doi/full/10.1111/adb.12660

Lawrence, L. (2017). *Opioid use increased among cancer survivors*. Retrieved 12 2, 2019, from https://cancernetwork.com/survivorship/opioid-use-increased-among -cancer-survivors

Lee, G., Grovey, B., Furnish, T., & Wallace, M. S. (2018). Medical cannabis for neuropathic pain. *Current Pain and Headache Reports*, 22(1), 8. Retrieved 11 9, 2019, from https://ncbi.nlm.nih.gov/pubmed/29388063

Lee, M., Silverman, S. M., Hansen, H., Patel, V. B., & Manchikanti, L. (2011 March-April). A comprehensive review of opioid-induced hyperalgesia. *Pain Physician*, 14(2), 145–161. Retrieved from https://www.ncbi.nlm.nih.gov/pubmed/21412369

Leweke, F., Piomelli, D., Pahlisch, F., Muhl, D., Gerth, C., Hoyer, C., ... Koethe, D. (2012). Cannabidiol enhances anandamide signaling and alleviates psychotic symptoms of schizophrenia. *Translational Psychiatry*, 2(3). Retrieved 8 26, 2019, from https://ncbi.nlm.nih.gov/pmc/articles/pmc3316151

Lotan, I., Treves, T. A., Roditi, Y., & Djaldetti, R. (2014). Cannabis (medical marijuana) treatment for motor and non-motor symptoms of Parkinson disease: An open-label observational study. *Clinical Neuropharmacology*, 37(2), 41–44. Retrieved 8 26, 2019, from https://ncbi.nlm.nih.gov/pubmed/24614667

Lowin, T., Schneider, M., & Pongratz, G. (2019). Joints for joints: Cannabinoids in the treatment of rheumatoid arthritis. *Current Opinion in Rheumatology*, 31(3), 271–278. Retrieved 11 9, 2019, from https://ncbi.nlm.nih.gov/pubmed/30920973

McAllister, S. D., Chan, C., Taft, R. J., Luu, T., Abood, M. E., Moore, D. H., ... Yount, G. (2005). Cannabinoids selectively inhibit proliferation and induce death of cultured human glioblastoma multiforme cells. *Journal of Neuro-Oncology*, 74(1), 31–40. Retrieved 11 9, 2019, from https://ncbi.nlm.nih.gov/ pubmed/16078104

McGuire, P., Robson, P., Cubała, W. J., Vasile, D., Morrison, P. D., Barron, R., ... Wright, S. (2017). Cannabidiol (CBD) as an adjunctive therapy in schizophrenia: A multicenter randomized controlled trial. *American Journal of Psychiatry*, 175(3), 225–231. Retrieved 8 26, 2019, from https://ajp.psychiatryonline.org/do i/10.1176/appi.ajp.2017.17030325

Murillo-Rodríguez, E., Millán-Aldaco, D., Palomero-Rivero, M., Mechoulam, R., & Drucker-Colín, R. (2008). The nonpsychoactive cannabis constituent cannabidiol is a wake-inducing agent. *Behavioral Neuroscience*, 122(6), 1378–1382. Retrieved 9 7, 2019, from https://ncbi.nlm.nih.gov/pubmed/19045957

Murillo-Rodríguez, E., Sarro-Ramírez, A., Sánchez, D., Mijangos-Moreno, S., Tejeda-Padrón, A., Poot-Aké, A., ... Arias-Carrión, O. (2014). Potential effects of cannabidiol as a wake-promoting agent. *Current Neuropharmacology*, 12(3), 269–272. Retrieved 9 7, 2019, from https://ncbi.nlm.nih.gov/pmc/articles/pm c4023456

Nicholson, A. N., Turner, C., Stone, B. M., & Robson, P. (2004). Effect of Delta-9-tetrahydrocannabinol and cannabidiol on nocturnal sleep and early-morning behavior in young adults. *Journal of Clinical Psychopharmacology*, 24(3), 305–313. Retrieved 9 5, 2019, from https://ncbi.nlm.nih.gov/pubmed/15118485

Pierre, J. M. (2017). Risks of increasingly potent cannabis: The joint effects of potency and frequency: As THC Levels Rise, the risk of psychosis, cognitive deficits, and structural brain changes increases. *Current Psychiatry*, *16*(2), 14. Retrieved 9 3, 2019, from https://questia.com/library/journal/1g1-486712020/risks-of-increasingly-potent-cannabis-the-joint-effects

Pierre, J. M., Gandal, M. J., & Son, M. (2016). Cannabis-induced psychosis associated with high potency "wax dabs". *Schizophrenia Research*, *172*(1), 211–212. Retrieved 11 9, 2019, from https://sciencedirect.com/science/article/pii/s09209996416300561

Pivik, R., Zarcone, V., Dement, W. C., & Hollister, L. E. (1972). Delta-9-tetrahydrocannabinol and synhexl: Effects on human sleep patterns. *Clinical Pharmacology and Therapeutics*, *13*(3), 426–435. Retrieved 9 5, 2019, from https://ncbi.nlm.nih.gov/pubmed/4337346

Portenoy, R. K., Ganae-Motan, E. D., Allende, S., Yanagihara, R., Shaiova, L., Weinstein, S., ... Fallon, M. T. (n.d.). Nabiximols for opioid-treated cancer patients with poorly-controlled chronic pain: A randomized, placebo-controlled, graded-dose trial. *The Journal of Pain*, *13*(5), 438–449.

Powell, D., Pacula, R. L., & Jacobson, M. (2015). Do medical marijuana laws reduce addictions and deaths related to pain killers. *Journal of Health Economics*, *58*, 29–42. Retrieved 11 20, 2019, from https://sciencedirect.com/science/article/pii/s0167629617311852

Retrieved from https://www.ncbi.nlm.nih.gov/pubmed/30670598

Retrieved from https://www.ncbi.nlm.nih.gov/pubmed/306705982019; http://cancerres.aacrjournals.org/content/68/2/339

Russo, E. B., Guy, G., & Robson, P. (2007). Cannabis, pain, and sleep: Lessons from therapeutic clinical trials of Sativex®, a cannabis-based medicine. *Chemistry and Biodiversity*, *4*(8), 1729–1743. Retrieved 9 3, 2019, from https://ncbi.nlm.nih.gov/pubmed/17712817

Taha, T., Meiri, D., Talhamy, S., Wollner, M., Peer, A., & Bar-Sela, G. (2019, April 24). Cannabis impacts tumor response rate to nivolumab in patients with advanced malignancies. *Oncologist*, *4*(4), 549–557.

Takakuwa, K. M., Hergenrather, J. Y., Shofer, F. S., & Schears, R. M. (2019). The impact of medical cannabis on intermittent and chronic opioid users with back pain: How cannabis diminished prescription opioid usage. *Cannabis and Cannabinoid Research*. doi:10.1089/can.2019.0039

Ward, K., Ramzan, A. A., Sheeder, J., Fischer, S., & Lefkowits, C. (2019). Persistent opioid use after radiation therapy in opioid-naive cervical cancer survivors. *International Journal of Gynecological Cancer*, *29*(7), 1105–1109. Retrieved 12 2, 2019, from https://ijgc.bmj.com/content/29/7/1105

Wilsey, B. L., Marcotte, T. D., Deutsch, R., Gouaux, B., Sakai, S., & Donaghe, H. E. (2013). Low dose vaporized cannabis significantly improves neuropathic pain. *The Journal of Pain*, *14*(2), 136–148. Retrieved 11 9, 2019, from https://ncbi.nlm.nih.gov/pubmed/23237736

Zajicek, J., Hobart, J., Slade, A., Barnes, D., Mattison, P., & MUSEC Research Group (2012). Multiple sclerosis and Extract of cannabis: Results of the MUSEC trial. *Journal of Neurology, Neurosurgery, and Psychiatry*, *83*(11), 1125–1132. Retrieved 8 26, 2019, from https://jnnp.bmj.com/content/83/11/1125

Medical Cannabis and Palliative Care in the Elderly with Acute and Chronic Illnesses

Lynn McNall and Kimberly Balko

Introduction

Recently, due to legalization in several states, the use of medical cannabis has come to the forefront of healthcare as a frequently requested medical therapy for the management of debilitating effects of a variety of acute and chronic effects of illness and associated treatments. In view of this shift, combined with the reality of an aging population in the United States, this chapter focuses on the concept of Palliative Care (PC) in conjunction with the use of medical cannabis as a complementary therapy/treatment that can be included in a plan of care—often at the request of an acutely or chronically ill elderly patient. The potential benefits and disadvantages that may arise when medical cannabis is used in the PC setting will be considered, including physical and psychosocial aspects for the geriatric PC patient associated with life-threatening diseases, chronic illness, and end-of-life care. Barriers such as stigma, lack of understanding, poor communication, and the importance of safe access to this medication will also be analyzed.

The Aging Population

According to the Institute of Medicine (2008) "by 2030 the number of adults in the United States who are 65 years old or older is expected to be almost double what it was in 2005, and the nation is not prepared to meet their social and health care needs" (p. 15). Baby Boomers born between 1946 and 1964 are now becoming Senior Boomers, and this change will not only affect their social and health care needs; it will change the business and lifestyle landscape in the United States (Potter, 2017).

The aging population has a higher prevalence of chronic diseases and acute illnesses, are vulnerable to injuries related to falls and have more limitations of their activities of daily living. Therefore, health professionals should be concerned with the shortfall of care that the elderly population will have now and into the future. Reports of current or projected health care and workforce shortages reveal the following:

- The shortage of direct care workers is a critical issue in 29 of 38 states (Harmuth & Dyson, 2005).
- The current shortage of 12,000 geriatricians will climb to 28,000 by 2030 (Association of Directors of Geriatric Academic Programs, 2007; Alliance for Aging Research, 2002).
- By 2025 there is a projected shortage of 100,000 physicians (Association of American Medical Colleges, 2007).
- The Registered Nurse shortage is projected at 808,000 by 2020 (Auerbach, Buerhasu, & Staiger, 2007; Health Resources and Services Administration, 2002).

Palliative Care

Palliative Care is an approach to provide comfort and support to patients and their families when dealing with the diagnosis of a chronic or life-threatening illness. Specific PC measures encompass ways to manage the psychosocial, physical, spiritual, and social concerns that often arise during illnesses (City of Hope, n.d.).

The National Coalition for Hospice and Palliative Care (2013) defines PC as "patient- and family-centered care that optimizes quality of life by anticipating, preventing, and treating suffering. PC, throughout the continuum of illness, involves addressing physical, intellectual, emotional, social, and spiritual needs and facilitating patient autonomy, access to information, and choice" (p. 9). It provides expert medical care for patients of any age diagnosed with chronic and/or acute complex illnesses which include but are not limited to cancer, heart disease, lung disease, kidney failure, multiple sclerosis, HIV/AIDS, and cystic fibrosis (National Institutes of Health, 2018). It focuses on providing patients with relief from symptoms, pain, and emotional stress during the trajectory of their illness.

The goal of PC is to improve quality of life for both the elderly patient and their support system and is delivered in a variety of settings such as the hospital, patient's home, nursing home, or physician offices. PC should not be confused with Hospice care which has strict admission criteria: The patient needs to be within six months of dying. PC is not about dying. It is about living as long as one can for as long as one is able (Meier as cited in Volandes, 2015, p. 174). The patient's rationale for seeking PC services is different from their reasons for seeking Hospice care. PC should be initiated at the time of diagnosis and does not depend on the possible trajectory of the diagnosed disease. Instead, it helps to promote "quality of life, mood, and prolong survival" (National Institutes of Health, 2017). Per the World Health Organization (WHO) (2019): "Palliative care provides relief from pain and other distressing symptoms; affirms life and regards dying as a normal process; intends neither to hasten or postpone death; integrates the psychological and spiritual aspects of patient care; offers a support system to help patients live as actively as possible until death; offers a support system to help the family cope during the patient's illness and in their own bereavement; uses a team approach to address the needs of patients and their families, including bereavement counseling, if indicated; will enhance quality of life, and may also positively influence the course of illness; is applicable early in the course of illness, in conjunction with other therapies that are intended to prolong life, such as chemotherapy or radiation therapy; and includes those investigations needed to better understand and manage distressing clinical complications" (para. 1). Matzo and Witt-Sherman (2015) state, "Excellent palliative care embraces cultural, ethnic, faith differences and preferences while interweaving the principles of ethics, humanities, and human values into every patient and family care experience" (p. 3).

The PC team approach to patient-centered care incorporates the extensive work of physicians, nurses, pharmacists, spiritual advisors, nutritionists, counselors, and social workers (Patient Quality of Life Coalition, n.d.). These professionals work together to improve the patient's quality of life by handling debilitating side effects of disease and treatment by providing "expert management of complex physical and emotional symptoms, including complex pain, anxiety, fatigue, shortness of breath, constipation, nausea, loss of appetite, and difficulty sleeping" (Centers to Advance Palliative Care, 2018, para. 5). Frequent communication is encouraged among patients, healthcare providers, and support systems to make certain that the patient receives the care they need and want. These discussions are related to physical changes as disease progresses, emotional support for both the patient and their caregiver, and access to requested spiritual care (National Institutes of Health, 2017).

Quality of Life Model in PC

Palliative care is a "comprehensive treatment of the discomfort, symptoms and stress of serious illness. The goal is to prevent and ease suffering and improve QOL" (National Institute of Nursing Research, 2018, p.1; Peat, 2010, p. 481). The term Quality of Life (QOL) is a subjective concept that can only be observed by others, can only be "understood from the patient's perspective" and therefore can only be defined by the patient (Connor, 2009, p. 191). A patient's QOL incorporates a variety of "dimensions of life" which includes a patient's past life experiences, interpersonal relationships and connections with others, functional ability related to their baseline health, intellectual and perceptual abilities, and insight into one's own well-being related to the management of the course of disease and side effects of treatment, and their insight into transcendence/spirituality to guarantee that all of the patient's concerns, wishes and "unresolved issues are addressed" (Connor, 2009, p. 192).

When a patient's QOL is assessed in the PC setting, the information obtained determines whether the care is effective, identifies all areas that

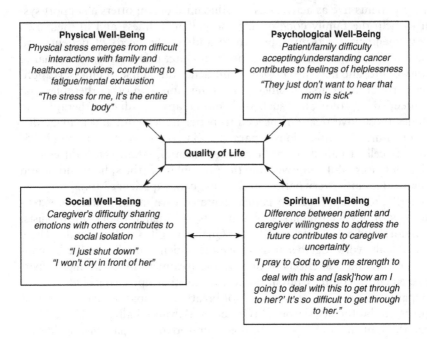

Figure 8.1 The City of Hope Quality of Life Model (City of Hope, n.d.)

the patient feels is important to them, and all areas that may still be of concern (Lawerence & Clancy, 2003). The City of Hope Quality of Life Model (below) is based on the assessment of certain forces that validates a patient's physical, psychological, social, and spiritual well-being. It measures how patients define satisfaction with aspects of their life they feel are most significant. It also incorporates the importance of the family in the process to achieve QOL for the patient (Lavdaniti & Tsitsis, 2015).

Autonomy, Empowerment, and Medical Cannabis in PC

Patients find themselves vulnerable while coping with serious medical conditions and making important treatment choices provide them with a sense of empowerment and autonomy. An autonomous patient is capable of making their own decisions that align with and promote the personal plan of care they have chosen. Decisions made solely by the patient, without any controlling, will define positive intentional actions (Beauchamp & Childress, 2012). Each patient is a vital and "unique" human being, entitled to treatment that is respectful of their human dignity and reduces their suffering (Matzo & Witt-Sherman 2015, p. 39; Norlander, 2014, pp. 86–87). Acknowledgment of the patient's concerns, through listening and observing for non-verbal clues, are important ways to understand the patient's concerns and provides an opportunity to find ways of "honoring the patient's wishes" (Matzo & Witt-Sherman, 2015, p. 39). A sense of autonomy is restored for patients when the physician provides safe access to medical cannabis and acceptance is shown by the family/support system. The patient would then be able to manage their medications and control their symptoms with the freedom to self-titrate, without the concern for overdosing, which provides a way for the patient to retain a sense of empowerment at a critical point when the ability to control many aspects of their care and lives may be out of reach (Spencer et al. 2016a).

Stigma Associated with Use of Medical Cannabis

Medical cannabis often carries the burden of stigma related to its controversial reputation of being a prohibited, illegal drug since 1937 and its well-known "psychoactive components" (Clark, 2018, E2; Johanningman & Eschiti, 2013, p. 360; Spencer et al., 2016b, p. 507). When requested by patients, the request is often met with shock and disbelief and disregard for the patient's wishes. Spencer et al. (2016a) state, a "70-year-old grandmother does not fit society's image of a cannabis user [which] may prevent such a patient from requesting medical cannabis and/or doctors from authorizing it for her" (p. 527).

Palliative care patients and their families often struggle with issues around "acceptance and hope." They look toward their healthcare providers to answer questions and provide education related to their treatment and symptom management. Professionals must listen and try to understand that patients and families are on their own personal journeys and a balance is needed between sharing accurate scientific information while sustaining a supportive and therapeutic relationship. This is achieved from establishing and maintaining an "open and honest communication." In this way, patients' and families' needs are being met while they are being gently guided toward making informed, safe decisions (Clark, 2018, p. E1; Spencer et al., 2016a).

Bultman and Kingsley (2014) state, the "medical field is changing, and the use of medical cannabis is now being accepted as an alternative, holistic, homeopathic and/or naturalistic medicine" (p. 39). By breaking down the wall surrounding medical cannabis, medical cannabis will find a steadfast place in today's health care community. Research opportunities would contribute to safety, dosing, access, and eliminating barriers that block access for patients in need. Advancing research would pave a way toward approval and coverage by insurance companies and would eliminate out-of-pocket expenses for the patients (Spencer et al., 2016a, p. 527).

Eliminating stigma would break down barriers and lead to open communication between patients and their health care providers. If patients are comfortable asking for cannabis to be a part of their medication regimen, it ensures this medication would not be obtained from an unsuitable source where the medication contains pollutants and could place patients at risk (Spencer et al., 2016a).

Advantages and Disadvantages of Medical Cannabis

When elderly patients are diagnosed with an acute or chronic disease, they often seek for ways to meet their own individualized needs. They strive to control the side effects associated with both disease and/or treatments, to improve their health and QOL, to promote "a holistic health philosophy or desire a transformational experience that changes their worldview" and/or to seek a greater sense of "control over their lives" (Matzo & Witt-Sherman, 2015, p. 237).

Recently the use of medical cannabis has been associated with the effective management of symptoms of certain diseases and management of a variety of treatment-related side effects (see Table 8.2). As patients learn the potential benefits of introducing cannabis into their medication regimen, physicians are now being asked to prescribe this medication to help alleviate distressing symptoms, promote comfort, and eventually to meet the patient's QOL goals. This allows patients to benefit from taking one medication as opposed to taking many medications, each with its own list of potentially dangerous side effects (Spencer et al., 2016a).

Per the National Academies of Sciences (2017), certain conclusions have been reached from the most recent research findings. Many aspects such as dosing, most effective routes of administration, best possible ways to control symptoms, potential long-term side effects, etc. still need to be investigated and documented. Table 8.1 compares the advantages and disadvantages of medical cannabis and shows what is known from the research thus far.

Palliative Care, Medical Cannabis, and Concerns of the Elderly

When utilizing palliative care, common issues surrounding the use of medical cannabis are in question. This section will discuss the common questions asked by patients in their quest for symptom relief.

Will Healthcare Providers Prescribe Medical Cannabis to the Elderly?

When an elderly patient is thinking about using cannabis as part of their prescription regimen it is important to first have this discussion with their physician and the palliative care team. Finding a physician to write a recommendation for patients to have cannabis who qualify based on state guidelines can be difficult. Asking the palliative care team about medical cannabis

Table 8.1 Advantages and disadvantages of medical cannabis

Medical Cannabis	Advantages	Disadvantages

Indications for Treatment	• Acute, chronic, neuropathic pain
	  • Fibromyalgia
	  • Rheumatoid Arthritis
	  • Sickle cell Disease
	  • Chronic Cystitis
	  • HIV/AIDS
	• Chemotherapy-induced nausea/vomiting (CINV)
	• Depression, anxiety
	• Sleep Disturbances
	• Multiple Sclerosis spasticity
	• Seizures
	• PTSD
	• Loss of appetite
	• Weight loss
	• Social anxiety disorders
	• Tourette Syndrome
	• Decreases polypharmacy
	• Addresses multiple symptoms with only one medication
	• Less diversion of cannabis related to opioid diversion
	
	Maida & Daeninck, 2016, p. 400
	National Academies of Science, 2017, p. 14
	Peat, 2010, p. 482
	Strouse, 2017, p. 639
	Spencer et al., 2016a, p. 526
		• Lack of documented research findings from randomized controlled studies for indications/ curative effects
		• Not recommended for treatment of post-op pain
		• Potential synergistic effect with opioid use
		• Out-of-pocket costs
		
		Clark, 2018, p. E2–3
		Johanningman & Eschiti, 2013, p. 361
		Maida & Daeninck, 2016, p. 399
		Spencer et al., 2016a, p. 526
		Strouse, 2017, p. 693

is a good first step because they might have a list of physicians that do use medical cannabis as a form of treatment and are willing to complete the required paperwork.

Patients, caregivers, and healthcare providers need to acknowledge that patients have a right to control their care and seek treatments that are effective without ever experiencing stigma or related embarrassment.

Is Medical Cannabis Safe When Utilizing Palliative Care?

In general, medical cannabis is safe when used appropriately. In palliative care, patients use cannabis for pain control, nausea, muscle spasms, depression, anxiety, insomnia, and anorexia/cachexia (Spencer et al., 2016a). Cannabis helps create a positive mood with an intent for healing by boosting energy, reinforcing sleep habits, and enhancing social interactions (Rahn, 2015). Cannabis has also been growing as a drug of choice, especially for some diseases such as multiple sclerosis, Alzheimer's disease, dementia, dystonia, Huntington's disease, Parkinson's disease, post-traumatic stress disorder, psychosis, Tourette syndrome, epilepsy, and others (Abuhasira et al., 2018).

There are two broad cannabis strains that are used, each with different levels of THC and CBD. It is up to the physician and palliative team to coordinate and communicate which strain would be most effective for a patient's condition.

Safety education should include ways to safeguard children and others against accidental exposure to cannabis in the PC setting. Safety guidelines for cannabis storage should be the same as those used when storing opioids and other controlled substances in the home (Strouse, 2017).

Education should encompass patient safety precautions, which include the risk of falling related the patient's physical condition and driving concerns (Strouse, 2017).

What Dose Would a Patient Take When Starting Medical Cannabis?

Overall, it is up to the patient to make a final decision on what he/she would like to use. Since everyone can react differently to the effect of medical cannabis, the rule is to "start low and go slow" (Spencer et al., 2016a; Childs, Lutz, & de Wit, 2017; Blesching, 2015). Starting low with a small measured amount and increasing the dose slowly by the same measured amount to gradually reach a "subjective therapeutic window" is suggested. Utilizing cannabis in this manner will help the patient achieve the greatest improvement in symptom control, function, and quality of life, with the fewest adverse effects (MacCallum & Russo, 2018; Blesching, 2015, p. 20; Maida & Daeninck, 2016, p. 399, 402; Spencer et al., 2016a, p. 526). This is especially important when attempting to reach successful palliative doses while trying newer strains of cannabis (Childs et al., 2017).

How is Medical Cannabis Supplied if Prescribed by the Healthcare Providers?

Medical cannabis is available in variety of forms: pills, smoke, vapor, tea, food, oils, sprays, or rectal suppository. The timing of the action of the medication depends on the route of administration. For example, smoking is a way to receive the benefits of the medication quickly as opposed to taking the medication orally. Route also depends on the symptom being treated. For example, cannabis may not be taken orally if nausea and vomiting are the symptoms being treated. It is important to follow the protocol and instructions from the health provider for obtaining, administering, and dosing the different forms of cannabis (Clark, 2018, pE3).

Medical cannabis also comes in a variety of strains. It is a "trial and error" process to find the strain that is most effective for a particular patient. If a patient experiences continued side effects, related to a particular strain, a different strain may be needed to achieve the desired effect and provide relief of their symptoms (Clark, 2018, p. E3).

What Adverse Effects Could Patients Experience When Taking Medical Cannabis?

Adverse effects vary greatly depending on the amount of cannabis being used. In palliative care, cannabis use starts low and slow to decrease the risk of adverse effects. Potential short-term and long-term effects are shown inTable 8.2. The most common side effects are not a cause for nonuse of the drug. MacCallum and Russo (2018) suggest that a person record their response or efficacy for each cannabis product and for any symptoms they display to keep the physician informed in determining treatment response (Table 8.2).

Is the Use of Medical Cannabis Addictive?

Addiction, according to Ivker (2017), is a "chronic disease of brain reward, motivation, memory, and related circuitry" (p. 29). Addiction occurs when the person cannot "consistently abstain, [by demonstrating] impairment in behavior control, craving, diminished recognition of significant problems with one's behaviors and interpersonal relationships, and a dysfunctional emotion response" (p. 29). Commonly prescribed drugs such as opioids (morphine, hydrocodone, oxycodone, and fentanyl) are powerful pain killers and highly addictive. According to Ivker, (2017) "in 2014, there were fifty-two deaths every day from opioid overdose" (p. 4). This has caused a public health crisis in America due to the over-prescribing, misuse, and abuse of opioids to our youth, younger adults, and the elderly. One study by Lucus (2012) suggested that reduction of opioid use can happen with cannabis as a replacement. In this way, the patient is mainly using cannabis and fewer tablets of prescription opioids to achieve the same level of pain relief. Cannabis is not addictive and has fewer side effects. Cannabis use also prevents opioid withdrawal from occurring (Potter, 2017).

What if the Patient is on Multiple Medications?

The physician would need to know what medications the patient is presently taking and if there are any issues of depression, cardiovascular issues, and

Table 8.2 Potential side effects of medical cannabis use

Medical Cannabis	Advantages	Disadvantages

Potential Side Effects	• Well tolerated
	• Lower risk for serious side effects/fatalities as compared to opioid use
	• Positive mood enhancer
	• Encourages an aim for self-healing
	• Energy booster
	• Promotes positive sleep habits
	• Enhances social interactions
	• Anti-inflammatory properties
	• Ability to self-titrate with lower chance of overdose
	• Improved treatment compliance due to reduction of treatment-related side effects
	• Less damage done by diversion than opioids
	• Most serious potential side effects not concerning in PC setting
	
	Bachhuber, Saloner, Cunningham, & Barry, 2014
	Bultman & Kingsley, 2014Carter et al., 2011
	Clark, 2018, p. E3
	Maida & Daeninck, 2016, p. 398
	Spencer et al., 2016a, p. 526
	Strouse, 2017, p. 693
		• Anxiety/panic
		• Respiratory symptoms/cough
		• Decreased psychomotor performance
		• Hyperemesis Syndrome
		• Dry mouth
		• Fatigue/tiredness
		• Aural/visual hallucinations
		• Increased heart rate (Tachycardia)
		• Lightheadedness/dizziness
		• Distorted perception of time
		• Red, irritated eyes
		• Impaired clarity
		• Potentiate psychiatric conditions
		  • Potential Long-Term Effects
		  • Severe/Chronic bronchitis
		  • Cognitive deficits (reversible with nonuse)
		  • Decline in receptor density (development of tolerance over time)
		• Withdrawal syndrome
		• Addiction
		• Lung Cancer
		
		Carter et al., 2011Clark, 2018, p. E3
		Johanningman & Eschiti, 2013, p.361
		Maida & Daeninck, 2016, p. 399
		Spencer et al., 2016a, p. 526
		Strouse, 2017, p. 693

or mental health concerns. It has been noted that "cannabis has a synergistic effect with opioids and may enhance opioid effectiveness"; therefore, caution should be encouraged when taking these medications together (Clark et al., 2018, p. E3). Further research is needed to document the potential interactions of cannabis with other medications.

Why Is It Important to Obtain Medical Cannabis from a Reputable Source (Licensed Dispensary)?

States have different laws and regulations; therefore, it is important for patients to understand the process and know if their condition qualifies them for a Medical Marijuana Certification Program. Obtaining an approved registry card provides patients access to a registered dispensary licensed within their state. Obtaining cannabis legally would enhance safety for patients by eliminating the need to purchase products from sources that lack quality-controlled conditions and would eradicate the need to use unreliable, non-reproducible products with inaccurate labeling. Products obtained outside of the licensed dispensaries are not processed to meet individual patients' needs and are often dangerously tainted. Also, legally obtaining this medication would reduce stigma-related issues that concern patients and the healthcare provider would have all the needed information for appropriately managing the patient's care (Clark et al., 2018, p. E3; Johanningman & Eschiti, 2013, p. 361; Maida & Daeninck, 2016, p. 399; Spencer et al., 2016a, pp. 526-7; Strouse, 2017, p. 693).

How Would a Patient Pay for a Medical Cannabis Prescription?

The National Council for Aging Care (2015) stated that approximately $650 per year is spent per patient using medical cannabis, compared to approximately $3,000 per year spent per patient taking prescription drugs. Therefore, information related to the status of legalization of marijuana on a federal level should be provided to patients and their families. This could contribute to lowering costs for patients as lack of insurance coverage for medical cannabis leads to high out-of-pocket expenses and could contribute to decreasing the stigma associated with cannabis use for medical care (National Council for Aging Care, 2018).

Case Study

G.D. is a 72-year-old widowed male. He lives with his 68-year-old sister who is working full time, transports G.D. to all appointments, is responsible for shopping, meal preparation, and provides company for her brother. He has been a widower for one year and has felt sad and lonely since the loss of his wife due to a long illness with cancer.

G.D. was diagnosed with a slowly progressing Parkinson's disease four years ago. G.D.'s sister met with the physician and expressed her concerns for his health and safety. He has become less steady upon his feet and is having difficulty urinating. He presents with tremors, rigidity, muscle weakness, and peripheral neuropathy in both feet. The tremors are treated with the oral medication, Levodopa. The foot pain, related to the neuropathy, is being treated with Gabapentin, Tramadol, and Codeine. Some days are worse than others for G.D.: he is unsteady upon his feet and the pain is uncontrolled with increased doses of the pain medications. His ability to complete his activities of daily living (ADLs) have diminished, especially on days he is experiencing increased pain. He is experiencing mental changes, increased lethargy, and fatigue also related to the need for increased pain medications. He is experiencing side effects from taking the pain medications, which include constipation resulting in decreased appetite and weight loss, as well as urinary retention.

The primary care physician consulted the Palliative Care (PC) consult to evaluate his physical, psychological, social, and spiritual well-being. The PC team identified that physically G.D. experiences significant mobility issues on the days of uncontrolled foot pain. They identified he is experiencing constipation, urinary retention, and decreased appetite with resultant weight loss of 10 lbs during the past two months. A low dose of antidepressant medication was ordered to treat his depression since the death of his wife and the progression of his Parkinson symptoms. The PC team suggested using medical cannabis as an alternative to the narcotic therapy because some of the symptoms G.D. is experiencing are related to the narcotic. G.D.'s safety and mobility concerns will be met by bringing in a healthcare aid to monitor his safety, help with his ADLs, and provide a companion during the day. Spiritual concerns will be met by a bi-weekly visit from the priest of the church G.D. and his family routinely attends. The patient agreed to all suggestions made by the PC team.

When the plan of care was presented to G.D.'s sister, the introduction of medical cannabis was met with shock and disbelief. She refused, stating she did not want him "stoned" in her home. She expressed safety concerns regarding the storage of the medication because her grandchildren visit regularly. The PC team provided education about the advantages, disadvantages, and safety procedures related to the addition of medical cannabis as part of G.D.'s plan of care. The sister agreed to a trial use of medical cannabis for her brother's plan.

The PC team contacted G.D.'s primary care physician who was unsure of the procedure of ordering medical cannabis and requested that the patient be referred to a qualifying practitioner who would guide the patient and the PC team to complete and submit the patient registration application to the Department of Health for approval. Because medical cannabis has found a role in PC, medical professionals and nurses have discovered there is a lack of evidence-based knowledge regarding its use as a medicinal treatment. Per Mastrian et al. (2011), learners are responsible for their own learning and for the decisions they make in the problem-solving process. Learning about new and innovative treatments requested by patients should be collaborative and incorporate all members of the team (p. 4). The use of medical cannabis in pain management allows medical professionals to meet the needs of their patients in a compassionate way that incorporates pain assessment and pain management to prevent suffering by patients and their families.

G.D. was started on a very low dose of medical cannabis with the expectation that he would begin to wean off the opioid medication. He was instructed to document his experiences and dosing schedule. The physician following him will monitor his reaction to the medical cannabis and titrate doses and order different strains as needed. G.D. is being closely followed by the PC team assessing the patient for symptom management of urinary retention, mental changes, and constipation related to the opioid therapy. They are also assessing G.D. for effective pain management, peripheral neuropathies, and mental health effects from the antidepressant therapy.

In this scenario, medical cannabis is being used to treat the acute and chronic symptoms of G.D.'s illness related to Parkinson's disease. There are documented studies that show benefits of its use in other acute and chronic illnesses under the PC umbrella, as noted in Table 8.1.

Conclusion

Medical cannabis is finding a place in the care of patients receiving PC for the treatment of a variety of symptoms and side effects experienced from acute and chronic diseases and associated medical treatments. Patients are learning more about its positive effects and are requesting its use from their healthcare providers. Research is needed to confirm both positive and negative effects through controlled studies conducted in a variety of disease states because currently most of the information known is anecdotal and obtained from patient's experiences. Healthcare providers need to be educated about how their patients can legally obtain medical cannabis, manage dosing schedules and potential side effects, and demonstrate continued acceptance to avoid having their elderly patients experience stigma or embarrassment when requesting this medication. Providing patients with a sense of autonomy and empowering them to be in control of their lives and medical plan of care is the utmost goal in providing patient care today.

References

Abuhasira, R., Schleider, L. B. L., Mechoulam, R., & Novack, V. (2018). Epidemiological characteristics, safety and efficacy of medical cannabis in the elderly. *European Journal of Internal Medicine, 49*, 44–50.

Alliance for Aging Research (2002). *Medical never-never land: Ten reasons why America is not ready for the coming age boom.* Washington, DC: Alliance for Aging Research.

Association of American Medical Colleges (AAMC) (2007). *2007 State physician workforce data book.* Washington, DC: AAMC.

Association of Directors of Geriatric Academic Programs (ADGAP) (2007). Fellows in geriatric medicine and geriatric psychiatry programs. *Training and Practice Update, 5*(1), 1–7.

Auerbach, D. I., Buerhaus, P. I., & Staiger, D. O. (2007). Better late than never: Workforce supply implications of later entry into nursing. *Health Affairs, 26*(1), 178–185.

Bachhuber, M. A., Saloner, B., Cunningham, C. O., & Barry, C. L. (2014). Medical cannabis laws and opioid analgesic overdose mortality in the United States, 1999–2010. *JAMA Internal Medicine, 174*(10), 1875. doi:10.1001/jamainternmed.2014.4005

Beauchamp, T., & Childress, J. (2012). *Principles of biomedical ethics* (7th ed.). New York: Oxford University Press.

Blesching, U. (2015). *Cannabis health index.* Berkeley, CA: Logo Publishing House.

Bultman, L., & Kingsley, K. (2014). *Medical cannabis primer: For healthcare professionals.* Middleton, MD: Minnesota Medical Solutions.

Carter, G. T., Flanagan, A. M., Earlywine, M., Abrams, D. I., Aggarwal, S. K., & Grinspoon, L. (2011). Cannabis in palliative medicine: Improving care and reducing opioid-related morbidity. *American Journal of Hospice and Palliative Medicine, 28*(5), 297–303.

Centers to Advance Palliative Care (CAPC) (2018). *Growth of palliative care in U.S. Hospitals.* Retrieved from https://www.capc.org/about/palliative-care/

Childs, E., Lutz, J. A., & de Wit, H. (2017). Dose-related effects of delta-9-THC on emotional responses to acute psychosocial stress. *Drug and Alcohol Dependence, 177*, 136–144.

City of Hope (n.d.). *Quality of life model.* Retrieved from https://www.google.com/search?client=firefox-b-1-d&tbm=isch&sa=1&ei=FrteXaq7DImL5wLE67MY&q=city+of+hope+qol+model&oq=city+of+hope+qol+model&gs_l=img.3...878.6332..7636...1.0..1.600.2086.4j7j1j5-1......0....1..gws-wiz-img.......0j0i67j0i24.n84iUCfM1mo&ved=0ahUKEwiqnt7R65bkAhWJxVkKHcT1DAMQ4dUDCAY&uact=5#imgrc=YplDB9wieqSGGM

Clark, C. S. (2018). Medical cannabis: The oncology nurse's role in patient education about the effects of marijuana on cancer palliation. *Clinical Journal of Oncology Nursing, 22*(1), E1–E6.

Connor, S. R. (2009). Hospice and palliative care. *The essential guide* (2nd ed.). New York: Routledge.

Harmuth, S., & Dyson, S. (2005). *Results of the 2005 national survey of state initiatives on the long-term care direct-care workforce.* New York: The National Clearinghouse on the Direct Care Workforce and the Direct Care Workers Association of North Carolina.

Health Resources and Services Administration (HRSA) (2002). *Projected supply, demand, and shortages of registered nurses: 2000–2020.* Rockville, MD.

Institute of Medicine (2008). *Retooling for an aging America: Building the health care workforce.* Washington, DC: National Academy Press.

Ivker, R. (2017). *Cannabis for chronic pain: A proven prescription for using marijuana to relieve your pain and heal your life.* New York: Touchstone.

Johanningman, S., & Eschiti, V. (2013). Medical use of marijuana in palliative care. *Clinical Journal of Oncology Nursing, 17*(4), 360–362.

Lavdaniti, & Tsitsis (2015). Definitions and conceptual models of quality of life in cancer patients. *Health Science Journal, 9*(2), 1–4.

Lawerence, W., & Clancy, C. (2003). Health outcomes assessment in cancer. *Disease Management and Health Outcomes, 11*(11), 709–721.

Lucus, P. (2012). Cannabis as an adjunct to or substitute for opiates in the treatment of chronic pain. *Journal of Psychoactive Drugs, 44*(2), 125–133.

MacCallum, C. A., & Russo, E. B. (2018). Practical considerations in medical cannabis administration and dosing. *European Journal of Internal Medicine, 49*, 12–19.

Maida, V., & Daeninck, P. J. (2016). The user's guide to cannabinoid therapies. *Current Oncology, 23*(6), 398–406.

Mastrian, K., McGonigle, D., Mahan, W. L., & Bixler, B. (2011). *Integrating technology in nursing education: Tools for the knowledge era.* Sudbury, MA: Jones and Bartlett Publishers.

Matzo, M., & Witt-Sherman, D. (2015). *Palliative care nursing. Quality care to the end of life.* New York: Springer.

National Academies of Science (2017). *The health effects of cannabis and cannabinoids: The current state of evidence and recommendations for research.* National Academies of Science. Retrieved from www.nap.edu

National Coalition for Hospice and Palliative Care (2013). *The National Consensus Project for quality palliative care clinical practice guidelines for quality palliative care* (3rd ed.). Retrieved from http://www.nationalcoalitionhpc.org/guidelines-2013/

National Council for Aging Care (2018). *The complete guide to medical marijuana for seniors.* Retrieved from https://www.aging.com/the-complete-guide-to-medical-marijuana-for-seniors/

National Institutes of Health (NIH) (2017). *Palliative care in cancer.* Retrieved from https://www.cancer.gov/about-cancer/advanced-cancer/care-choices/palliative-care-fact-sheet

National Institute of Nursing Research (NINR) (2018). *Palliative care: The relief you need when you have a serious illness (Booklet).* Retrieved from https://www.ninr.nih.gov/sites/files/docs/palliative-care-brochure.pdf

Norlander, L. (2014). *To comfort always: A nurse's guide to end of life.* Indianapolis, IN: Sigma Theta Tau International.

Patient Quality of Life Coalition (n.d.). *Palliative Care at a glance.* Retrieved from http://patientqualityoflife.org/wp-content/uploads/2019/02/Palliative-Care-At-A-Glance_April2018.pdf

Peat, S. (2010). Using cannabinoids in pain and palliative care. *International Journal of Palliative Nursing, 16*(10), 481–485.

Potter, B. A. (2017). *Cannabis for seniors.* Oakland, CA: Ronin Publishing.

Rahn, B. (2015). *What are the best cannabis strains for cancer-related symptoms?* Retrieved from https://www.leafly.com/news/strains-products/what-are-the-best-strains-for-cancer-related-symptoms

Spencer, N., Shaw, E., & Slaven, M. (2016a). Finding comfort beyond your comfort zone: Defining medical cannabis' place in palliative care. *Journal of Pain Management, 9*(4), 525–528.

Spencer, N., Shaw, E., & Slaven, M. (2016b). Medical cannabis use in an outpatient palliative care clinic: A retrospective chart review. *Journal of Pain Management*, 9(4), 525–528.

Strouse, T. B., & Associate Editor (2017). Cannabinoids in palliative medicine. *Journal of Palliative Medicine*, 20(7), 692–694.

Volandes, A. E. (2015). *The conversation: A revolutionary plan for end-of-life care*. New York: Sheridan Press.

World Health Organization (WHO) (2019). *Cancer*. Retrieved from https://www. who.int/cancer/palliative/definition/en/

Chapter 9

Risk and Protective Factors for Cannabis Abuse

Cathleen A. Lewandowski

Is cannabis harmful? Is it addictive? Even before the days of "Reefer Madness" of the 1950s and continuing to the present, these are questions that have circled around the discussion of cannabis; likely ever since humankind first discovered cannabis' mind-altering qualities (Sloman, 1998). While perhaps always known anecdotally, research is now seeking to demonstrate the health and mental health benefits of cannabis. Nonetheless, in spite of a dearth of systematic research demonstrating the medicinal properties of cannabis, cannabis has rapidly been legalized across the United States for medical use. While research on the medical benefits of cannabis is increasingly being conducted, there is also research pointing to its harmful effects. As its medicinal benefits are promoted, it cannot be forgotten that cannabis is a psychoactive substance, meaning that individuals may develop a dependence, even to the extent to meet DSM V criteria for cannabis use disorder.

This chapter will explore the potential harmful and addictive properties of cannabis. The chapter examines the risk and protective factors for cannabis misuse and dependence, and the progression from experimenting and recreational use of cannabis to misuse and/or dependence. The chapter concludes with recommendations for future research.

Risk and Protective Factors for Cannabis Misuse

Research has demonstrated that the "addictive personality" does not exist. While a considerable amount of research has been conducted to identify the "addictive personality," the overwhelming conclusion is that the addictive personality is a myth. Instead there is a plethora of factors including trauma early in life, and one's genetic make-up, that contribute to an individual developing a dependence on cannabis or other psychoactive substances. Based on accumulated research, one's genes account for about 50% of addiction, regardless of the substance (Szalavitz, 2015). It is also important to note that 50% of addiction is caused by individual, social, and environmental factors, which allows for a great deal of variation between individuals. Overall, children and adolescents are at greatest risk for developing a habit of cannabis misuse, as they are continuing to develop both physically, socially, and emotionally. Early exposure to cannabis or other psychoactive substances is associated with an impaired prefrontal cortex, which may enhance an individual's neurological susceptibility to being impulsive and to engaging in impulsive drug use (Feingold et al., 2020).

When considering the potential emotional, social, and environmental factors, childhood trauma, such as exposure to violence and abuse is a predictive factor for early onset of cannabis use among youth (Feingold et al., 2020). A recent study identified substance use classes among adolescents and found differences by both gender and race/ethnicity. Males were more likely than females to use e-cigarettes for both tobacco and marijuana, as well as all products in general. Female adolescents were more likely to use marijuana and alcohol only. Black and Latino adolescents were more likely than White adolescents to use marijuana exclusively (Morean et al., 2016).

At least one study suggests that children and youth can be screened to identify youth who may be at risk for beginning substance use at an early age and experiencing adverse outcomes as a result of such use. The ABCD Study developed a brief screening assessment to identify those youth who are at risk for early-onset marijuana use by ages 14–15. Four social, or "externalizing," problems were identified: destroys things belonging to his/her family or others; disobedience at school; lying or cheating; steals outside the home; and parental smoking. Interestingly, children and youth's emotional or "internalizing problems" did not improve the predictive utility of the screening instrument (Loeber et al., 2018). Social, biological, and/or emotional factors may underlie these externalizing or behavioral factors "externalizing" factors. Nonetheless, based on this research, the external factors appear to be most predictive, suggesting that children and youth who experience emotional or social concerns but do not exhibit externalizing factors may be less at risk than those who exhibit such behaviors.

How marijuana is consumed is an additional risk factor that may contribute to whether an individual develops a cannabis dependence. Cannabis can be ingested by inhalation, sublingually, orally, and topically. When consumed orally, it is ingested in the form of edibles, tinctures, capsules or oils. Marijuana can also enter the blood stream when placed under the tongue and held in the mouth. There are several blood vessels under the tongue which can absorb cannabinoids. Common examples of these types of products include dissolvable strips, sublingual sprays, or medicated lozenges or tinctures.

The onset for oral ingestion is slower and the effects are stronger and last longer than with inhalation. Marijuana may also be ingested through topical applications, such as in the form of lotions, salves, bath salts, and oils that are applied to the skin. The skin has a relatively complex absorption process that is based on a chemical's ability to dissolve in water. The cannabinoids penetrate the skin and work to reduce pain and inflammation. This method is very popular with older consumers because it works on localized pain and is non-psychoactive.

Inhalation is the most common form of ingestion and most individuals prefer to use marijuana this way. When a consumer inhales marijuana, the majority of cannabinoids enter the body through the lungs where they are passed along directly into the consumer's blood stream. The effect is almost instantaneous. Cannabis, or marijuana when inhaled, can be consumed as a roll, using a joint, a blunt, or a spliff. A joint contains marijuana only and is rolled with a loose paper. Blunts are rolled with tobacco paper and also contain marijuana only. Spliffs are rolled with loose joint paper but are hybrids, part marijuana and part tobacco (Williams, 2015).

Research suggests that adolescents and young adults who are blunt smokers had significantly higher odds of being dependent on marijuana and tobacco than those who reported smoking joints. Such use is moderated by social norms, and a sub-culture of blunt smokers among adolescents reflected the importance of social factors in developing a dependence on cannabis during adolescence. For adolescents, their perceptions of enhancement, craving expectancies, alcohol use, and having peers who use marijuana are additional significant risk factors (Timberlake, 2009).

Protective factors for adolescents are negative behavior expectancies and social anxiety. Social anxiety may protect adolescents from initiating cannabis use. In contrast to research cited earlier, this study supports the benefit of identifying an internalizing profile of adolescents for prevention or treatment (Schmits et al., 2015). Additionally, recreational physical activity and sports participation appear to be protective factors for marijuana use among female adolescents but not males. In contrast, recreational physical activity and sports participation appear to be risk factors for alcohol use behaviors among males (Dunn, 2014). Though not discussed in the research, these differences may be attributable to differences in norms for group behavior between male and female adolescents who engage in sports.

Of import for clinicians is the relationship between cannabis use and mental health disorders in adolescence. One study found significant associations between the frequency of cannabis use and the presence of psychotic and depressive symptoms in late adolescence and early adulthood (Rhew et al., 2017). This association extended into later adulthood and included an association with anxiety as well. For individuals experiencing depression and psychotic symptoms, reducing cannabis use may improve mood, the presence of psychotic symptoms, and possibly overall functioning at all ages.

Cannabis Use Disorder

In 2015, the Centers for Medicare and Medicaid services required that all providers transition to the ICD-10 codes to maintain HIPAA compliance on claims submissions (US Department of Health and Human Services,

2009). Given this mandate, understanding the extent that the DSM V and the ICD-10 are comparable is essential, as it has implications for assessment, diagnosis, treatment selection, billing, and reimbursement. Using data from routine assessments, Proctor and colleagues discuss the diagnostic differentials between DSM IV and ICD-10 in a study conducted among 6,871 male and 801 female prisoners admitted to a state prison between 2000 and 2003. In their analyses of how prisoners were diagnosed, the researchers found that the DSM V mapped well to the ICD-10 when there was no diagnosis. Similarly, the DSM V diagnosis of severe CUD mapped well to the ICD-10 diagnosis of dependence. However, about half of the sample who received a moderate diagnosis in the DSM V received an ICD-10 code of dependence, while the other half received a harmful use diagnosis. Given these findings, it is unclear whether the DSM V categories of mild and moderate actually represent distinct groups from a clinical point of view, and if the ICD-10 codes for harmful use and dependence are appropriate (Proctor et al., 2016).

Individuals who use cannabis daily are at higher risk for developing Cannabis Use Disorder (CUD) due to frequent use and recent increases in cannabis potency (ElSohly et al., 2016). A recent study suggests that one in four individuals who use cannabis will develop CUD over the course of their life. The progression from use to CUD is more common among men than women. Those with a co-occurring disorder as well as individuals with another substance abuse disorder are also more likely to develop CUD. Individuals who begin to use cannabis at an early age are more than twice as likely to transition from use to CUD as individuals who begin to use CUD at a later age (Feingold et al., 2020).

Using data from the National Survey on Drug Use and Health (NSDUH) the prevalence of CUD among people reporting daily or almost daily use decreased between 2002 and 2016. Tolerance is one item that did not decrease over time in any age group (Santaella-Tenorio et al., 2019). At the same time, the number of individuals who use marijuana has increased across all age groups, excepting individuals aged 12–17, as indicated by the 2017–2018 NSDUH survey (Substance Abuse and Mental Health Services Administration, 2019). Table 9.1 illustrates this change.

Cannabis Use Disorder (CUD) may be under diagnosed among adults as the DSM V does not include a cannabis use quantity or frequency measure. The NSDUH does not ask about daily cannabis use, reflecting the DSM IV and DSM V criteria. However, with the increase in legalization of cannabis, many adults are reporting daily use without reporting a CUD when responding to the NSDUH survey. The extent that CUD is self-reported could be impacted by the increase in medical and recreational cannabis legalization, the related decrease in stigma associated with daily use, and the decrease in perceived harmfulness of cannabis. When comparing cannabis use in 2002–2017 in the NSDUH, cannabis use in the past year, initiation of use, and frequency of use increased, consistent with increases in cannabis

Table 9.1 Percent of individuals reporting marijuana use, 2008–2009 and 2017–2018

Age Category	2008–2009 (%)	2017–2018 (%)	P Value Test of Difference in Percent (%)
12–17	7.03	6.56	.056
18–25	17.42	22.12	0.00
26 +	4.42	8.25	0.00
18 +	6.33	10.16	0.00

Source: NSDUH, 2019

legalization. Approximate CUD (based on 2 of 9 DSM V criteria, and mild CUD increased. Thus, new measures to assess the severity, quantity and frequency of cannabis use are urgently needed.

Medical Marijuana and Commercialization: Impact on Trends

Recent changes in the national cannabis policy environment may have reduced the stigma as well as the perception of harm associated with cannabis use (Cerda et al., 2017; Compton et al., 2016). These laws could in turn be associated with changes in social attitudes toward cannabis use, resulting in fewer conflicts with family and friends. Further, individuals who use cannabis may now be experiencing fewer problems with the law. According to Hasin et. al., the criterion of "recurrent cannabis use and related legal problems has been removed from the DSM V because of its poor fit with other substance use disorder criteria" (Hasin et al., 2013).

While the increased acceptability of cannabis use may have contributed to reduced social and legal concerns, the legalization of cannabis has potential downsides as well. Researchers are now starting to analyze trends in marijuana use and associated risk factors pre- and post-commercialization. For example, Colorado hospitals have seen an increase in marijuana detected in patients being treated for injury post-commercialization. There has also been a higher increase in the proportion of fatal motor vehicle accidents associated with using marijuana, since marijuana has been commercialized in Colorado (Chung et al., 2019). Similarly, a study was conducted of at-risk adolescents diagnosed with DSM IV cannabis use disorder to assess whether having a cannabis use disorder was predictive of obtaining a medical marijuana card in young adulthood. Results showed that 16% of the sample self-reported that they had a medical marijuana card in young adulthood (Kim et al., 2018). Physicians were cautioned to consider past and current cannabis addiction when conducting an evaluation for medical marijuana. However, a meta-analysis of studies examining the impact of legalization did not support the hypothesis that the laws led to an increase in adolescent marijuana use (Sarvet et al., 2018).

Cannabis and the Brain

Regarding cannabis and its impact on the brain, there is strong evidence that chronic cannabis use causes cognitive impairment and damage to the brain, especially in white matter where cannabinoid 1 receptors abound (National Academies of Sciences Engineering and Medicine 2017). In fact, there is some evidence that prolonged cannabis use may cause neuroanatomical changes in several areas of the brain that are associated with memory function (Mandelbaum & de la Monte, 2017). Contrary to the popular perception that cannabis is harmless and even beneficial, there are few objective data supporting a preference of cannabis over conventional therapy for restoration of the central nervous system (CNS). This includes brain functioning in disease states such as multiple sclerosis, epilepsy, or schizophrenia.

While there have not been any large randomized-control studies examining cannabis and epilepsy two meta-analytic studies have recently been published to assess the benefits and potential adverse effects of medicinal cannabis for epilepsy. One meta-analysis focused on epilepsy with adults who suffered from intractable epilepsy (de Carvalho Reis et al., 2020), and the other addressed treatment-resistant epilepsy among children and youth (Ben-Zeev, 2020). Conclusions from both these meta-analyses suggest that while there is some benefit to using cannabis to treat epilepsy, there are also some possible adverse effects.

Inclusion criteria for the studies in the adult meta-analysis were clinical studies with a longitudinal observational design and intervention using cannabinoid derivatives. Using this inclusion criteria, researchers reviewed 16 studies for descriptive analyses, and four studies for the meta-analysis. The result for the adult meta-analysis showed that cannabidiols were more effective than placebo, regardless of the etiology of the epileptic syndromes and dosage (de Carvalho Reis, 2020). Adverse events were more prevalent under short-term compared with long-term CBD treatment. Study limitations of this meta-analysis are the low number of studies, with a total of four meeting the inclusion criteria. Further, the four papers in the meta-analysis were from the same research group, and it is not clear whether the different research articles were derived from overlapping samples.

For youth, one meta-analysis suggests that children and youth should receive as low a dose as possible, to control epileptic seizures among youth with treatment-resistant epilepsy. This is largely due to the potential short and long-term side effects, especially its impact on memory and cognition in a brain that is still developing. A cautionary note for parents and medical personnel who are considering using cannabinoids with youth is that one study found that 9 out of 14 samples studied had concentrations that were different than the declared content on the package. Thus, parents may not always be assured of the dose their child is receiving. The conclusion of the meta-analysis was that the actual response of cannabinoid was comparable to other anti-epileptic drugs that have been prescribed to youth (Ben-Zeev, 2020). Parents and caregivers of children with intractable epilepsy should weigh the potential benefits of cannabinoid in treating their child's epilepsy with its potential effects on their child's developing brain.

In sum, there is some evidence supporting the benefits of cannabinoids as a treatment for epilepsy, with the cautionary note that there could be side effects, especially for children. Chronic cannabis use can cause damage to the brain contributing to cognitive impairment. As illustrated by the recent meta-analyses (Ben-Zeev, 2020; de Carvalho Reis et al., 2020) there are few studies which meet inclusion criteria for a meta-analysis. In addition to epilepsy, more research is needed to determine whether there are subsets of individuals with a range of neurological and psychiatric diseases who might benefit from cannabis (Mandelbaum & de la Monte, 2017).

Cannabis and Veterans with PTSD

Many veterans, especially veterans who have served in a combat zone, and who suffer from PTSD symptoms related to their military experience, use cannabis as a coping mechanism. In fact, veterans with PTSD are increasingly turning to cannabis to alleviate their PTSD symptoms, such as insomnia and anxiety (Betthauser et al., 2015). Some researchers suggest that Expectancy Theory may explain the perceived benefits of marijuana among veterans with PTSD. As the name suggests, Expectancy Theory posits that individuals are motivated to select certain behaviors over others due to what they expect the result of that behavior to be (Oliver, 1974). A recent study of combat veterans who self-reported using marijuana to cope found that veterans' marijuana use increased as the magnitude of their PTSD symptoms increased along with their expectancy of marijuana-induced relief of these symptoms. This seemed to lead to a feedback loop where, as self-reported symptoms increased, so did veterans' expectations for marijuana-induced relief, leading to more marijuana consumption (Earleywine & Bolles, 2014).

Overall, the benefits of marijuana or cannabis for mental health concerns such as depression, PTSD, psychotic symptoms, and anxiety are mixed. Some individuals may find that cannabis use may have little effect on their depression, anxiety, or other mental health concerns. For others, cannabis may have similar effects as conventional pharmacotherapies, though much still needs to be learned about its safety and efficacy. Little is known about the effect of cannabis use on use of common treatments for depression, when compared to standard treatments such as SSRIs and CBT (Leadbeater et al., 2018). When compared to conventional pharmacotherapies, cannabis may be less addictive. It is important to point out that all pharmacotherapies carry some known risks. More research is needed on the effects of cannabis use on mental health, especially in treating veterans with PTSD.

Cannabis and Psychosis

There is some emerging research suggesting that regular cannabis use among individuals with psychosis can contribute to treatment failure and to poorer treatment outcomes overall. For example, anti-psychotic medications, such as Clozapine, are dopamine antagonists, in line with research suggesting that elevated presynaptic dopamine function contributes to individuals' psychosis. Regular cannabis use counters the impact of the dopamine antagonist effects by down-regulating the dopaminergic system (Sami & Bhattacharyya, 2018; Bloomfield, 2014; Sami, 2015). Thus, continued cannabis use can contribute to significant worsening in ratings of psychotic symptoms (Clausen et al., 2014; Seddon et al., 2016), as well as individuals' ratings of their depressive symptoms (González-Ortega, 2015). Regular cannabis use may also interfere with individuals' ability to regularly adhere to the regimen of their anti-psychotic prescription medication, as prolonged cannabis use has been associated with changes in memory function (Batalia et al., 2013; Lorenzetti et al., 2020). Providers may suggest intermittent cannabis use for individuals who use anti-psychotic medication and who appear to be unlikely to abstain from cannabis. Using a less potent strain of cannabis may also be beneficial (González Ortega et al., 2015).

Cannabis and the Lungs

While there are many routes for cannabis use, smoking has generally been the most common route, though other routes are becoming increasingly more common. Overall, there is some indication that smoking cannabis, especially over a period of several years, may be harmful to lung health. When smoked, cannabis, like tobacco, produces a tar that leaves a potentially carcinogenic residue in pipes and other devices that are used for inhalation. Over time, smoking cannabis can have a cumulative effect on the lungs. Chronic bronchitis is common among people smoking marijuana for a number of years. Among those who smoke cannabis for more than twenty years, limitation of air flow in the lungs is often found (Schwartz, 2018). Smoking cannabis has also been associated with lung cancer. A systematic review and meta-analysis of studies examining the effects of cannabis smoking on the lungs found that cannabis smoking increased individuals' risk for lung cancer in the future (Bouti et al., 2014). More recent research suggests that the data studying cannabis and lung cancer are limited to small studies and further, that it is difficult to rule out other parallel risk factors, such as chronic tobacco use (Jett et al., 2018).

Vaping cannabis has become an increasingly more common route for cannabis, especially among adolescents and young adults. Recently, more than 200 individuals who vaped cannabis developed severe and mysterious lung illnesses. For several stricken individuals, the malady was tied to E acetate, an ingredient found in cannabis-containing vapor products (Edney, 2019). While E acetate has been found to be directly associated with these respiratory conditions, the short and long-term effects of using vaping devices and vape liquid cannabis oil are poorly understood (Abeles et al., 2020). Thus, it is important that individuals be aware that vaping cannabis may pose health risks, even when E acetate is removed.

Cannabis and Pregnant Women

Based on 2007 to 2012 NSDUH data, research suggests that approximately 10% of pregnant women used cannabis when pregnant, most of them reported using cannabis daily. Many of these women met criteria for cannabis abuse or dependence, and a good number used multiple substances (Ko et al., 2015). Cannabis, when consumed by pregnant women, may pose severe threats to the developing fetus. Maternal cannabis use has long-term impacts on children's physical and behavioral development. Prenatal cannabis exposure was found to have a significant effect on children's sleep, cognitive functions, including memory and scholastic skills, as well as on executive functions located in the frontal lobe, including reasoning, attention, impulsivity, and motivation. Symptoms of depression and anxiety were evidence throughout a child's stages of development (Day et al., 2011).

While some researchers suggest that the effect of prenatal exposure to cannabis is unclear, there does seem to be a body of research indicating that prenatal exposure may be harmful to brain development and function. Based on accumulated published data and clinical experiences with many young adult psychiatric patients who were exposed to cannabis in utero, some researchers are now hypothesizing the existence of fetal cannabis spectrum disorder (Schreiber and Pick, 2019; Stone et al., 2012). Given the trend toward increased legalization of cannabis, further research is needed to assess whether fetal cannabis spectrum disorder emerges as a valid diagnosis (Alpar et al., 2016).

Cannabis and Injury or Death

According to the National Academies of Science's report on the health effects of cannabis, there is no significant association between all-cause mortality and cannabis use. However, the authors of this report conclude that there is insufficient evidence to have confidence in this conclusion. One study indicated that cannabis use disorder, encompassing intoxication, withdrawal, and dependence criteria for diagnosis, accounted for two million of disability-adjusted life years (DALY) globally, with the United States being the country with the highest age-standardized DALY rates (Degenhardt et al., 2018).

Research does suggest that there is a substantial statistical association between cannabis use and increased motor vehicle accidents. Across age cohorts, children are at-risk for cannabis overdose injuries and respiratory distress in states where cannabis is legal. To address the risk of accidental overdose among children, Colorado requires that medical and retail marijuana be sold in child-resistant packages, and that the container display several warning statements. One such warning states that ingested forms of cannabis can have different effects from smoked cannabis (Ko et al., 2015).

Conclusion and Recommendations

The increase in the number of states that have legalized marijuana both for recreational and medical use, along with hype and marketing of its benefits and relative lack of risks may contribute to individuals' tendency to believe cannabis is effective for a range of physical and emotional/mental concerns (Fitzcharles et al., 2019). There is some indication that increased legalization trends are associated with a concomitant increase in problematic cannabis use. The epidemiology of CUD is shifting, due to cannabis itself evolving, shifting attitudes toward cannabis, and the increasing legalization across states (Lopez & Blanco, 2019).

Future research should study cannabis use and all-cause and cause-specific mortality, among large representative populations and among specific demographic and clinical sub-groups. Such groups may include the elderly, persons with mental illness, working adolescents, minority groups, and women. Research should also focus on how the form of cannabis, such as edibles, flowers, and concentrates, affect the risk of overdose and the accidental or intentional overdose in children and adults. In addition, further research is needed on the impact the route of cannabis use has on health, such as smoking, vaping, and ingesting.

Given that the legalization of cannabis in states has contributed to an increase in motor vehicle accidents, studies should focus on the degree of acute cannabis intoxication among U.S. drivers (National Academies of Sciences, Engineering, and Medicine, 2017). Researchers and practitioners both have an ethical obligation to scientifically study the benefits, potential drawbacks, and limitations of cannabis in support of patients' health and well-being.

References

Abeles, M., Valsamis, C., Webb, A., Halaby, C., Pirzada, M., Popofsky, S., & Wen, A. (2020). Vaping-associated lung injury caused by inhalation of cannabis oil. *Pediatric Pulmonology*, 55(1), 226–228. doi:10.1002/ppul.24579

Alpar, A., Di Marzo, V., & Harkany, T. (2016). At the tip of an iceberg: Prenatal marijuana and its possible relation to neuropsychiatric outcome in the offspring. *Biological Psychiatry*, 22, 283–290. doi:10.1016/j.biopsych.2015.09.009.

Batalia, A., Bhattacharyya, S., Yucel, M., Fusar-Poli, P., Crippa, J. A., Nogue, S. (2013). Structural and functional imging studies in chronic cannabis users: A systematic review of adolescent and adult findings. *PLOS ONE*, 8(2), e55821.

Ben-Zeev, B. (2020). Medical cannabis for intractable epilepsy in childhood: A review. *Rambam Maimonides Medical Journal*, 11(1), 1. Complementary Index.

Betthauser, K., Pilz, J., & Vollmer, L. E. (2015). Use and effects of cannabinoids in military veterans with posttraumatic stress disorder. *American Journal of Health-System Pharmacy*, 72(15), 1279–1284. CINAHL Plus with Full Text. doi:10.2146/ajhp140523

Bouti, K., Borki, R., Harrak, L., & Fenane, H. (2014). Cannabis smoking and risk of lung cancer—A systematic review and meta-analysis. *International Journal of Medicine and Surgery*. https://doi.org/10.15342/ijms.v1i2.57

Cerda, M., Wall, M., Feng, T., Keyes, Sarvet, A., Schulenberg, J., … Hasin, D. S. (2017). Association of state recreational marijuana laws with adolescent marijuana use. *JAMA Pediatrics*, 171(2), 142–149.

Chung, C., Salottolo, K., Tanner, A., Carrick, M. M., Madayag, R., Berg, B., … Bar-Or, D. (2019). The impact of recreational marijuana commercialization on traumatic injury. *Injury Epidemiology*, 1, 1. doi:10.1186/s40621-019-0180-4

Clausen, L., Hortoj, C. R., Thorup, A., Jeppesen, A., Petersen, P., Bertelsen, L., … Nordentoft, M. (2014). Change in cannabis use, clinical symptoms and social functioning among patients with first-episode psychosis: A 5-year follow-up study of patients in the OPUS trial. *Psychological Medicine (Print)*, 1, 117.

Compton, Han, B., Jones, C. M., Blanco, C., & Hughes, A. (2016). Marijuana use and use disorders in adults in the USA, 2002–14. *Lancet Psychiatry*, 3(10), 954–964.

Day, N. L., Leech, S. L., Goldschmidt, L., Singer, L. T., & Richardson, G. A. (2011). The effects of prenatal marijuana exposure on delinquent behaviors are mediated by measures of neurocognitive functioning. *Understanding Developmental Consequences of Prenatal Drug Exposure: Biological and Environmental Effects and Their Interactions: Special Issue in Honor or Dr. Vincent Smerglio, Psychological Medicine*, 1, 129.

de Carvalho Reis, R., Almeida, K. J., da Silva Lopes, L., de Melo Mendes, C. M., & Bor-Seng-Shu, E. (2020). Efficacy and adverse event profile of cannabidiol and medicinal cannabis for treatment-resistant epilepsy: Systematic review and meta-analysis. *Epilepsy and Behavior*, 102. APA PsycInfo. https://doi.org/10.1016/j.yebeh.2019.106635

Degenhardt, L., Bharat, C., Bruno, R., Glantz, M. D., Sampson, N. A., Lago, L., … Kessler, R. C. (2018). Concordance between the diagnostic guidelines for alcohol and cannabis use disorders in the draft icd-11 and other classification systems: Analysis of data from the who's world mental health surveys. *Addiction*, 114(3), 534–552. doi:10.1111/add.14482

Dunn, M. (2014). Association between physical activity and substance use behaviors among high school students participating in the 2009 youth risk-behavior survey. *Psychological Reports*, 114(3), 675–685.

Earleywine, M., & Bolles, J. R. (2014). Marijuana, expectancies, and post-traumatic stress symptoms: A preliminary investigation. *Journal of Psychoactive Drugs*, 46(3), 171–177. Academic Search Complete.

Edney, A. (2019). Vaping lung illness tied to cannabis products, New York says. Bloomberg.Com.

ElSohly, M. A., Mehmedic, Z., Foster, S., Gon, C., Chandra, S., & Church, J. C. (2016). Changes in cannabis potency over the last 2 decades (1995–2014): Analysis of current data in the United States. *Biological Psychiatry*, 79(7), 613–619.

Feingold, D., Livne, O., Rehm, J., & Lev-Ran, S. (2020). Probability and correlates of transition from cannabis use to DSM-5 cannabis use disorder: Results from a large-scale nationally representative study. *Drug and Alcohol Review*, 2(2), 142. doi:10.1111/dar.13031

Fitzcharles, M.-A., Shir, Y., & Hauser, W. (2019). Medical cannabis: Strengthening evidence in the face of hype and public pressure. *CMAJ: Canadian Medical Association Journal*, 33, 907. doi:10.1503/cmaj.190509

Hasin, D. S., O'Brien, C. P., Auriacombe, M., Borges, G., Bucholz, K., Budney, A., ... Grant, B. F. (2013). DSM-5 criteria for substance use disorders: Recommendations and rationale. *American Journal of Psychiatry*, 170(8), 834–851. doi:10.1176/appi.ajp.2013.12060782

Jett, J., Stone, E., Warren, G., & Cummings, K. M. (2018). Cannabis use, lung cancer, and related issues. *Journal of Thoracic Oncology : Official Publication of the International Association for the Study of Lung Cancer*, 13(4), 480–487. doi:10.1016/j.jtho.2017.12.013

Kim, J., Coors, M. E., Young, S. E., Raymond, K. M., Hopfer, C. J., Wall, T. L., ... Sakai, J. T. (2018). Cannabis use disorder and male sex predict medical cannabis card status in a sample of high risk adolescents. *Drug and Alcohol Dependence*, 25–33. doi:10.1016/j.drugalcdep.2017.11.007

Ko, J. Y., Farr, S. L., Tong, V. T., Creanga, A. A., & Callaghan, W. M. (2015). Prevalence and patterns of marijuana use among pregnant and nonpregnant women of reproductive age. *American Journal of Obstetrics and Gynecology*, 2(2), 201.e1. doi:10.1016/j.ajog.2015.03.021

Leadbeater, B. J., Ames, M. E., & Linden-Carmichael, A. N. (2018). Age-varying effects of cannabis use frequency and disorder on symptoms of psychosis, depression and anxiety in adolescents and adults. *Addiction*, https://doi.org/10.1111/add.14459

Loeber, R., Clark, D. B., Ahonen, L., FitzGerald, D., Trucco, E. M., & Zucker, R. A. (2018). A brief validated screen to identify boys and girls at risk for early marijuana use. *Developmental Cognitive Neuroscience*, 32, 23–29.

Lopez, M., & Blanco, C. (2019). Epidemiology of cannabis use disorder. In D. Montoya & S. R. B. Weiss (Eds.), *Cannabis use disorders, I* (pp. 7–12). Berlin: Springer. doi:10.1007/978-3-319-90365-1

Lorenzetti, V., Chye, Y., Suo, C., Walterfang, M., Lubman, D. I., Takagi, M., ... Solowij, N. (2020). Neuroanatomical alterations in people with high and low cannabis dependence. *Australian and New Zealand Journal of Psychiatry*, 54(1), 68–75. doi:10.1177/0004867419859077

Mandelbaum, D. E., & de la Monte, S. M. (2017). Adverse structural and functional effects of marijuana on the brain: Evidence reviewed. *Pediatric Neurology*, 66, 12–20.

Morean, M. E., Kong, G., Camenga, D. R., Cavallo, D. A., Simon, P., & Krishnan-Sarin, S. (2016). Latent class analysis of current e-cigarette and other substance use in high school students. *Drug and Alcohol Dependence, 161,* 292–297.

National Academies of Sciences, Engineering, and Medicine (2017). *The health effects of cannabis and Cannabinoids: The current state of evidence and recommendations for research* (p. 486). Washington, DC: The National Academies Press. doi:10.17226/24625

Oliver, R. L. (1974). Expectancy theory predictions of salesmen's performance. *Journal of Marketing Research, 11*(3), 243–253.

Proctor, S. L., Williams, D. C., Kopak, A. M., Voluse, A. C., Connolly, K. M., & Hoffmann, N. G. (2016). Diagnostic concordance between DSM-5 and ICD-10 cannabis use disorders. *Addictive Behaviors, 58,* 117–122.

Rhew, I. C., Fleming, C. B., Vander Stoep, A., Nicodimos, S., Zheng, C., & McCauley, E. (2017). Examination of cumulative effects of early adolescent depression on cannabis and alcohol use disorder in late adolescence in a community-based cohort. *Addiction, 11*(11), 1952. doi:10.1111/add.13907

Sami, M. B., & Bhattacharyya, S. (2018). Are cannabis-using and non-using patients different groups? Towards understanding the neurobiology of cannabis use in psychotic disorders. *Journal of Psychopharmacology, 32*(8), 825–849. doi:10.1177/0269881118760662

Santaella-Tenorio, J., Levy, N. S., Segura, L. E., Mauro, P. M., & Martins, S. S. (2019). Cannabis use disorder among people using cannabis daily/almost daily in the United States, 2002–2016. *Drug and Alcohol Dependence, 205.* Retrieved from http://proxy.ulib.csuohio.edu:2050/login?url=http://search.ebscohost.com/login.aspx?direct=true&db=edselp&AN=S0376871619303989&site=eds-live&scope=site

Sarvet, A. L., Wall, M. M., Fink, D. S., Greene, E., Le, A., Boustead, A. E., ... Hasin, D. S. (2018). Medical marijuana laws and adolescent marijuana use in the United States: A systematic review and meta-analysis. *Addiction, 113*(6), 1003–1016. doi: 10.1111/add.14136

Schmits, E., Mathys, C., & Quertemont, E. (2015). A longitudinal study of cannabis use initiation among high school students: Effects of social anxiety, expectancies, peers and alcohol. *Journal of Adolescence, 41,* 43–52.

Schreiber, S., & Pick, C. G. (2019). Cannabis use during pregnancy: Are we at the verge of defining a "fetal cannabis spectrum disorder"? *Medical Hypotheses, 124,* 53–55.

Schwartz, D. A. (2018). Cannabis and the lung. *International Journal of Mental Health and Addiction, 16*(4), 797–800. doi:10.1007/s11469-018-9902-z

Seddon, J. L., Birchwood, M., Copello, A., Everard, L., Jones, P. B., Fowler, D., ... Singh, S. P. (2016). *Cannabis use is associated with increased psychotic symptoms and poorer psychosocial functioning in first-episode psychosis: A report from the UK National Eden Study.* https://doi.org/10.1093/schbul/sbv154

Sloman, L. (1998). *Reefer madness: The history of marijuana in America.* (Ohio University; 1st St. Martin's Griffin ed.). St. Martin's Griffin; cat02507a. Retrieved from http://proxy.ulib.csuohio.edu:2050/login?url=http://search.ebscohost.com/login.aspx?direct=true&db=cat02507a&AN=ohiolink.b18909241&site=eds-live&scope=site

Substance Abuse and Mental Health Services Administration (2019). *Comparison of 2008–2009 and 2017–2018 population percentages (50 states and the District of Columbia)*. National Institute of Health. Retrieved from http://www.samhsa.go v/data/report/comparison-2008-2009-and-2017-2018-nsduh-state-prevalence-est imates

Szalavitz, M. (2015). Genetics: No more addictive personality. *Nature, 522*(s7557), S48–S49.

Timberlake, D. S. (2009). A comparison of drug use and dependence between blunt smokers and other cannabis users. *Substance Use and Misuse, 44*(3), 401–415.

Williams, K. (2015, January 7). What's the difference between joints, blunts and spliffs? Leafly. Retrieved from https://www.leafly.com/news/cannabis-101/what s-the-difference-between-joints-blunts-and-spliffs

Part Three

In Their Own Voice

Chapter 10

Lessons from Realm of Caring Foundation

Case Studies, Research and Practical Knowledge

Heather Jackson and Courtney Collins

Imagine finally getting to know your child after a decade of daily seizures and the negative effects of heavy pharmaceuticals that did little to control episodes. What if you had to make the controversial decision to try and save your child's life using cannabis? Would you do it? If not, why not? What previous notions would you bring to the table while making that decision, and are those ideas based on science or stigma?

This chapter takes a look at problems and barriers for medical cannabis consumers and how those barriers led to a movement to change access and opinions around this often-controversial topic. It will also delve into some solutions and a summary of initiatives, mostly driven by consumers and caregivers, that have and are taking place. It will also help social service professionals be able to identify problems that individuals and families face when traditional approaches to medicine have been exhausted and they choose to turn to medical cannabis. Additionally, social service professionals will recognize historical and current struggles of medical cannabis consumers and caregivers who cope with the toll of misinformation, disease, cost, disability, and stigma, and identify personal bias, if it exists, in the treatment and course of action with the families with whom they come in contact. Sprinkled throughout, are opportunities to examine case studies of resilience and empowerment in communities, including grassroots political action, legislative advocacy, the creation of self-help organizations and outreach, as well as stories about human services professionals challenged by negative attitudes about medical cannabis.

All names, with the exception of one of the authors of this chapter, have been changed to protect the privacy of the participants in the case studies (Levine, 2019).

Public Health Considerations for Medical Cannabis Use

The public health ramifications of medicinal cannabis legalization warrant considerable attention and investment; meanwhile, the effects of cannabis use on public health are still being measured. Prior studies have documented modest increases in cannabis use at the population level following legalization, particularly among older adults, despite a decrease in the rate of cannabis use (Hasin et al., 2017; Hasin et al., 2015). Prior studies have documented modest increases in cannabis use at the population level following legalization, particularly among older adults, despite a decrease in the rate of Cannabis Use Disorder among users (Hasin et al., 2017; Hasin et al., 2015). Mixed results have been observed with respect to opioid-sparing effects of medicinal cannabis legalization (Bachhuber et al., 2014; Campbell et al., 2018; Salomonsen-Sautel et al; 2014; Shover et al. (2019). Within states that have legalized cannabis, motor vehicle accidents and emergency department (ED) visits have increased (Kim et al., 2016; Liang et al., 2018). However, the impact of medicinal cannabis legalization at the level of individual cannabis users is inadequately understood.

There is an apparent lack of evidence-based education and misinformation in abundance. One of the biggest challenges is a lack of trained medical professionals to guide patients on using cannabis safely and effectively. We lack best practices and protocols for administration and monitoring both short- and long-term use. This can leave consumers seeking the advice of "bud tenders" in local dispensaries to make medical decisions. They are neither trained appropriately nor have the scientific knowledge of mechanism of action, potential harms, and contraindications to inform consumers appropriately. A study conducted (Dickson, et. al., 2018) to characterize recommendations given to pregnant women by Colorado cannabis dispensaries regarding use of cannabis products for nausea during the first trimester of pregnancy resulted in some shocking results. This was a statewide cross-sectional study in which advice about cannabis product use was requested using a "mystery caller" approach. The caller stated she was eight weeks pregnant and experiencing morning sickness. Dispensaries were randomly selected from the Colorado Department of Revenue Enforcement Division website.

The primary outcome was the proportion of marijuana dispensaries that recommended a cannabis product for use during pregnancy. Of the 400 dispensaries contacted, 37% were licensed for medical sale (n=148), 28% for retail (n=111), and 35% for both (n=141). The majority, 69% (277/400), recommended treatment of morning sickness with cannabis products (95% CI 64–74%). Frequency of recommendations differed by license type (medical 83.1%, retail 60.4%, both 61.7%, P<.001). Recommendations for use were similar for dispensary location (urban 71% versus nonurban 63%, P=.18). The majority (65%) based their recommendation for use in pregnancy on personal opinion, and 36% stated cannabis use is safe in pregnancy. Ultimately, 81.5% of dispensaries recommended discussion with a health care provider; however, only 31.8% made this recommendation without prompting. As cannabis legalization and use expands, policy and education efforts should involve dispensaries since they are often the "first line of defense" for consumers.

Dilemmas Faced When Traditional Medical Options Have Been Exhausted

"My name is Heather Jackson and I am "just a mom" who tried to save her son from an intractable medical condition when all else failed. I went on to co-found and serve as CEO of Realm of Caring Foundation, a nonprofit that conducts research so that it can aid consumers, medical professionals, and inform policy on medical cannabis and hemp. Almost eight years later I now serve as Board President. The foundation has become a learning lab where we gain valuable insights from the over 60,000 families and 1,500 medical professionals that we serve from all over the world. We conduct research with the United States' top universities to discover trends and outcomes of cannabis users and nonusers (controls). I hope these experiences will enable an appreciation into the complexities of the human experience traversing this often difficult path and a special comprehension that other human services professionals may lack. The opening account is my personal experience."

The scream. 3:30 AM. Again. Startled, Heather Jackson is awoken from what hasn't been a peaceful night's sleep in almost a decade. Her son Zaki is having another seizure. These early morning seizures start with a scream, and within a minute, Zaki's lips are grey, and the tips of his fingers begin to appear to have been dipped in blueberry syrup. He is not breathing. Although a regular occurrence, Heather will never get used to these life-threatening seizures and will not cease looking for a solution to stop them. The year is 2011 and Zaki is 8 years old and receiving hospice palliative services through a waiver in their home state of Colorado after 17 pharmaceuticals have failed Zaki, leaving his development delayed. His seizures, numbering in the hundreds daily, are devastating for the family: They cannot bring themselves to give up on treatment options even if those treatments are unconventional. They have just returned from their Make-A-Wish trip, and Heather promised herself when that was over, she would get more serious about researching cannabis, something her hospice social worker mentioned prior to their trip. The message was discreetly delivered, handwritten on a piece of scratch paper, with a warning that the social worker could lose her job if the agency knew she was offering such a suggestion. This was monumental enough for Heather to realize the controversy of this decision that weighed on the family.

One of the first things Heather had to consider was the legality of marijuana for a child in the state of Colorado, and in her city specifically. She discovered that it is a Schedule I substance federally, which means marijuana has no currently accepted medical use and a high potential for abuse. Schedule I drugs are considered the most dangerous drugs of all the drug schedules with potentially severe psychological or physical dependence. Heroin and LSD also make this list. By contrast, cocaine is a Schedule II. Her son was medically fragile. She wanted to ease his suffering and did not want to hurt him in any way. In light of the warnings that accompany a Schedule I drug, she wondered where she could find research about the obvious medical use of cannabis. She was able to find lethal dose ratings that showed it was less toxic than caffeine. She even found a United States government patent on cannabinoids as neuroprotectants and antioxidants. This was all quite confusing (Table 10.1).

Despite all of this, in Colorado medical cannabis was legal for her son with an epilepsy diagnosis, if she could get two doctors to make a recommendation for him to use it. She approached their neurologist for one of the recommendations. Zaki had been under the supervision of this neurologist his whole life, and the doctor would allow it, stating they had "nothing to lose" but was not going to be able to help with dosing because it was against the policy of his affiliated network to make such a recommendation. Now what? He did it anyway. The second doctor was a medical cannabis doctor who had built an entire practice on making these recommendations, but she had only made one other recommendation for a child and was also not able to advise on dosing. Furthermore, the Colorado Department of Public Health and Environment (CDPHE) never issued the medical cannabis license for the previous child even though she had a qualifying condition and two doctors had made the recommendation. Even though Heather also found two doctors to make the recommendation, CDPHE could still deny issuing the license allowing the use of cannabis, thereby denying the ability of their family to

Table 10.1 Toxicity Rating of Cannabis Compared to Other Substances

Substances used to make drugs are classified into five distinct categories or schedules depending upon their acceptable medical use and the potential for abuse or dependency [3].

CONTROLLED SUBSTANCES

In July of 2011, the DEA proposed the addition of a new drug code to the CSA, titled "Marihuana Extract", which specifically included the term "Cannabidiols". Oddly enough, the DEA did not present any evidence or scientific merit that would prove Cannabidiol is toxic, addictive, or otherwise presents any potential for abuse.

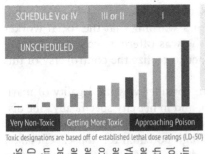

Toxic designations are based off of established lethal dose ratings (LD-50)

Although the term "Cannabidiol" is not specifically listed in the Controlled Substances Act (CSA), it is currently considered to be a Schedule I substance by the DEA because cannabidiol is derived from the Cannabis plant species, which is included in the CSA under the term "Marihuana".

In October 2003, the United States federal government obtained US Patent 6630507 titled, "Cannabinoids as antioxidants and neuroprotectants [4]." The patent claims:

shop at a dispensary, the only legal way to obtain it in Colorado at the time. Many hoops had to be jumped through, appointments made, and money expended, all while caring full time for Zaki and not knowing if this would even work or if the hassle would pay off in the end. Heather could not see any other options, so she persisted. Her final audit was calling the Colorado Department of Human Services prior to administration of cannabis to ensure that she would not jeopardize her parental rights. They affirmed that if the doctors' recommendations were sought, and Zaki had his medical cannabis license, they would not be able to interfere with this treatment course.

Zaki began to use a form of cannabis high in cannabidiol (CBD) and low in tetrahydrocannabinol (THC) in July 2012. CBD is not intoxicating, and THC is. Both have documented medicinal properties. With no existing course charted, Heather embarked on a carefully regimented and thought-out plan, leaned on the few other families she could talk to, and found sparse existing research in regard to CBD and epilepsy carried out over the previous 30 years. She did not change anything else in his treatment regimen to avoid confusion about pending results. She used cannabis that was laboratory tested so she knew exactly the number of milligrams of both CBD and THC she was giving her son and that it was free from contaminants like molds, pesticides, and residual solvents. She documented everything as she had done with all his previous medical interventions so they could assess the efficacy of this new option. Within three months Zaki's seizures went into remission.

His neurologist was regularly checking the blood serum levels of the pharmaceuticals that Zaki was on, and the family communicated with their neurologist to get a wean schedule of the current medications he was on, which were not working before starting cannabis. Their plan was to slowly remove previous medications. Zaki who was previously incontinent, not having much meaningful retainable academic success, and emotionally challenged along with other difficulties, was seeing a huge shift in his development. With the seizures at bay and the sedating pharmaceuticals being reduced, Heather, who was very skeptical of this working, was shocked with his positive response.

Zaki was not expected to make it into adulthood, and now the seizures were in remission. Three single acts of bravery: a hospice social worker who had another family she was seeing with great success, so much so that she would not have forgiven herself if she didn't pass that scrap paper that day; a doctor who challenged the status quo and his affiliation's regulations; and a mother who did not give up on finding a treatment option for her son no matter how unconventional.

Realm of Caring Foundation Was Established

Within months Heather began to publicly discuss what was working for her and a handful of other families; a movement was born, and Realm of Caring Foundation, Inc. (RoC) was founded. The foundation is a 501c3 nonprofit

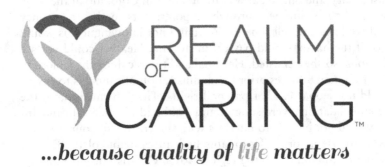

Figure 10.1 Realm of Caring Foundation Logo

organization headquartered in Colorado Springs, Colorado and now serves over 60,000 families living with intractable medical diagnoses of all types. They focus on conducting research with university partners and educating the community, medical professionals, and government about cannabis use. They operate the only call center on medical cannabis, and can field as many as 10,000 inquiries a month from all over the country and the world. They do not manufacture any cannabis products, nor do they make any money off of the sale of cannabis products—they offer grants to families in financial need. Realm of Caring is also enrolling in several studies, the largest of which is a registry in collaboration with Johns Hopkins University looking at health outcomes and quality of life outcomes for both cannabis and non-cannabis users that the foundation serves. Heather was determined that no one should have to start at square one when using cannabis like she had to (Figure 10.1).

Realm of Caring: Research and Practical Knowledge

Although historically cannabis has been used medically for thousands of years (Russo, 2007), there is quite a bit of stigma that consumers, caregivers, medical professionals, and social services professionals face when starting use or supporting someone with a treatment regimen that includes this plant. Additionally, it was not that long ago that we had no viable data on safety, dosing, potential interactions, and contraindications of cannabis use for consumers using products available via mail order or from dispensaries. It is hard to make an informed decision without all of the relevant data. Consumers should be able to have these conversations with their medical teams and not be judged or marginalized by them, society, or social service professionals. However, that can be difficult based on the lack of double-blind placebo-controlled studies on cannabis which are made almost impossible by the federal scheduling of the drug as level I. Thus, there is a circular dichotomy: Not enough research and the extreme classification prohibits the study of it. Despite all that, there are more than 20,000 peer-reviewed research articles in PubMed, the United States National Library of Medicine maintained by the National Institutes of Health and other organizations like the Realm of Caring dedicated to collecting data on cannabis use (see Appendix A).

One must remove emotionalism and look to the science that exists about cannabis and recognize that science is shifting constantly. It is impossible for us to find what we are *not* looking for. To put it another way, if the benefits of cannabis are not being researched then it is impossible to know the true potential of it or for whom it might be indicated or contraindicated.

Realm of Caring: Observational Research Registry

Realm of Caring has been conducting a longitudinal observational research registry that this chapter will reference repeatedly, presenting results and updated findings from this study (see Appendix). There are several sources to discover why people are using cannabis in published peer-reviewed clinical trials and surveys of what people are using cannabis for in their natural environment (Table 10.2).

Clinical cannabis studies, however, are not always able to help us gauge quality of life improvement and why someone may choose to continue to use cannabis even when it does not put their condition into remission, like Zaki in our opening narrative. This raises an important issue for consideration : How do we prioritize the success of a treatment that doesn't stop the disease course, but does drastically improve quality of life?" In most cases, the Diagnostic and Statistical Manual of Mental Disorders, Fifth Edition (DSM-5) has a scale that can specifically be administered to diagnose Substance Abuse and Cannabis Use Disorder (CUD).

Defining a Medical Refugee

The term medical refugee was coined by the media when droves of families were pouring into Colorado after hearing and witnessing some state residents having success with cannabis or seeing a documentary that was produced by CNN featuring medical correspondent Sanjay Gupta and Realm of Caring families. Even though it was 2013, zip codes truly dictated whether someone had the option to try medical cannabis with a sick loved one or for themselves. After arriving in a state that did have a medical cannabis program, people were then essentially landlocked, not being able to travel outside of the state and take what had become their medicine with them for fear of breaking the law. Families were looking for options, not trying to become criminals. It was difficult, but many

Appendix A Practical Tools and Resources for Human Services Professionals

Resource	Link
American Cannabis Nurses Association	https://cannabisnurses.org/
Colorado Caseworker Resources	https://www.coloradocwts.com/resources-f or-caseworkers/laws-and-rules
• Colorado Children's Code (Title 19 of the Colorado Revised Statutes) • Volume 7 of the Code of Colorado Regulations (Social Services Rules)	
Quality of Products	https://realmofcaring.org/resources/client-po rtal/printable-resources/
• Realm of Caring • U.S. Hemp Authority	https://www.ushempauthority.org/certified-com panies/
Realm of Caring Foundation	https://realmofcaring.org/ Telephone: 719-347-5400 Option 1
• Education and call center for • consumers and medical professionals • Discounts on cannabinoid products	Email: info@realmofcaring.org
• Research results dashboard (must make a client account)	https://realmofcaring.org/resources/client-po rtal/
• Cannabis Research Library (organized by condition and symptom)	https://realmofcaring.org/roc-research/resear ch-library/
• Cannabis laws state by state	https://realmofcaring.org/qualifying-conditions-fo r-a-medical-marijuana-card-by-state/
• Research Opportunities	https://realmofcaring.org/roc-research/partic ipate-in-research/
Society of Cannabis Clinicians	https://www.cannabisclinicians.org/

split up their families to provide relief for their loved one with one parent staying in the home state and the other going to the cannabis safe haven state. All of this had to be done before even knowing if this would even work as a treatment.

The number of outdated, antiquated, and incongruent rules, regulations, and laws regarding marijuana cultivation, consumption, commerce, and transportation are dizzying. These can change between city, county, state, and of course, federally. What laws are consumers to follow? How can they easily navigate this on top of their sometimes complex medical issues? Consumers and caregivers delicately and often secretly embark on this path with fear of medical and social services involvement—the very type of support that families should be able to depend on. Sometimes it is completely illegal to use medical cannabis in a city or state. Sometimes a move is needed, leaving individuals with no option but splitting up their families and leaving all the support systems they have established in their home state and becoming medical refugees.

Table 10.2 Primary Medical Condition for Participants Who Were or Were Not Considering Use of Cannabis (Cannabis Realm of Caring Observational Study)

	Cannabis Users (n=808)	Controls (n=468)	p-value
Primary Medical Condition Neurological, n (%)	307 (38)	170 (36)	.35
Chronic Pain, n (%)	204 (25)	108 (23)	-
Neuropsychiatric, n (%)	146 (18)	94 (20)	-
Autoimmune, n (%)	75 (9)	46 (10)	-
Cancer, n (%)	59 (7)	33 (7)	-
Insomnia, n (%)	6 (1)	10 (2)	-
Other, n (%)	11 (2)	7 (1)	-

The following two case studies illustrate examples of medical refugees and the lengths a parent will go to help their sick child.

Case Study One: Medical Refugee Family With Terminal Illness

Christina the matriarch of the Johnson family, also a psychiatric nurse practitioner with a PhD in health education, relocated their entire family for medical cannabis in 2013 from Florida to Colorado where a budding cannabis movement and community were already being built. Three of their biological family members were diagnosed with Dentatorubral-pallidoluysian atrophy (DRPLA), a progressive brain disorder that causes involuntary movements, mental and emotional problems, seizures, and a decline in thinking ability eventually leading to death. The average age of onset of DRPLA is 30 years old. Not only did Christina's husband present with this disease, her son and daughter had it as well with symptoms producing in early childhood. This is an extremely rare diagnosis, and there is no treatment or cure. Christina's Florida community began to talk to her about an hour-long CNN special called WEED that aired in August of 2013 hosted by Sanjay Gupta. Many families featured in the special were in the Realm of Caring community. A friend of Christina's reached out about the show, and she dismissed it. A self-professed conservative, she did not think that using cannabis medicinally was a viable option or that any research existed in regard to its medical use. But after several more friends reached out to her, she began to look at the existing research, got in touch with the Realm of Caring Foundation, and subsequently packed up her family and moved more than two thousand miles for access.

The family lost their son in 2016 to DRPLA. Her daughter uses Cannabidiol (CBD) a nonintoxicating hemp-based product as a neuroprotectant and antioxidant, and her husband uses various cannabis products to help with end-stage dementia, aggression, irritability, and insomnia which happens because his brain is starting to atrophy from the disease. Although cannabis is not ultimately going to save her loved ones, Christina says "Quality of life matters. Quality of life is not just hospice. It could be 10 or 20 years of decreased pain and not on opioids. You know? So, in all the stages of life, quality of life matters."

Relocation is a good example of a solution that exists when clients live in a place where medical cannabis is not permitted or if it is permitted but not for their particular medical indication. Although this is not possible for most individuals living with intractable and chronic health concerns, it is possible for some. As a human services professional, this could be a piece of advice given to families who want to access medical cannabis but are not able to.

Issues that families should consider before moving to a state where cannabis is legal are:

- Does the new state have a functioning and affordable medical cannabis program?
- Does the family have the financial resources to move including being some time without employment after their move?
- Is there a support system in the new state, colleagues, friends, and community?
- What support will the individual with the chronic health condition have? Are there support groups, medical waivers, appropriate schools, therapies, nursing agencies, specialists, and more?
- When they get there, now what? Will the family be able to keep up with the cost of living in the new state?

Helping clients to think through the long-term effects of a decision to relocate including doing their homework before moving is ideal.

State and Federal Incongruencies

Case Study Two: State and Federal Incongruencies for Medical Refugee Families

A more recent case highlights the challenges that families face when medical professionals and Child Protective Services lack sufficient knowledge of state and federal laws surrounding cannabinoid therapy. In Indianapolis, Indiana, six-month-old Julie Brown had her first seizure in 2017. As the months passed, the seizures increased to 30–40 a day. By 17 months old, a neurologist diagnosed Julie with Doose syndrome, or myoclonic-astatic epilepsy (MAE). Several pharmaceuticals were suggested, but Julie's parents, Susan and Jeff, were concerned about the side effects. While researching different medical approaches, the family came across Charlotte Figi's story on that same CNN special that the Johnsons saw. At first, the stigma of using medical cannabis caused Susan to hesitate, but after reading the potential side effects of all the epilepsy drugs, she was inclined to at least try CBD.

Meanwhile a family member suggested Julie see a functional medical professional; upon examination he gave her fish oil, a probiotic, a multivitamin, and CBD oil in the office that same day. Naturally, the Browns assumed CBD oil was legal since the provider sold it from his office. Gradually over the next two weeks, Julie's seizures decreased in duration, frequency, and severity, from 30–40 a day, down to five a day. Eventually, Julie's seizures were reduced by more than 90%, with an average range of 2 to 3 a day.

When the neurologist followed up weeks later and Julie returned for a checkup, Susan told the doctor about her daughter's successful seizure reduction using CBD; the doctor did not entertain discussing CBD, but instead recommended a pharmaceutical and potential brain surgery. Since CBD seemed to be working, this prompted the Browns to seek a second opinion. When seeking a second opinion from another neurologist, the nurse practitioner heard about the reduction of seizures as a result of CBD, yet she suggested a low dose of Keppra, an epilepsy pharmaceutical, which the family started. Within 48 hours, Julie's seizures increased, her appetite decreased, and her behavior became erratic. To make matters worse, Susan received a phone call from a social worker prompted by the second neurologist that reported their family to Child Protective Services (CPS) for medical neglect. CPS inquired about Julie's CBD use and demanded that the family follow up with a specific care plan: The family can only take Julie to one doctor, she had to stay on Keppra, and she must have lab draws once a week to prove she is taking Keppra. If they didn't comply, CPS threatened they would remove all of the Brown's children from their home.

Susan called Mark Messmer, an Indiana state senator, who assured her that Julie's CBD consumption was legal and helped the family resolve the case with CPS. However, a few months later, CPS visited the Brown's house several more times, accusing the family of medical neglect. CPS continued to visit, which according to the family, felt like harassment. The gross misunderstanding of the medical community and CPS caused the family to panic, fearing that at any moment, their children will be taken away. At this point, what are the Browns supposed to do? Do they follow the recommendation of the doctor even though Julie was getting worse? Should they stay in Indiana and endure the anxiety? Or do they flee?

Following their gut, Susan and Jeff relocated their entire family to Colorado Springs, Colorado, after being awarded a relocation grant from the Realm of Caring's Joy Fund. This fund was started after Joy Baldwin, a Realm of Caring client who used medical cannabis for her amyotrophic lateral sclerosis (ALS), donated to the foundation before succumbing to the disease in 2014. The Browns found comfort and support from families with similar cases of epilepsy and cannabinoid therapy use. As a result, Julie has thrived on CBD with the additional legal protections of a medical cannabis license recommended by local doctors.

Incongruencies among states and federal governments make this a difficult path to traverse. Not only must a family become the expert in their diagnoses, they must learn different regulatory structures, oftentimes limit their travel, and become landlocked in their residing state depending on the type of cannabinoid products they use, all while educating and defending themselves to their doctors and oftentimes social service workers.

Critical Issues for Consideration by Medical Cannabis Consumers

Stigma and Stereotypes

Unfortunately, whether cannabis is working or not, there is still a negative connotation that our society associates with cannabis use. In 2019, Columbia Broadcast System (CBS) rejected a Super Bowl commercial that would justify the benefits of cannabis, highlighting the medical outcomes of a struggling veteran and a toddler with seizures. The stigma surrounding cannabis continues to plague the daily facets of everyday life by stoking fear, deception, and falsehood. A recent Colorado study highlighted these themes from both medical and recreational cannabis use in older adults, and focus groups revealed a strong reluctance to discuss cannabis use openly due to the stigma attached to it (Bobitt et al., 2019).

In a preliminary thematic content analysis of Realm of Caring's observational research registry, 4% of the 541 medical cannabinoid users explicitly cited social stigma as a significant concern that affected their medical cannabinoid use. "I do experience some anxiety over feeling the stigma of its use. But my family and I had to choose quality of life over that fear," said one participant.

Human services professionals may also be affected by the stigma attached to cannabis. To counter this, they can think back to their personal drug education programs from middle school and high school and remember when they first learned about marijuana. They can recall if they developed a stigma or stereotype for those who used cannabis and if they still carry the same sentiment today. Our subconscious still tends to judge unfairly as a result of early misconceptions and astute propaganda. It is important for human service professionals to observe their visceral response when a client discloses they are using medical cannabis or giving their child medical cannabis. Yes, the plant can show up with a lot of baggage, so being aware of thoughts around this will provide the client and the professional with the best possible relationship.

In the following case study, we look at a United States veteran trying to overcome trauma, PTSD, and Traumatic Brain Injury.

Case Study Three: United States Military Veteran

Consider the case of Jeremy Wilson, a a military veteran who had served for 16 years, who medically retired due to a traumatic brain injury from a rocket-propelled grenade while stationed in Fallujah, Iraq in 2003. The repercussions from the injury led Jeremy to alcohol abuse as well as the use of several pharmaceuticals prescribed by Veterans Affairs. He recalls being prescribed upwards of ten drugs like mood stabilizers, opioids, steroids, and several other potentially lethal drugs. Tiredness, weakness, muscle and joint pain, dehydration, and frequent illness were just a few symptoms Jeremy experienced from his prescribed medications.

After leaving the military, he suffered from internal organ complications and elevated liver enzymes, which eventually led to the unnecessary removal of his gallbladder. As a result, he began to lose faith in Veteran Affairs. He took it into his own hands and gradually reduced his medications on his own schedule, lying to his VA doctors.

He turned to cannabis and noticed positive changes in his exercise, mood, pain, inflammation, recovery, and overall health. Additionally, cannabis sparked an innate sense of creativity. He was kind to others, and he engaged in conversations and developed a sense of empathy with family, friends, and strangers alike. Eventually he came clean and told the VA and colleagues about his cannabis use. "I'm not hiding it anymore and I help other veterans get the benefits that they deserve as well and I tell them about the laws and the memorandums that say they can use cannabis," he said.

Over time, the energy boost encouraged him to become an avid runner and he gradually weaned himself off of the prescription medications, eliminating their harrowing side effects; although, Jeremy admits that THC initially brought on "mental discomfort" and at times paranoia. Having a medical license gave him peace of mind; it reassured him that he was a law abiding citizen and exercising his rights. He worked through these side effects and now microdoses throughout the day to maintain positive results. Most surprising were his brain scans: Doctors reported that his damage had completely healed. His brain had recovered from the blast.

Jeremy is honest about the stigma associated with cannabis as a result of youth drug education programs, media, and character stereotypes. Although cannabis use is becoming more mainstream, there are many personal and communal barriers and, no matter what, some people will judge. Even doctors judged him for consuming it, lecturing him on all the negative side effects and disregarding his personal success with the plant. Unfortunately, not everyone is as forthcoming and candid about their cannabis use. Sometimes a reputation, a job, or honor is at stake if an individual comes forward and admits to consuming cannabis.

Jeremy points out that conversations, education, and research will normalize cannabis as a medical tool. In addition to being open about his use, he also speaks about legalities, especially around growing organic cannabis and developing a relationship with the plant with fellow veterans. The cultivation taught him how to care, heal, respect, and connect with his medicine, which in turn, he says helped him connect with others.

All in all, Jeremy reflected on his own experience and stressed the importance of human services professionals to keep an open mind and not make assumptions or quick judgments about a client's cannabis use. Even though he's a proponent of the plant, he believes that abuse can be present. In years to come, he believes cannabis use will be normalized. There will be freedom from shame, guilt, paranoia, and judgment. Overall, it is important to understand that maintaining a healthy balance and using cannabis in moderation is essential to its therapeutic use.

Quality of Cannabinoid Products Matters

Not everyone has the resources or the ability to grow their own cannabis like Jeremy Wilson; it is a sure way to know exactly what was used to grow the plants, keeping it safe from fungicides and pesticides, or growing it organically without using any chemicals at all. Even if someone can grow their own plants, how can they test it to know the cannabinoid, terpene, and other constituents of the final product they consume? Or perhaps consumers are prohibited from cultivating their own plants or live in a state where only hemp-based CBD products are available by mail order or in local stores. Perhaps they live in a state where medical cannabis is available through a dispensary, but the dispensary may or may not be required to carry tested products. If products are being tested, how does one know the testing facility is accurate and able to test for all the contaminants a consumer would need to discover? As described earlier, this creates a conundrum and another point of concern for families using cannabis.

Quality of cannabinoid products should be a top priority for consumers and the professionals who serve them. Depending on the state and the companies producing the final product, the quality can vary wildly. In one study by researchers on medical cannabis edibles in California, they discovered of the 75 products purchased (47 different brands), 17% were accurately labeled, 23% were under-labeled, and 60% were over-labeled with respect to THC content (Vandrey et al., 2015). Products that contain significantly more THC than labeled place patients at risk of experiencing adverse effects. Because medical cannabis is recommended for specific health conditions, regulation and quality assurance are needed. This study was not replicated in other medical cannabis states, and there are states with later legislative approval that have put many protections in place for consumers. It is important for consumers and social service professionals to know what is in cannabis products.

In a subsequent study, *Labeling Accuracy of Cannabidiol Extracts Sold Online*, researchers analyzed the content of 84 cannabidiol (CBD) products purchased on the internet and compared the results to their advertised concentrations (Bonn-Miller, 2017). Products were mislabeled with 26% containing less CBD than labeled and 43% containing more, indicating a high degree of variability and poor standardization of online products. In addition to CBD mislabeling, THC was detected in 21% of samples. This study also notes that products containing THC could have sufficient enough concentrations to produce intoxication in children (Bonn-Miller, 2017). The results of this study suggest that despite FDA warning letters going out in 2016, the online marketplace for CBD products at that time lacked standardization and had a high rate of mislabeling.

There is a great need for consistency and regulation of these products which in 2020 is being prioritized by the industry and federal government agencies. There are now organizations that certify the quality of products in the marketplace. Realm of Caring (see Appendix A), as a consumer-driven organization, has created standards and conducts quality reviews certifying quality products that they recommend in both medical cannabis and hemp-based CBD products. Another company is the U.S. Hemp Authority, which is creating guidance and certifying hemp-based CBD companies (see Appendix A). If a client would like to find their own product, the client needs to ensure they look to national standards such as the FDA's Current Good Manufacturing Practices (CGMP) and the American Herbal Products Association (AHPA) guidelines for botanical extracts or refer them to consumer based nonprofit organizations to help.

Another piece of the quality picture is checking if the company provides great customer service, and continued availability of a product. For example, if a particular product works, will they be able to continue to get that same product consistently over time? Where does the company source their raw product if they are not vertically integrated and do not grow their own? Do they have third party independent audits in their lab facility? Although it is challenging to find, assess, and ensure the quality of a product, it is not impossible, and there are several resources social service professionals can share with clients. Yes, clients' quality of life matters, and so does the quality of the products they use.

Cost of Cannabinoid Therapy as a Barrier

Another barrier to consumers of cannabis is cost. When facing an unpredictable and chronic health condition, one's socioeconomic status is compromised: Economic suffering forces families to make demanding decisions between care and everyday living expenses (Jeon et al., 2009). These decisions may cause less than optimal health outcomes and increased costs to the health system. The findings in this Australian study support the necessity of a critical analysis of health, social, and welfare policies to identify cross-sectoral strategies to alleviate such hardship and improve the affordability of managing chronic conditions (Jeon et al., 2009).

Another U.S. investigation examined family outcomes as a result of an unexpected health event. In that report data was collected from more than one hundred families with a child with cystic fibrosis. The study revealed a decline in finances in addition to psychological stress in the areas of family development, relationships, and management and decision making (Patterson & Mccubbin, 1983). In a climate of global economic instability, such research into the economic impact of chronic illness on individuals' health and well-being and their disease management capacity provides timely evidence to inform policy development.

Families cannot always consider treatments not covered by their insurance company. If they do, other financial needs can go unmet. Families of lower socioeconomic status may need assistance finding access to quality products and programs that educate and support them and their doctors throughout the process of considering if cannabis may be right for them. Realm of Caring is one such organization with a program to subsidize cannabinoid therapy for families in need. In Realm of Caring's observational research registry there were major themes and subthemes discovered in the analysis of the data.

In a subset of the registry that included 541 participants from April 2016 to February 2018, cost was the highest reported problem, with 14% of the respondents specifically stating it was a barrier for them to access this type of therapy or accessing it consistently. One of the respondents wrote: "I wish my insurance company would help cover the costs. It is so expensive in New Jersey. I can't always afford to use it. I don't work." This same study showed in the broader participation set of 1276 individuals that included controls (non-cannabis users) that cannabis users self-reported using statistically significant fewer prescription medications [RR=0.86; 95% CI, 0.77 to 0.96] and were less likely to have a past month emergency department (ED) visit [RR=0.61; 95% CI, 0.44 to 0.84] or hospital admissions [RR=0.54; 95% CI, 0.34 to 0.87]. Perhaps in the future landscape, cannabis or hemp-based CBD products will be covered by insurance companies, thus reducing costs directly to consumers and insurance companies through better health outcomes, lower pharmaceutical costs, and less hospital utilization.

Dawn's son Keenan has 11 diagnoses. She stated: "Unfortunately I am disabled myself, and financially it was very hard to come up with the money to try this for Keenan as this is our last resort. So I went into debt. Within a few weeks we saw a difference and it was well worth it. After joining Realm of Caring's financial aid program, this helped tremendously to cover the expense so that my son could once again have a life." Realm of Caring provided a monthly stipend of $150 dollars for a two-year grant cycle in 2017 to offset the cost of a therapy not covered by insurance.

It would be helpful to assist clients with appropriate budgeting to ensure their essentials are being taken care of while paying for a treatment not covered by insurance. Families accessing community financial gifts are sometimes a good option if a client has a strong support system of friends, family, and church members, for example. Connecting them to other financial aids like help with their utilities, food, clothing, and medical expenses, thereby allowing a budget to include the cost of cannabinoid therapy, should all be considered. Additionally, connecting them to programs already available, such as grants given by the Realm of Caring, combined with budgeting help, could all be effective support for clients (see Appendix A for cost-saving resources).

Challenges Faced by Human Services Professionals Serving Medical Cannabis Consumers

It is essential for human services professionals to be familiar with all facets of cannabinoid therapy. This is a challenging aspect of the job due to existing codes of ethics and legalities. When families and individuals exhaust traditional medical options, they will try all available avenues, including cannabis. If a child with intractable epilepsy finds seizure relief or other positive effects from using cannabis, is it considered abuse? Should the cannabis use of a child constitute abuse or neglect? As we learned from the Brown family, it is critical that Human Services Professionals receive factual and legal guidance in order to best serve their clients. Unfortunately, many of these cases operate in a grey space due to the complex variables. Federal funding further complicates matters in Colorado, because cannabis is still federally illegal under the Schedule I status, a higher category than a prescription drug. Therefore, Human Services Professionals must comply with federal and state regulations.

In the final case study, we examine the perspective of a human services professional who has had first-hand experience with children on cannabinoid therapy and the challenges she faced even in a medical cannabis state.

Case Study Four: Human Services Professional in a Legal Medical Cannabis State

Karen Williams specializes in Child Welfare Intake in the Department of Human Services in Colorado, a state with legal recreational cannabis. The rural, suburban, and urban settings deliver a diverse demographic of clientele; consequently, each subset possesses unique intricacies and challenges. Karen's sole mission is to ensure that children are safe and that families receive any services that they need. The Department follows a specific policy, Title 19, Colorado Children's Code, Volume 7, an overview of child welfare services (see Appendix A).

Karen points out that if a child is born exposed to cannabis, it meets the criteria for assessment because cannabis remains a Schedule I drug under federal law. If a caregiver consumes cannabis in the presence of minors,

Human Services Professionals must evaluate how it is impacting the child or children. For example, hospitals often contact the Department and work together to determine if there is physical evidence of cannabis in the mother or newborn baby. Cases of cannabis-exposed newborns are the most challenging for the Department. Once there is an official referral, professionals like Karen will assess these cases. Other referrals come from schools when, on occasion, a child goes to class and their backpack smells of cannabis. Karen notes it is important to consider the behavior of the child. How are they doing academically? Are there any physical, emotional, or social concerns? Is the child lethargic or falling asleep in class? Perhaps the caregiver consumed cannabis in the same room as the backpack while the child was not present. According to policy, there must be one sober caregiver, free of drug and alcohol consumption, who can care for the minor while the other caregiver is consuming, but not in the presence of children in the home. In such cases, the department assesses the home and car environment and interviews the children.

Ultimately, Human Services Professionals rely on medical professionals for evidence-based information regarding safe medical cannabis use; however, there can be conflicting medical opinions. Because cannabis is a Schedule I drug, there is little research available due to restrictions; therefore, health care professionals' knowledge is inconsistent. Karen explains how some doctors recommend breastfeeding mothers or pregnant women who are experiencing severe symptoms like nausea to try consuming cannabis rather than a pharmaceutical, while other doctors would not approve this course of treatment because of its potential harm to the fetus or baby. But what happens when that baby tests positive for THC? Inevitably, Karen would have to get involved and assess the safety of the newborn even if a doctor made the recommendation of cannabis use.

Karen mentions how confusing cannabis use can be and where to draw the line. For example, is it acceptable for a mother to take CBD oil, which is known for its therapeutic benefits? What about vaping or dabbing (smoking a concentrate) of THC? At what point is cannabis unlawful? When the caregiver or child is using some form of cannabis and has doctor approval, do human services professionals really need to assess the safety profile of the family? In most cases, it points back to the importance of research and education about what constitutes proven therapeutic uses for CBD and THC. Karen believes their Department would benefit from more education and knowledge to understand these compounds, since they are not medical professionals, and some medical professionals do not understand it either. To best serve and support families, it would also help human services professionals evaluate children's safety.

Comprehending the functionality of cannabis would go a long way to help inform their community and their systems which are intertwined and work together. Often, irrelevant referrals based on stigma and stereotypes do not meet the criteria to open an investigation and the concern for abuse is repudiated. Accurate, quality, and comprehensive training from experts derived from evidence-based information is essential for this field. Many individuals are fearful of something they don't fully comprehend. What happens when the experts present personal bias and focus only on the abuse as opposed to the proven therapeutic value? Karen recalls attending a conference where anti-cannabis educators organized a training that shed a negative light on cannabis use. She points out that any kind of education should present balanced views backed by empirical evidence and specific cases in order to highlight practical applications.

Stigma around cannabis is prevalent and implicit bias is inevitable. False perceptions run rampant in the community; for example, just because cannabis is legal, it must be safe. Some teens believe, therefore that the drug is harmless and, as a result, there have been increased referrals of parents smoking cannabis with their kids. How is this any different than a parent drinking alcohol with their teenager? In response, Karen emphasizes the importance of cannabis training from the Department of Human Services. The lack of research and long-term effects of cannabis limits their ability to accept cannabis as a safe medical therapy. In addition to the drug itself, there are also questions about families that grow their own plants. Professionals must assess if the grow lights can cause a fire, if the excess water fosters mold, and if the fertilizers or pesticides contain harmful chemicals. It's important that the child's physical environment is not compromised by the plants either.

When human services professionals require drug testing, they confront another round of challenges. Testing for alcohol use is measured with a breathalyzer and blood alcohol content, whereas cannabis use requires more time and effort—urinalysis, hair analysis, and saliva tests may take days or weeks. The tests can lack validity and do not necessarily identify the level of impairment. Karen affirms that it is important to establish a baseline to determine if continued testing demonstrates increases or decreases of consumption. Typically, professionals do not open many cases based on reported cannabis use alone; there are other variables that contribute to the case, such as additional drug use/abuse and erratic behavior that compromises a child's safety. For example, should a caregiver be driving children after smoking or vaping? How does an individual know their limitations when consuming cannabis? As a result of these unspecified effects, are more state specific policies around cannabis use needed, especially in regard to driving? Consumption in these cases lack consistent and concrete guidelines and operate in grey areas.

The contradicting legalities of this plant on the state and federal level challenge human services professionals the most, in Karen's opinion. Cannabis is here to stay, and people are consuming it regardless of federal laws, so the state needs to accommodate for its use and define consumption levels, especially for caregivers. Research and technology need to catch up to how the Department determines impairment. The lack of baseline information makes Karen's job more difficult, for example, how to know if children's safety is at risk when their caregiver is consuming cannabis. Consistency within the medical and judicial communities will grant families the protection and support they deserve. As education and policies drag behind, professionals lack the tools to enact consistent safety measures for minors.

Table 10.3 presents a summary of the challenges and solutions of the case studies in this chapter.

Table 10.3 Summary of Human Service Professionals Challenges/Potential Solutions Specific to Cannabis Consumption

Challenges	Potential Solutions	Applicable Case Study
Determining level of impairment when consuming cannabis	Developing guidelines and tests that accurately and consistently regulate cannabis consumption in order to protect children's safety	4
Biases, Stigmas, Stereotypes, Misconceptions	Advancing evidence-based research and access to unbiased education	3, 4
Contrasting state and federal legalities of cannabis	Establishing clear state specific policies that help define individuals' rights	1, 2, 3, 4
Contrasting professional medical opinions	Advancing evidence-based research to support accredited continuing education opportunities	4
Assessing quality of life improvement	Predetermining success criteria with cannabinoid therapy that may include symptoms relief like sleep, life improvement not otherwise associated with remission of disease progression	1
Weighing moral and ethical decisions	Creating community, weighing pros and cons of cannabis use, science-based education	1, 3
Negative stigma and stereotype associated with cannabis use	Advancing evidence-based research and access to unbiased education	3
Determining quality cannabis products	Realm of Caring, U.S. Hemp Authority	NA
Cost of cannabinoid therapy	Connect clients to financial aids like help with their utilities, food, etc., thereby allowing a budget for cannabinoid therapy. Connect client to Realm of Caring	NA

Conclusion

Zaki has not had a seizure in which he has stopped breathing for more than eight years now. He is 17, doing basic math, receives help to write stories, (the last one about being a super spy), and is being tutored to hopefully learn to read. He has deep friendships and has a great sense of humor. He is continuing to heal; so is his family. His experience and the challenges and overcoming of others should serve as a silver lining to the abundance of barriers that exist for consumers to access medical cannabis and social services professionals who service them.

We hope this chapter leaves human services professionals with questions to ask themselves, beliefs to be challenged, and resources to help clients. Consider the advantage clients will have with a professional's unique understanding of their personal situation and an ability to help them with resources without bias. Supplying resources is not condoning use. Social workers are able to provide support without endorsing the use of medical cannabis which, after all, is a decision that can only be made by clients and their medical team. Although, remember the single act of bravery made by the hospice social worker who not only helped Zaki find quality of life, but also created a movement to change the way we see cannabis and the people who use it (Figure 10.2).

Having now met Zaki, the Johnsons, the Browns, Jeremy Wilson, and colleague Karen Williams, social workers can be empowered to effect real change and offer meaningful support during what could be that family's most challenging time.

Social service professionals must ask themselves how they can be prepared, informed, and taught to confidently support and advise clients when it comes to cannabinoid therapy use. Education and evidence-based research is a stepping stone to equip them with the necessary tools to fill a gap in their discipline. Increased cannabis knowledge will continue to identify best therapeutic practices as well as potential for abuse. There is a need

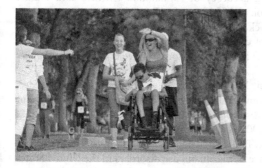

Figure 10.2 Realm of Caring Family at Fundraiser 5k

for researchers to bridge the gaps that exist between credible and evidence-based core cannabis knowledge and medical education. In order to aid the medical community and help shape public health policies, it is important that researchers receive the necessary funding to drive relevant studies so that social service professionals recognize the capabilities and limitations of this plant. Every day, peer-reviewed publications are building a bank of evidence-based knowledge that will be disseminated to all learners.

There are glimmers of hope that all will have equal access and support, despite the many challenges of cannabinoid therapy use among individuals and families highlighted in these case studies. Tenacious pioneers paved a path so others can navigate this rocky road. Their actions alleviated some pre-existing legal and societal barriers while shedding light on their daily struggles. As a result, a grassroots movement to access cannabis ignited communities to voice their concerns to politicians and move the legislative needle on reform. Over time, overwhelming public support has favored medical cannabis use, especially as families seek a better quality of life. Yet, continued advocacy is imperative to those who depend on this medicine and the future for absolute acceptance.

"It does not matter how slowly you go as long as you do not stop."
—Confucius

References

Bachhuber, M. A., Saloner, B., Cunningham, C. O., & Barry, C. L. (2014). Medical cannabis laws and opioidanalgesic overdose mortality in the United States, 1999–2010. *JAMA Internal Medicine*, 174(10), 1668–1673.

Bobitt, J., Qualls, S. H., Schuchman, M., Wickersham, R., Lum, H. D., Arora, K., ... Kaskie, B. (2019). Qualitative analysis of cannabis use among older adults in Colorado. *Drugs and Aging*, 36(7), 655–666. doi:10.1007/s40266-019-00665-w.

Bonn-Miller, M. O., Loflin, M. J., Thomas, B. F., Marcu, J. P., Hyke, T., & Vandrey, R. (2017, November). Labeling accuracy of cannabidiol extracts sold online. *JAMA*, 318(17), 1708–1709. doi:10.1001/jama.2017.11909

Campbell, G., Hall, W. D., Peacock, A., Lintzeris, N., Bruno, R., Larance, B., ... Degenhardt, L. (2018). Effect of cannabis use in people with chronic noncancer pain prescribed opioids: Findings from a 4-year prospective cohort study. *Lancet Public Health*, 3(7), 341–350.

Dickson, B., Mansfield, C., Guiahi, M., Allshouse, A. A., Borgelt, L. M., Sheeder, J., ... Metz, T. D. (2018). Recommendations from cannabis dispensaries about first trimester cannabis use. *Obstetrics and Gynecology*, 131(6), 1031–1038. doi:10.1097/AOG.0000000000002619

Hasin, D. S., Saha, T. D., Kerridge, B. T., Goldstein, R. B., Chou, S. P., Zhang, H., ... Grant, B. F. (2015). Prevalence of marijuana use disorders in the United States between 2001–2002 and 2012–2013. *JAMA Psychiatry*, 72(12), 1235–1242.

Hasin, D. S., Sarvet, A. L., Cerda, M., Keyes, K. M., Stohl, M., Galea, S., & Wall, M. M. (2017). US adult illicit cannabis use, cannabis use disorder, and medical marijuana laws: 1991–1992 To 2012–2013. *JAMA Psychiatry, 74*(6), 579–588.

Jeon, Y. H., Essue, B., Jan, S., Wells, R., & Whitworth, J. A. (2009). Economic hardship associated with managing chronic illness: A qualitative inquiry. *BMC Health Services Research, 9*, 182. doi:10.1186/1472-6963-9-182

Kim, H. S., Hall, K. E., Genco, E. K., Van Dyke, M., Barker, E., & Monte, A. A. (2016). Marijuana tourism and Emergency Department visits in Colorado. *The New England Journal of Medicine, 374*(8), 797–798.

Levine, J. (2019). *In their own voices: Interviews with medical cannabis refugees, caregivers, and consumers.* Unpublished raw data.

Liang, D., Bao, Y., Wallace, M., Grant, I., & Shi, Y. (2018). Medical cannabis legalization and opioid prescriptions: Evidence on US Medicaid enrollees during 1993–2014. *Addiction (Abingdon, England), 113*(11), 2060–2070.

Patterson, J., & Mccubbin, H. (1983). The impact of family life events and changes on the health of a chronically ill child. *Family Relations, 32*(2), 255–264. doi:10.2307/584685

Russo, E. B. (2007). History of cannabis and its preparations in saga, science, and sobriquet. *Chemistry & Biodiversit, 4*(8), 2624–2648.

Salomonsen-Sautel, S., Min, S. J., Sakai, J. T., Thurstone, C., & Hopfer, C. (2014). Trends in fatal motor vehicle crashes before and after marijuana commercialization in Colorado. *Drug and Alcohol Dependence, 140*, 137–144.

Shover, C. L., Davis, C. S., Gordon, S. C., & Humphreys, K. (2019). Association between medical cannabis laws and opioid overdose mortality has reversed over time. *Proceedings of the National Academy of Sciences of the United States of America, 116*(26), 12624–12626.

Vandrey, R., Raber, J. C., Raber, M. E., Douglass, B., Miller, C., & Bonn-Miller, M. O. (2015). Cannabinoid dose and label accuracy in edible medical cannabis products. *JAMA, 313*(24), 2491–2493. doi:10.1001/jama.2015.6613

Appendix

Practical Tools and Resources for Human Service Professionals

Resource	Link
American Cannabis Nurses Association	https://cannabisnurses.org/
Colorado Caseworker Resources	https://www.coloradocwts.com/resources-for-caseworkers/laws-and-rules
• Colorado Children's Code (Title 19 of the Colorado Revised Statutes) • Volume 7 of the Code of Colorado Regulations (Social Services Rules)	
Quality of Products	https://realmofcaring.org/resources/client-portal/printable-resources/
• Realm of Caring • U.S. Hemp Authority	https://www.ushempauthority.org/certified-companies/
Realm of Caring Foundation	https://realmofcaring.org/ Telephone: 719-347-5400 Option 1
• Education and call center for consumers and medical professionals • Discounts on cannabinoid products	Email: info@realmofcaring.org
• Research results dashboard (must make a client account) • Cannabis Research Library (organized by condition and symptom) • Cannabis laws state by state • Research Opportunities	https://realmofcaring.org/resources/client-portal/ https://realmofcaring.org/roc-research/research-library/ https://realmofcaring.org/qualifying-conditions-for-a-medical-marijuana-card-by-state/ https://realmofcaring.org/roc-research/participate-in-research/
Society of Cannabis Clinicians	https://www.cannabisclinicians.org/

Glossary[1]

Sherry Yafai

CBD   Cannabinol, one of the major phytocannabinoids of *Cannabis sativa* L. This is the nonintoxicating chemical in the plant, and it was recently part of a major study for a new drug, Epidiolex (See below).

Endocannabinoids   The naturally occurring molecules in multiple organ systems that parallel the plant's phytocannabinoids. The most well-known are anandamide and 2AG.

Endocannabinoid System   The body's natural system that responds to phytocannabinoids and endocannabinoids. This includes the receptors CB1 (cannabinoid), CB2, and a host of receptors involved in other physiologic responses (see: Front Behav Neurosci. 2012; 6:9, http://bit.ly/2PXYBbS.) This system generally tends toward homeostasis.

Epidiolex   A plant-based CBD oil that is both DEA and FDA approved for treating severe seizure disorders, Lenox-Gestalt and Dravet Syndrome. This CBD is more concentrated and suggested starting dose is much larger than typical CBD. Notable side effects and drug-drug interactions in the literature with other CYP450 medications.

Hemp   The *Cannabis sativa* L. plant that is grown primarily for its stalk and fiber. The plant has to have less than 0.3 percent of THC to classify as hemp.

Lethality   There is no known lethal dose for *Cannabis sativa* L.

Marijuana   Mexican slang for the plant *Cannabis sativa* L. This term gained popularity as Mexicans immigrated into the United States in the 1920s and 1930s and was used to create fear around the plant and the immigrants. This slang term was ultimately used by the DEA as a Schedule I drug.

Metabolism   Phytocannabinoids are generally broken down through the liver by the cytochrome P450 pathway. Endocannabinoids are broken down locally. Be aware of exacerbating effects if a patient is taking another medication metabolized through the same pathway as phytocannabinoids. CBD is a much greater inhibitor of CYP P450 than THC. Organ transplant patients taking tacrolimus, for example, should not use CBD, but THC is OK because of the weak inhibition of CYP P450.

Antiepileptic medications are also frequently metabolized through the CYP P450 pathway and there has been increased concern about drug-drug interaction with Epidiolex (plant-based CBD) now on the market.

Organ Systems   Multiple organ systems are involved, including the brain, muscle, skin and soft tissue, GI system, cardiovascular system, and immune system, which is why this medication can affect so many diseases and illnesses. Of note, there are no receptors in the medulla (where breathing is regulated). This lack of receptor presence is the reason that there is no acute respiratory death (a common side effect of narcotics). There have been two pediatric cases (only one published) of acute cardiac pause as a complication of an acute accidental ingestion of a large amount of THC which resolved without any interventions.

Phytocannabinoids   The cannabinoids that come from the plant *Cannabis sativa* L. This begins with the identification of THC and CBD, the **major cannabinoids**. But the **minor cannabinoids** are being evaluated and research is beginning, including CBDA, THCA, CBG, CBGA, CBN, and CBDV.

Synthetic Cannabinoids   Marinol is a synthetic THC product available at the hospital and through prescriptions. Spice, K2, and bath salts cause acute psychosis and some cannibalistic behaviors.

Terpenes   The essential oils of the plant, which can also be chemically active or sedating. This is what differentiates many of the plant types from one another, in addition to the major and minor cannabinoids in the plant. Think of lavender, lemon, basil, etc., as some of the "additional" elements that are terpenes.

THC   Tetrahydrocannabinol, another major phytocannabinoids of *Cannabis sativa* L. This is the intoxicating chemical in the plant. It has a number of other major activities including increasing appetite, pain management, and treating nausea and vomiting related to chemotherapy.

Note

1   Adapted from   Yafai, S. (2020). The A to Z of Cannabis. *Emergency Medicine News, 42*(1), 1–24. https://doi.org/10.1097/01.EEM.0000651016.96829.63

Index

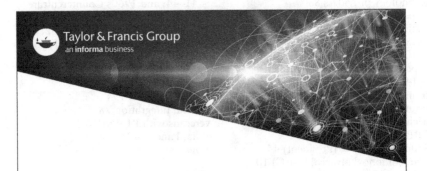

Printed in the United States
by Bookmasters

Printed in the United States
By Bookmasters